Immune Functions of the Vessel Wall

Advances in Vascular Biology

A series of books bringing together important advances and reviewing all areas of vascular biology.

Edited by *Mathew A. Vadas, The Hanson Centre for Cancer Research, Adelaide, South Australia* and *John Harlan, Division of Hematology, University of Washington, Seattle, USA.*

Volume One
Vascular Control of Hemostasis
   edited by *Victor W.M. van Hinsbergh*

Volume Two
Immune Functions of the Vessel Wall
   edited by *Göran K. Hansson* and *Peter Libby*

Volumes in Preparation

Platelets, Thrombosis and the Vessel Wall
   edited by *M.C. Berndt*

The Selectins: Initiators of Leukocyte-Endothelial Adhesion
   edited by *D. Vestweber*

Structure and Function of Endothelial Cell to Cell Junctions
   edited by *E. Dejana*

The Early Atherosclerotic Plaque: Viral, Mutagenic and Developmental Mechanisms

---

Immune Functions of the Vessel Wall

edited by

Göran K. Hansson

Karolinska Institute,
Karolinska Hospital,
Stockholm,
Sweden

and

Peter Libby

Brigham & Women's Hospital, and
Harvard Medical School,
Boston,
United States of America

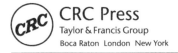

CRC Press
Taylor & Francis Group
Boca Raton London New York

CRC Press is an imprint of the
Taylor & Francis Group, an **informa** business

CONTENTS

SERIES PREFACE

It is our privilege to live at a time when scientific discoveries are providing insights into human biology at an unprecedented rate. It is also a time when the sheer quantity of information tends to obscure underlying principles, and when hypotheses or insights that simplify and unify may be relegated to the shadow of hard data.

The driving force for editing a series of books on Vascular Biology was to partially redress this balance. In inviting editors of excellence and experience, it is our aim to draw together important facts, in particular areas of vascular biology, and to allow the generation of hypotheses and principles that unite an area and define newer horizons. We also anticipate that, as is often the case in biology, the formulation and application of these principles will interrelate with other disciplines.

Vascular biology is a frontier that has been recognised since at least the time of Cohnheim and Metchikoff, but has really come into prominence over the last 10–15 years, once the molecules that mediate the essential functions of the blood vessel started to be defined. The boundaries of this discipline are, however, not clear. There are intersections, for example, with hypertension and atherogenesis that bring in, respectively, neuroendocrine control of vessel tone and lipid biochemistry which exist as separate bodies of knowledge. Moreover, it would be surprising if some regional vascular biology (for example, pulmonary, renal, etc.) were not to emerge as subgroups in the future. Our aims for the moment, however, are to concentrate on areas of vascular biology that have wide impact.

It is our hope to publish two books each year for the next 3–4 years. Indeed the first five books have been commissioned and address areas primarily in endothelial biology (hemostasis and thrombosis), immunology, leukocyte adhesion molecules, platelet adhesion molecules, adhesion molecules that mediate cell–cell contact. Subsequent volumes will cover the physiology and pathology of other vascular cells as well as developmental vascular biology.

We thank the editors and contributors for their very hard work.

Mathew VADAS
John HARLAN

LIST OF CONTRIBUTORS

Allavena, P.
Istituto di Ricerche Farmacologiche
Mario Negri
Via Eritrea 62
I-20157 Milano
Italy

Amberger, A.
Institute for Biomedical Aging Research
University of Innsbruck, Medical School
Fritz-Pregl-Strasse 3/IV
6020 Innsbruck
Austria

Bach, F.H.
Sandoz Center and Dept. Surgery and
Pathology
New England Deaconess Hospital
Harvard Medical School
Boston, MA. 02215
United States of America

Cohen Tervaert, J.W.
Department of Clinical Immunology
University Hospital
Oostersingel 59
9713 EZ Groningen
The Netherlands

Colotta, F.
Istituto di Ricerche Farmacologiche
Mario Negri
Via Eritrea 62
I-20157 Milano
Italy

Dietrich, H.
Institute for General and Experimental
Pathology
University of Innsbruck, Medical School
Fritz-Pregl-Strasse 3/IV
6020 Innsbruck
Austria

Fabry, Z.
Department of Pathology
(Division of Neuropathology)
University of Iowa College of Medicine
Iowa City, Iowa 52242
United States of America

Fujiyama, J.
Department of Pathology
Tohoku University School of Medicine
1-1-2 chome, Katahira
Aoba-Ku, Sendai 980
Japan

Hancock, W.W.
Sandoz Center and Dept. Surgery and
Pathology
New England Deaconess Hospital
Harvard Medical School
Boston, MA. 02215
United States of America

Hansson, G.K.
King Gustaf V Research Institute
Karolinska Hospital
S-171 76 Stockholm
Sweden

Hart, M.N.
Department of Pathology
(Division of Neuropathology)
University of Iowa College of Medicine
Iowa City, Iowa 52242
United States of America

Itoh, J.
Department of Pathology
Tohoku University School of Medicine
1-1-2-chome, Katahira
Aoba-Ku, Sendai 980
Japan

Kallenberg, C.G.M.
Department of Clinical Immunology
University Hospital
Oostersingel 59
9713 EZ Groningen
The Netherlands

Kato, M.
Department of Pathology
Tohoku University School of Medicine
1-1-2-chome, Katahira
Aoba-Ku, Sendai 980
Japan

Kleindienst, R.
Institute for Biomedical Aging Research
University of Innsbruck, Medical School
Fritz-Pregl-Strasse 3/IV
6020 Innsbruck
Austria

Kyogoku, M.
Otsuka Pharmaceutical Co Ltd
Fujii Memorial Research Institute
Karasaki 1-11-1
Otsu 520-01
Japan

Libby, P.
Vascular Medicine and Atherosclerosis
Unit
Brigham and Women's Hospital
221 Longwood Avenue
Boston, Massachusetts
United States of America

Mantovani, A.
Istituto di Ricerche Farmacologiche
Mario Negri
Via Eritrea 62
I-20157 Milano
Italy

Miyazawa, M.
Department of Pathology
Tohoku University School of Medicine
1-1-2-chome, Katahira
Aoba-Ku, Sendai 980
Japan

Murakami, K.
Department of Pathology
Tohoku University School of Medicine
1-1-2-chome, Katahira
Aoba-Ku, Sendai 980
Japan

Nose, M.
Department of Pathology
Tohoku University School of Medicine
1-1-2-chome, Katahira
Aoba-Ku, Sendai 980
Japan

Palinski, W.
University of California, San Diego
Department of Medicine, 0682
La Jolla
CA 92093-0682
United States of America

Pober, J.S.
Boyer Center for Molecular Medicine
Yale University School of Medicine
295 Congress Avenue
New Haven, Connecticut 06536-0812
United States of America

Robson, S.C.
Sandoz Center and Dept. Surgery and
Pathology
New England Deaconess Hospital
Harvard Medical School
Boston, MA. 02215
United States of America

Schett, G.
Institute for Biomedical Aging Research
University of Innsbruck, Medical School
Fritz-Pregl-Strasse 3/IV
6020 Innsbruck
Austria

Seitz, C.
Institute for Biomedical Aging Research
University of Innsbruck, Medical School
Fritz-Pregl-Strasse 3/IV
6020 Innsbruck
Austria

Sozzani, S.
Istituto di Ricerche Farmacologiche
Mario Negri
Via Eritrea 62
I-20157 Milano
Italy

Wick, G.
Insitute for General and Experimental
Pathology
University of Innsbruck, Medical School
Fritz-Pregl-Strasse 3/IV
6020 Innsbruck
Austria

Witztum, J.L.
University of California, San Diego
Department of Medicine, 0682
La Jolla
CA 92093-0682
United States of America

Xu, Q.
Institute for Biomedical Aging Research
University of Innsbruck, Medical School
Fritz-Pregl-Strasse 3/IV
6020 Innsbruck
Austria

VOLUME PREFACE

THE VESSEL WALL AS AN IMMUNE ORGAN

Twenty years ago, many immunologists viewed the blood vessels as a system of inert tubing. Its only immunologic function was thought to be to serve as a conduit for the immunocompetent cells and macromolecules *en route* between lymphoid organs. Cardiovascular physiologists, on the other hand, often seemed to look upon lymphocytes merely as particles that disturbed the laminar blood flow in the vessels.

Today, the picture is entirely different. There is a continuous flow of information between the vascular cells and those of the immune system. The endothelium is known to be an important antigen-presenting cell directly involved in the activation of immune responses. Vascular endothelial and smooth muscle cells actively participate in the inflammatory response that is often associated with immune activation, by both responding to and producing the cytokine signals that govern this process. Finally, the differentiation of the immunocompetent cells themselves depends on their migration from central to peripheral lymphoid organs, a process that is now known to be mediated by addressins on the endothelial surface which permit the binding of lymphocytes equipped with appropriate homing receptors.

Not surprisingly, this intricate network is perturbed in several pathological conditions. The vasculitides are characterized by pathological inflammation in the vessel wall, which is often initiated by autoimmune attacks on vascular cells. Hyperacute rejection of organ transplants is largely effectuated by complement-activating antibodies to endothelial antigens, while chronic rejection involves a lymphocyte-dependent, proliferative arterial disease process. Finally, atherosclerosis, which is the most common lethal disease of the Western world, is characterized by infiltration of monocyte-derived macrophages and T lymphocytes into the arterial intima, where they secrete cytokines that modulate cell proliferation and lipid metabolism. The important role played by the immune system in all these diseases suggests that intervention with immunologic mechanisms may turn out to be a successful therapeutic strategy. Because of this and because of the significant role played by vascular cells in basic immunologic functions, there is currently a huge interest in vascular immunology throughout the scientific world.

The time is therefore ripe for a book dedicated to vascular immunology. This volume is an attempt to summarize information that is presently available in the field. Jordan Pober provides an overview of the antigen-presenting and immune-regulatory functions of the vascular endothelium and Zsuzsanna Fabry and Michael Hart discuss the interactions between vascular smooth muscle cells and lymphocytes. The immune-vascular cytokine network is dissected by Peter Libby and Alberto Mantovani and his colleagues give a vascular biologic perspective on chemotaxis-regulating chemokines. Leukocyte-endothelial adhesion, an important part of vascular immunology, will be covered in a separate volume in this series, and is therefore discussed only briefly and in the context of other aspects in this volume.

The physiologically oriented chapters are followed by a section examining pathology and pathophysiology. The immunopathology of the vasculitides is described by Matsuhiro Kogota and his colleagues and the role of myeloid lyosomal enzymes as important autoantigens in these diseases is addressed by Jan Willem Cohen Tervaert and Cees Kallenberg. Fritz Bach and co-authors evaluate the importance of immune-induced vascular injury in the rejection of xenografts, an area where vascular-immune reactions remain major obstacles to progress into the clinical arena. Atherosclerosis, finally, is the topic of the last three chapters. Göran Hansson analyzes the involvement of immuno-competent cells and points out the possibility that autoantigens may be involved in the disease process. Two potentially important antigens, oxidized lipoproteins and heat shock proteins, are discussed in separate chapters by Joseph Witztum and Wulf Palinski and by Georg Wick and colleagues.

We are convinced that this book on vascular immunology will be followed by others that may be able to provide a more comprehensive picture of the field than it is possible to do at the moment. However, we also believe that the present volume, which is the first of its kind, should be attractive for many scientists and physicians interested in immunology, inflammation, and cardiovascular diseases. We are indebted to our co-authors, who have so generously devoted their time, energy and knowledge to the creation of this book. We would also like to acknowledge the support and patience of our publishers, the Gordon and Breach Publishing Group.

Göran K. Hansson   Peter Libby

1 The Endothelium as an Antigen Presenting Cell

Jordan S. Pober, M.D., Ph.D.

Director, Molecular Cardiobiology Program, Professor of Pathology, Immunobiology and Biology, Boyer Center for Molecular Medicine, Yale University School of Medicine, 295 Congress Avenue, New Haven, Connecticut 06536–0812

INTRODUCTION

The central question that will be addressed in this chapter is, can vascular endothelial cells present foreign antigens to circulating T cells, leading to intravascular T cell activation at a local site of antigen challenge (e.g. at a site of infection)? This question must be addressed in the more general context of what is currently understood about how T cells recognize and become activated by antigen. The introduction of this chapter will therefore be a recapitulation of current concepts in this field. Relevant aspects of this subject have been extensively reviewed elsewhere (Bierer *et al.*, 1989; Bjorkman and Parham, 1990; Halloran and Madrenas, 1990; Janeway, 1992; Jorgensen *et al.*, 1992; Reth, 1992; Fitch *et al.*, 1993; Germain and Margulies, 1993; Gray, 1993; Linsley *et al.*, 1993; Minami *et al.*, 1993; Sherman and Chattopadhyay, 1993; Berke, 1994; Crabtree and Clipstone, 1994; Cresswell, 1994; Trowbridge and Thomas, 1994). Key findings will be briefly summarized and readers wishing more detailed information may refer to these review articles as an introduction to the primary literature.

T Cell Recognition of and Activation by Antigen

Specific Antigen Recognition by T cells

The principal function of the immune system is to protect an individual host against infection. It does so by mobilizing an array of destructive defense mechanisms that serve to eliminate foreign microbes or parasites. A cardinal feature of the protective immune response is that it is highly specific for foreign organisms, sparing host tissues from the worst of the assault. Specificity is provided by lymphocytes, including both T and B cells. The basis of this remarkable specificity is now understood in molecular terms (Jorgensen, *et al.*, 1992; Reth, 1992). Each developing lymphocyte generates (and expresses many copies of) a unique antigen receptor through several interacting mechanisms including selective but random expression of one of many germline genes, genetic recombination with random diversification at recombination junctions, and (in the case of antibody-producing B cells) random somatic mutation. The number of possible different antigen receptors that can be generated by these mechanisms is very large (i.e. greater than 1×10^{16} different receptors), but the maturing lymphocytes (especially T cells) are subjected to selection processes (both positive and negative) that limit the number of receptors that are utilized. As a result, about 1×10^{13} different T cell receptors and 1×10^{11} different B cell receptors are actually expressed on mature lymphocytes and each different lymphocyte (and its clonal progeny) expresses a receptor that can specifically bind only one or a few closely related chemical structures called "antigenic determinants". The collection of antigen receptors displayed by the population of mature lymphocytes is called the "repertoire". The normal T cell repertoire has been shaped by selection to specifically recognize a large variety of possible foreign antigenic determinants but generally not self antigens.

Recent molecular studies have also defined the form of antigens recognized by lymphocytes. B cells, which use antibody molecules as their antigen receptors, recognize both native and denatured macromolecules of all classes (eg. protein, lipid, complex carbohydrate, and nucleic acid) as well as a wide variety of different types of small molecules. T cells, the principal initiator and regulator of immune reactions, almost exclusively recognize linear amino acid sequences (i.e. peptides) derived from the partial degradation of proteins. Most T cells express an antigen receptor consisting of selectively expressed, somatically recombined, and junctionally diversified α and β polypeptide heterodimers associated with a complex of invariant polypeptides (eg. CD3γ, δ and ε) and other proteins involved in signal transduction. (A minor population of T cells express an alternative receptor of γ and δ heterodimers that are also expressed on the T cell surface in association with CD3γ, δ and ε and other signalling proteins; less is known about the functions of this class of T cells or about their antigen specificities and these cells will not be discussed further.) During T cell maturation in the thymus, the $\alpha\beta$ T cell receptors are selected to recognize a molecular complex of a specific peptide sequence bound to a specialized cell surface peptide-binding protein. These cell surface peptide-binding proteins are encoded by genes of the major histocompatibility complex (MHC) and are called MHC molecules. Both the peptide and the MHC molecule contact the T cell receptor and contribute to the antigenic determinant recognized by the T cell.

MHC molecules may be divided on the basis of structure into two classes (Bjorkman and Parham, 1990; Cresswell, 1994). Class I molecules contain a single, approximately 44 kD, transmembrane MHC-encoded polypeptide that is expressed in non-convalent association with a small 12 kD polypeptide, called β_2 microglobulin, that is encoded by a gene outside the MHC. The peptide binding site is formed by folding the 180 extracellular amino terminal amino acid residues of the class I heavy chain. Structurally, this site consists of a floor base of eight β-pleated strands supporting two parallel α-helical walls. The resultant structure contains a cleft between the α-helices that is able to accommodate peptides of nine to eleven amino acid residues. The genes encoding class I heavy chains are extraordinarily polymorphic; over 100 alleles are commonly expressed in the population. The amino acid differences among class I alleles are concentrated in the α-helical walls and β-strand floor of the peptide binding cleft, producing protrusions and/or pockets that define the subset of different possible peptides that can bind to each allelic form. This specificity is not highly stringent; perhaps 100 or more different peptides may be bound by a particular allelic form of a class I MHC molecule (although any individual molecule can only bind one peptide at a time). Every individual human has three class I gene loci (called HLA-A, B and C) and, if heterozygous at each locus, each individual will therefore express six different class I heavy chains, allowing for the binding of nearly 1000 distinct peptides. (There are also additional MHC loci that encode non-polymorphic class I — like molecules; it is not certain whether these unconventional molecules, sometimes called class Ib molecules, are involved in antigen presentation.) Since each foreign protein can be cleaved into many different overlapping peptides, very few foreign proteins can escape T cell recognition by failing to contain sequences able to bind to at least one of the six class I MHC molecules expressed by any individual. About one third of circulating mature $\alpha\beta$ T cells recognize peptides associated with class I MHC molecules. Each individual T cell recognizes only one specific peptide (or a few closely related peptides) bound to one allelic form of a class I heavy chain. This form of antigen recognition is called "class I MHC-restricted," meaning that T cell recognition is restricted to recognition of peptide on the surface of cells expressing the relevant class I allele.

The remaining two thirds of circulating $\alpha\beta$ T cells recognize peptides associated with class II MHC molecules. Class II molecules are cell surface heterodimers consisting of two approximately 30 kD transmembrane polypeptides (called α and β), each encoded by separate MHC genes. A peptide binding site similar to that in class I molecules is formed by an interaction between the extracellular amino terminal 90 amino acid residues of each class II peptide chain. The class II peptide-binding site is longer than the class I binding site and the size of peptides accommodated by the class II cleft is therefore larger; class II-associated peptides average fourteen to seventeen amino acid residues in length. The genes encoding class II molecules are also highly polymorphic and the variable residues are also clustered in the peptide binding site, providing specificity for peptide binding. Each human individual expresses class II heterodimers encoded by at least three class II loci (HLA-DR, DP and DQ); each locus encodes one α chain and one or more β chains so that in a heterozygous individual, more than six different class II molecules may be expressed. (Heterodimers between α chains from one locus and β chains from another are uncommon.) Consequently, each individual can form class II MHC complexes with over a thousand different peptides. Each individual T cell recognizes only one specific peptide (or a few closely related peptides) bound to a particular allelic form of a class II MHC molecule. This form of antigen recognition is called "class II MHC-restricted."

Transplantation presents a special case of T cell recognition of antigen (Sherman and Chattopadhyay, 1993). In this setting, T cells encounter non-self allelic forms of MHC molecules. Many (if not all) T cells that are specific for a complex of a particular foreign peptide bound to a particular self allelic form of a class I or class II MHC molecule will cross-react and recognize the antigenic determinant formed by some peptide (often derived from a self protein) bound to the foreign MHC molecule. This cross-reaction is called "direct recognition" of allogeneic MHC molecules, as opposed to indirect recognition which would involve presentation of non-self peptides derived from the foreign MHC molecules in a complex with self-encoded MHC molecules. Each foreign MHC molecule, like self MHC molecules, can bind 100 or more different peptides, and each peptide MHC complex can involve cross-reactions with different clones of T cells. Consequently the frequency of T cells that directly recognize each specific foreign MHC molecule is typically a hundred to a thousand-fold higher than the frequency of T cells that can recognize a specific foreign protein in the form of peptide associated with a self MHC molecule.

Antigen Processing

As the preceding discussion makes clear, $\alpha\beta$ T cells recognize non-self peptides (derived from foreign proteins) that are bound in a complex to self class I or class II MHC molecules. This conclusion raises two new but related questions: (1) how is the complex of foreign peptide with MHC molecule generated? and (2) where is the complex made available to T cells? The generation of a peptide — MHC molecule complex is called "antigen processing" and the display of the complex is called "antigen presentation."

Antigen processing is fundamentally different for peptides destined to associate with each of the two classes of MHC molecules (Germain and Margulies, 1993). Class I MHC molecules associate with peptides during assembly of newly translated polypeptides in the endoplasmic reticulum. The major source of these peptides is protein degradation in the cytosolic compartment, probably by proteosomes. Peptides generated in the cytosol are transported into the endoplasmic reticulum by a peptide "pump" called the transporter in antigen processing (or TAP). TAP is believed to function as a heterodimer of TAP-1 and TAP-2 MHC-encoded polypeptides. Recent evidence suggests that TAP binds newly translated class I heavy chains within the endoplasmic reticulum and "loads" them with peptides as they fold. (Such heavy chains are already proteolytically cleaved to remove the leader sequence and glycosylated, since these processes occur co-translationally.) The association of β_2 microglobulin with the class I heavy chain, which also occurs within the endoplasmic reticulum complex, stabilizes the peptide-heavy chain complex. Empty class I molecules do not efficiently exit from the endoplasmic reticulum and may be preferentially degraded within it in a process involving the protein calnexin. Indeed, a second source of peptides for MHC molecules may be proteolysis within the endoplasmic reticulum, e.g. from leader sequences that are normally cleaved during protein translation or from defective proteins, such as empty class I, that are degraded with the endoplasmic reticulum. Once peptide and β_2 microglobulin are bound to the heavy chain, the class I molecule complex is transported to the Golgi apparatus (for carbohydrate processing) and then to the cell surface.

Neither the provision of peptides to newly translated class I molecules nor the assembly of class I molecules is thought to favor peptides derived from foreign proteins over peptides derived from self proteins. Indeed, both self peptides and non-self peptides (when present) are simultaneously displayed in complexes with class I MHC molecules on the cell surface. Instead, the specificity of the immune response for non-self peptide resides exclusively in the specificity of $\alpha\beta$ antigen receptors found on mature T cells. This specificity exists because self-reactive T cells were eliminated or made unresponsive during maturation through processes of selection. Non-self peptides are, by definition, not normally present. Those foreign proteins that do give rise to peptides associated with class I are generally synthesized in the cytosol of the cell eg. during a viral infection.

Class II MHC molecules associate with peptides in a membrane-enclosed compartment that is reached only after transit of newly synthesized molecules through the Golgi apparatus. The peptide binding cleft of class II molecules is blocked in the endoplasmic reticulum and Golgi apparatus by the binding of a non-polymorphic class II binding protein, called invariant chain. The occupancy of the cleft by invariant chain prevents peptide binding so that class II molecules usually do not associate with the set of peptides found in the endoplasmic reticulum that are normally associated with class I molecules. The invariant chain is dissociated from class II molecules (and probably degraded) in a post-Golgi vacuolar compartment. Extracellular proteins, taken into the cell by various forms of endocytosis (eg. pinocytosis, phagocytosis, or receptor-mediated endocytosis) are also brought to this same compartment. Such proteins are partly degraded just before or after their encounter with class II MHC molecules, generating peptides. These peptides may bind to the newly liberated (from invariant chain) class II molecules, and the class II-peptide complex is then transported to the cell surface. Consequently, class II associated peptides are generally derived from proteins found in the extracellular milieu.

As in the case of class I-peptide binding, peptide generation from extracellularly derived proteins and the binding of peptide to class II MHC molecules are not able to discriminate between self and foreign proteins. Again the specificity of the response for foreign molecules resides in the T cell repertoire, resulting from the elimination of T cells bearing $\alpha\beta$ antigen receptors reactive with self peptides. Class II molecules occupied by self and (when present) non-self peptides are simultaneously expressed on the cell surface. The source of foreign proteins that give rise to peptides associated with class II MHC molecules is principally extracellular bacteria and parasites.

Antigen Presentation to T Cells

As noted above, the antigen receptors of $\alpha\beta$ T cells recognize foreign peptides that are bound to self-allelic forms of MHC molecules. Implied in this statement is the fact that these complexes are recognized on a cell surface because that is where MHC molecules are normally expressed. Remarkably, the complex recognized by a particular T cell through its antigen receptor must reside on the surface of another cell; in other words, there appear to be no interactions between T cell receptors and peptide-MHC molecule complexes on the surface of an individual T cell despite the fact that T cells co-express T cell receptors for antigen and peptide-MHC molecules. The cell that displays a peptide-MHC complex to a specific T cell is said to "present the antigen", and is referred to as an "antigen presenting cell" (APC). The term APC is often restricted to cells that present peptide-class II MHC complexes to a subset of T cells that initiate immune reactions (called helper T lymphocytes or HTL), but the same processes are involved in presentation of peptide-class I MHC complexes to T cells and the cell that displays this complex is, in fact, acting as an APC.

The capacity to present antigen requires at a minimum that a cell synthesize and express MHC molecules. Expression of class I and class II MHC molecules is differentially regulated (Halloran and Madrenas, 1990). Class I MHC molecules are constitutively synthesized by almost all nucleated cell types, neurons being a notable exception. Synthesis and expression of class I molecules are increased by pro-inflammatory cytokines, particularly tumor necrosis factor (TNF) and the structurally related cytokine lymphotoxin (LT), type 1 interferons (IFN) (i.e. IFN-α and IFN-β, and type 2 interferon, (i.e. IFN-γ). TNF or LT acts synergistically with either type 1 or type 2 IFN to increase class I molecule expression. Class II MHC molecules are expressed less widely. Human T cells express class II molecules upon activation by antigen. B cells express class II molecules constitutively and the level of expression is increased by interleukin 4 (IL-4) and, at certain developmental stages, by IFN-γ. Dendritic cells, which specialize in antigen presentation, express a very high level of class II MHC molecules, but this may depend upon prior exposure (during maturation) to IFN-γ or granulocyte/monocyte-colony stimulating factor (GM-CSF). Mononuclear phagocytes express little class II constitutively but increase expression in response to IFN-γ or GM-CSF. Type 1 IFN and IL10 inhibit class II expression on mononuclear phagocytes. Most tissue cells, including vascular endothelial cells (EC), express class II molecules only in response to IFN-γ. Type I IFN (but probably not IL-10) inhibits class II expression on tissue cells. TNF or LT may either inhibit or enhance class II expression, depending on the cell type.

Based on these patterns of regulation of MHC molecule expression, it follows that most cell types generate class I-associated peptide complexes and this ability is increased by pro-inflammatory cytokines. Few cell types generate class II-associated peptide complexes under basal conditions, but most can do so after exposure to pro-inflammatory cytokines (especially to IFN-γ).

T Cell Activation by Antigen: The Requirement for Costimulation

The primary event on a T cell when it encounters specific peptide-MHC molecule complexes on the surface of an APC is the clustering of T cell receptors at the point of cell contact. Each T cell may express over 10,000 antigen receptor molecules, but only a few hundred must be clustered to initiate a response. The clustering of antigen receptors triggers a cascade of intracellular events leading to T cell activation and proliferation (Crabtree and Clipstone, 1994). The primary intercellular events appear to be activation of cytoplasmic protein tyrosine kinases that are associated with the receptor, namely fyn and ZAP 70. The ultimate events in this T cell response to antigen are new gene transcription (see below) and entry into cell cycle. The intervening pathways connecting receptor-associated tyrosine kinases to transcription and cell proliferation are not fully worked out. The T cell response to antigen can be mimicked by manipulations other than recognition of antigen that cause clustering of T cell antigen receptors, e.g. with antibodies to the α or β receptor polypeptide chains, with antibodies to the associated CD3 polypeptides, or with lectins that bind to carbohydrate moieties attached to the T cell receptor polypeptides such as phytohemagglutinin (PHA) or concanavalin A (Con A). "Superantigens", i.e. bacterial or viral proteins that bind to class II MHC molecules on APC and to a large subset of T cell receptor β chains, can also mimic the events provoked by recognition of specific peptide-MHC complexes. When large numbers of T cell receptors are clustered, as can happen with tetravalent plant lectins, superantigens, or with immobilized (e.g. bead- or plate-bound) anti-receptor antibodies, no additional signals are needed to cause T cell gene transcription and proliferation. However, this "one signal" pathway is non-physiological. APC simply do not express sufficient numbers of specific peptide-MHC complexes to cause enough receptor clustering to fully trigger activation. APC overcome this problem by providing antigen-independent signals, called "costimulators," that increase the sensitivity of T cells to a lower level of receptor clustering. Many of these costimulator signals have been identified. For example, all mature $\alpha\beta$ T cells express either CD4 polypeptides or CD8 polypeptides on their cell surface (Janeway, 1992). CD4 binds to class II MHC molecules on the APC at a site distinct from that involved in peptide-MHC complex interaction with the T cell receptor. When T cells recognize peptide-class II MHC complexes with their specific antigen receptor, T cell CD4 molecules are drawn into the cluster of antigen receptors. Each CD4 molecule is associated intracellularly with a cytoplasmic protein tyrosine kinase (lck) that interacts and increases the signals provided by the receptor-associated protein tyrosine kinases fyn and ZAP 70. CD8 binds to class I MHC molecules and is also associated with lck. The expression of CD4 or CD8 is co-selected with antigen specificity during T cell matura-tion. Consequently, CD4$^+$ T cells constitute the two thirds of $\alpha\beta$ T cells that are MHC class II-restricted (and respond primarily to foreign protein antigens that are acquired through endocytosis) whereas CD8$^+$ T cells constitute the one third of $\alpha\beta$ T cells that are MHC class I-restricted (and respond primarily to foreign proteins that are synthesized within the cytoplasm of the APC).

CD45 is another T cell polypeptide that contributes to activation (Trowbridge and Thomas, 1994). The cytoplasmic domains of this protein have protein tyrosine phos-phatase activity. Paradoxically, CD45 action is thought to increase net protein tyrosine kinase activity within the activated T cell by removing phosphates from certain tyrosine residues within the protein tyrosine kinases that normally inhibit enzyme activity. The extracellular regions of CD45 contain three polypeptide sequences that can be removed by alternative mRNA splicing out of the exons (denoted A,B and C) that code for them. Mature $\alpha\beta$ T cells that have never encountered their specific antigen (called "naive" or "virgin" T cells) express an isoform of CD45 that contains all three of these variable exons; this form of CD45 is usually detected on human T cells by an antibody reactive with sequences in exon A and is called CD45RA. Mature T cells that have encountered their specific antigen usually alternatively splice out exons A,B and C from CD45 mRNA and either coexpress different isoforms or express exclusively the form lacking exon A-encoded sequence. The isoform lacking A,B and C sequences is called CD45RO. The structure of the associated carbohydrate moieties on CD45 molecules also change upon activation, and the CD45RO isoform can be recognized on human T cells by a specific mouse antibody (UCHL-1) that reacts with these altered carbohydrate structures. T cells recognized by this antibody are designated CD45RO$^+$. Some CD45RO$^+$ T cells, i.e. those that have recently encountered specific antigen, are in active cell cycle; more have left the cell cycle and returned to a resting state. These resting T cells may remain in the cir-culation as long lived memory T cells. Resting CD45RO$^+$ memory $\alpha\beta$ T cells are easier to activate in response to antigen than resting CD45RA$^+$RO$^-$ naive $\alpha\beta$ T cells. It is likely that the different CD45 isoforms contribute to this difference.

Several other T cell surface ligands contribute to activation i.e. act as costimulators. Two systems are thought to be particularly important: CD28 and CD2. The CD28 system consists of at least five proteins (Linsley, *et al.*, 1993). The T cell may express CD28 in its resting state and, upon activation, may express a structurally related protein called cytolytic T lymphocyte antigen (CTLA)-4. Both molecules bind the same ligands. CD28 delivers positive stimulation to T cells and is a strong costimulator; CTLA-4 binds with higher affinity to its ligands than CD28 but delivers inhibitory signals. Thus activated T cells may synthesize and express CTLA-4 as a mechanism to shut off signals through this pathway. CD28 signals may augment gene transcription but the major role of CD28-mediated signals may be to stabilize certain mRNAs, especially IL-2 mRNA. The ligands recognized by both CD28 and CTLA-4 have been designated B7.1 and B7.2; indirect evidence exists for a third ligand, called B7.3. These molecules are absent from resting B cells or monocytes, but are induced after interactions with T cells, possibly involving a contact-dependent pathway involving CD40 on the APC and a ligand for CD40, called gp39, on the activated T cell. Dendritic cells may constitutively express CD28 ligands (although this may require prior exposure of immature dendritic cells to IFN-γ or GM-CSF). The requirement for induction of the ligands suggests that this system may act late in T cell activation.

The CD2 pathway involves at least five polypeptides (Bierer, *et al.*, 1989). CD2 is the major T cell receptor for signals. Extensive clustering of CD2 can directly activate T cells, producing new transcription and entry into the cell cycle, bypassing the T cell antigen receptor. Physiologically, more likely this system augments signals provided by the T cell receptor and strongly synergizes with signals from the CD28 system. Three APC ligands for the CD2 pathway have been identified: lymphocyte function-associated antigen (LFA)-3 or CD58), CD59 and CD48. LFA-3 is the principal signaling ligand. CD59, which also functions as a complement regulatory protein, can augment CD58 signals but is less or not active by itself. CD48 is the principal murine ligand for CD2 (where LFA-3 may be absent); it is not clear to what extent CD48 delivers functional signals. The CD2 pathway can also involve CD44, a hyauloronic acid receptor. CD44 may strengthen attachments so that CD2 signaling improves or it may signal directly. CD44 is usually expressed by both the T cell and the APC and it is not clear whether CD44 on both cells is required for these interactions.

Two other kinds of molecules need to be considered in costimulation: adhesion proteins (Springer, 1990) and cytokines. As noted above for one of the proposed roles of CD44, increased adhesion between the T cell and the APC may increase the efficiency of stimulation and costimulation through other molecules. Adhesive interactions of T cells with APC are mediated predominantly by integrins. T cells use LFA-1 (CD11aCD18), a $\beta2$ (or CD18) integrin to recognize three APC ligands: intercellular adhesion molecule (ICAM)-1, 2 and 3. ICAM-1 and 3 are found constitutively on leukocytes. Expression of ICAM-1 is increased on tissue cells (including endothelium) by proinflammatory cytokines (notably TNF, IL-1 and IFN-γ). ICAM-2 is constitutively expressed by endothelial cells and is not known to be regulated. T cells also use $\beta1$ (or CD29) integrins to recognize APC and matrix proteins. Very late activation (VLA) antigen-4 (CD49dCD29) is used to recognize vascular cell adhesion molecule (VCAM)-1 on cytokine-treated endothelium and other cells; VLA-4 and VLA-5 (CD49eCD29) recognize different regions of fibronectin and VLA-6 (CD49fCD29) recognizes laminin. The VLA-4 α chain (CD49d) may also combine with a $\beta7$ integrin chain to recognize an endothelial ligand found on gut vessels, called mucosal addressin cell adhesion molecule (MadCAM)-1. Interference with these interactions (eg. with competing monoclonal antibodies) may inhibit antigen presentation. Although these effects are primarily attributed to adhesion, engagement of T cell integrins may also deliver signals that directly provide costimulation. Non-integrin adhesive interactions may involve selectins and immunoglobulin-like molecules. T cell L-selectin (CD62L) can interact with glycoproteins on cytokine-treated EC and activated EC express E-selectin (CD62E) and P-selectin (CD62P) that can interact with T cell glycoproteins, especially on a subset of CD45RO[+] memory cells. T cell platelet-endothelial cell adhesion molecule (PECAM)-1 (CD31) may interact with PECAM-1 on endothelial cells and other APC.

Cytokines were identified as the first costimulators. IL-1, once called lymphocyte activation factor, can act as a costimulator for thymocytes (i.e. immature T cells in the thymus) and certain differentiated mouse T cell clones (i.e. those designated T helper 2 that produce IL-4 but not IL-2). However, IL-1 seems to have no role in the activation of resting human $\alpha\beta$ T cells isolated from peripheral blood. IL-6 may also costimulate thymocytes and may act on resting blood T cells. TNF or LT may act as a growth factor for thymocytes and for activated T cells. Recently, it has been appreciated that T cells, either resting or activated, express a number of proteins homologous to the receptors for TNF, including Fas, CD27 and CD30. APC may express surface-bound ligands for these proteins that can deliver costimulatory signals to resting T cells. It is too early to determine the importance of cytokine-like contact-dependent signals as physiological costimulators. However it is generally agreed that soluble cytokines are less important as costimulators for resting mature T cells than are contact-dependent pathways, especially those involving CD28 and CD2.

T Cell Activation by Antigen: Post-Activation Responses

The activation of resting T cells is defined by new gene transcription and entry into cell cycle. Many of the genes that are newly transcribed in activated T cells encode proteins that are involved with transcription of other genes (eg. c-fos or c-myc). Another important class of genes that are activated are cytokines and, in some cases, cytokine receptors. The details of the response made by mature $\alpha\beta$ T cells upon encounter with specific antigen depends upon the precise developmental status of T cell and upon the costimulatory signals received. Naive $\alpha\beta$ T cells produce only small quantities of cytokines and even this response is only seen in the presence of strong costimulators, such as ligands for CD28. The key cytokine produced by naive T cells upon activation is IL-2. IL-2 is an autocrine and paracrine growth factor for T cells, and the principal action of IL-2 at physiological concentrations is to drive recently activated T cells through the cell cycle, i.e. IL-2 acts as a progression factor. At sufficiently high (i.e. pharmacological) concentrations, IL-2 can also activate resting T cells to enter cell cycle, acting as a competence factor as well.

T cells are the only cell type that normally synthesizes IL-2. The inducible regulation of IL-2 synthesis has been studied in great detail, (Crabtree and Clipstone, 1994), although almost exclusively in T cell tumor lines that may not be accurate models for regulation in naive T cells. In brief, resting T cells do not transcribe the gene for IL-2. Clustering of the T cell antigen receptor causes tyrosine phosphorylation of γ isoforms of phosphotidylinositol-specific phospholipase C (PI-PLCγ), activating enzymatic activity. Activated PI-PLCγ cleaves membrane phosphatidylinositol into inositol triphosphate, a signal for elevating cytosolic calcium, and diacyl glycerol, a signal that activates certain protein kinase C isoforms in the presence of elevated calcium. Cytosolic calcium binds to calmodulin and the calcium/calmodulin complex activates the enzymatic activity of calcineurin, as protein serine/threonine phosphatase. Activated calcineurin dephosphorylates one or more cytosolic proteins, the most important of which are called nuclear factor of activated T cells pre-existing (NFAT$_p$) or nuclear factor of activated T cells, cytoplasmic (NFAT$_c$). Dephosphorylated NFAT$_p$ and NFAT$_c$ translocate from the cytosol to the nucleus where they combine with newly synthesized proteins, notably c-fos/c-jun heterodimers.

This heterotrimeric complex of $NFAT_{p/c}$, c-fos, and c-jun, called NFAT, binds to each of two different cis regulatory sequences in the IL-2 promoter, contributing to the onset of IL-2 gene transcription. Other transcriptional activating factors are recruited to act in concert with NFAT. For example, synergistic induction of IL-2 transcription has been observed between NFAT and nuclear proteins that bind to a nearby tetrahydrophorbol response element (TRE). The principal TRE-binding protein is activating protein (AP)-1 which is comprised of c-fos and c-jun (i.e. the same proteins that form part of NFAT). In resting T cells, AP-1 synthesis is induced primarily through protein kinase C signals. IL-2 transcription can be initiated by a combination of calcium ionophore and synthetic protein kinase C activators, leading to both NFAT and AP-1 formation, respectively. Other important transcription factors include nuclear factor kappa B (NF-κB) and octomer activating factor (OAF) which binds to constitutively expressed octomer binding protein (Oct)-1. Optimal IL-2 transcription depends on cooperation between all of these factors. Once transcribed, the mRNA is translated and IL-2 protein is secreted. IL-2 mRNA is usually unstable, but signals generated through the CD28 pathway may prevent mRNA degradation, increasing and prolonging IL-2 synthesis and secretion.

IL-2 acts on T cells. Resting T cells express a heterodimeric IL-2 receptor composed of a 70kD subunit (β) and a 60kD subunit (γ) (Minami *et al.*, 1993). $\beta\gamma$ receptors bind IL-2 with moderate affinity ($K_d \approx 10^{-9}$M); such T cells are generally unable to respond to concentrations of IL-2 produced in response to antigen. Upon activation, T cells synthesize and express an additional 55kD IL-2 binding polypeptide (also called T activation or Tac antigen). The α subunit does not signal but, in combination with $\beta\gamma$, improves IL-2 binding ($K_d = 1 \times 10^{-11}$M) so that T cells readily respond to physiologically-generated levels of IL-2. Naive T cells make both IL-2 and IL-2Rα upon activation, and they can proliferate through an autocrine pathway. IL-2Rα expression is induced primarily through signals induced by clustering of the T cell antigen receptor, but IL-2Rα expression may also be induced in response to T cell-derived cytokines. Consequently some T cells not activated by antigen, particularly those adjacent to antigen-activated IL-2-secreting cells, may respond in a paracrine manner and also proliferate.

In most experimental systems, the quantity of IL-2 produced is a critical determinant of the outcome of a primary immune response. If insufficient IL-2 is generated, antigen-specific naive T cells enter cell cycle but fail to progress. Such T cells may die or may become refractory to further stimulation, entering a state called "clonal anergy". In other systems, such T cells may revert to a resting state as if they never encountered antigen, referred to as "immunologic ignorance." In the presence of adequate IL-2, the antigen-stimulated and cytokine-stimulated naive T cells expand; naive T cells are relatively (compared to memory T cells) adept at proliferation. Because naive T cells have very strong costimulator requirements, IL-2 concentrations adequate to stimulate proliferation is probably only generated when antigen is presented by specialized APC such as dendritic cells. These encounters of naive T cells with dendritic cells generally occur in lymph nodes and other secondary lymphoid organs, where antigen (collected through afferent lymphatics) and naive T cells (recirculating between blood and node) are efficiently brought together. Naive T cells express adhesion molecules (especially L-selectin) that favor extravasation at the high endothelial venules of secondary lymphoid organs; these cells are not adept at interacting with endothelium at sites of peripheral inflammation. After several population doublings within the lymph node stroma, some antigen-activated T cells may become overly sensitive to IL-2 and undergo programmed cell death. Other antigen-stimulated T cells eventually leave the cell cycle and return to the circulation as memory T cells.

Memory $\alpha\beta$ T cells are less adept at proliferation than naive T cells but better able to generate sizable quantities of cytokines, including IL-2. IL-2, secreted by memory T cells, appears to be the primary determinant of the outcome of secondary as well as primary immune responses. Memory T cells express a range of surface adhesion molecules that reduce their tendency to migrate to lymph nodes compared to naive cells, but increase their ability to migrate to peripheral sites of inflammation, marked by activated EC that express increased levels of ICAM-1, VCAM-1 and E-selectin. Memory T cells also have less stringent requirements for costimulators than naive cells, allowing for efficient activation on a broader range of APC types. Cumulatively, these properties favor the activation of memory cells by antigen at peripheral tissue sites, as is commonly seen in secondary responses to foreign antigen. The identity of the most important APC at these sites is not known. However resting memory cells still exhibit a requirement for costimulators (albeit less than for naive T cells) and not every cell type is capable of presenting antigen in a manner that can efficiently activate memory T cells from their resting states. In other words, secondary responses, like primary responses, are initiated by specialized APC, but cells other than dendritic cells (e.g. mononuclear phagocytes, B cells or, as will be discussed, vascular endothelial cells) may serve this role.

Some memory T cells, upon activation by antigen, acquire differentiated effector functions. Many CD8$^+$ T cells develop an exocytotic vacuole system that contain a pore-forming protein (called "perforin" or "cytolysin") and a number of serine proteases (called "granzymes"). Such T cells can mediate lysis of other cells and are called "cytolytic T lymphocytes" (CTL) (Berke, 1994). Upon recognition of peptide-MHC complexes on the surface of another cell, CTL release the contents of some of these vacuoles on the surface of the cell displaying antigen, killing the target cell by causing increased membrane permeability and/or DNA fragmentation. Some CTL can also injure target cells through membrane protein interactions independent of exocytosis, mediated by protein such as Fas ligand or membrane-associated TNF. Because killing is initiated and localized by peptide-MHC complex recognition, CTL can kill specific targets without causing injury of bystander cells.

Many newly activated CD4$^+$ memory T cells become "helper T lymphocytes" (HTL) that specialize in cytokine secretion (Fitch *et al.*, 1993). These HTL make a panoply of cytokines including IL-2, IL-4, IL-5, IL-6, IL-10, IL-13, IFN-γ, TNF, LT and GM-CSF, and are designated as T helper type 0 (T$_H$0) cells. Upon repeated stimulation by antigen, some of the T$_H$0 cells may further differentiate into subsets of HTL (T$_H$1) that secrete IL-2, IFN-γ, and LT but not IL-4, IL-5, IL-6, IL-10 and IL-13 or HTL (T$_H$2) that serete only the reciprocal subset of cytokines. The cytokines made by T$_H$1 cells favor immune reactions involving neutrophils, activated macrophages and isotypes of antibody that bind to F$_c\gamma$ receptors on leukocytes. The cytokines made by T$_H$2 cells favor reactions involving eosinophils and isotypes of antibody that activate mast cells (IgE and IgG4). (Note that this separation of T$_H$1 and T$_H$2 functions differs from an earlier notion that T$_H$1 cells favor cell-mediated immunity and T$_H$2 cells favor humoral immunity).

T$_H$1 and T$_H$2 cells may be preferentially activated by different types of APC. In addition, it has been proposed that different types of APC may favor differentiation of T$_H$0 cells into either T$_H$1 or T$_H$2 phenotypes. In particular, APC that produce IL-12 may favor

T_H1 differentiation. However, it is not known precisely what types of APC contribute to such differentiation and whether these events are likely to occur in peripheral tissues or lymphoid organs.

Endothelium as an Antigen Presenting Cell

The preceeding discussion of antigen presentation to T cells may be summarized as three points: (1) T cell activation, measured by entry into cell cycle and synthesis of IL-2 and other cytokines, depends upon both T cell receptor recognition of a specific antigen signal (i.e. a specific peptide-MHC complex) and engagement of antigen-independent costimulator molecules, both of which are provided by an APC; (2) different cell types will differ in their capacities to act as APC depending upon the level of MHC molecule expression and upon the ability to provide costimulator signals such as ligands for CD28 and CD2; and (3) that T cells at different stages of differentiation will have different requirements for costimulators and may preferentially respond to different types of APC. Thus it is possible (and likely) that EC will present antigen to T cells only at certain stages of T cell differentiation. Human vascular EC appear less able to activate naive T cells than are specialized APC of bone marrow origin (e.g. dendritic cells). On the other hand, EC have better costimulator functions than most tissue cells and appear very efficient at activating resting memory T cells. Less is known about the capacities of EC to interact with or cause differentiation of T cells into CTL or into specialized T helper cells.

There are teleological reasons to endow EC with the capacity to activate resting memory T cells, namely increased speed and efficiency of a secondary response. Memory T cells circulate for the purpose of mounting immune reactions at peripheral sites with sufficient rapidity as to contain the invading microbe at the local site (Gray, 1993). Although memory T cells are expanded by their previous encounter with antigen, memory T cells specific for a particular antigen are still not very abundant; typical frequencies may range from one in ten thousand to one in one hundred thousand circulating T cells (compared to one in one hundred thousand to one in one million naive T cells). Thus the host is faced with the problem of fostering encounters of rare T cells with their specific antigens in a timely manner. There are two non-exclusive solutions to this problem: (1) memory T cells may be non-selectively but efficiently recruited into sites of infection by the inflammation that develops in response to local production of pro-inflammatory cytokines and expression of cytokine-induced endothelial adhesion molecules such as ICAM-1, VCAM-1 and E-selectin on the local microvessels; or (2) antigen-specific memory T cells may be selectively activated and recruited by recognition of specific peptide-MHC complexes expressed on the luminal surface of the local microvascular EC. The second mechanism can significantly increase the efficiency and speed of the protective response compared to the first mechanism. At present, the best evidence to support the hypothesis of presentation of antigen occurs on the luminal surface of EC is indirect, namely that recall (secondary) responses are initiated with astonishing rapidity. Human and baboon responses to protein antigens can be detected histologically within 2–3 hours or less of intradermal antigen injection, (Dumonde *et al.*, 1982; Munro *et al.*, 1989) which seems much too rapid for non-specific recruitment of memory T cells. This being said, it must be emphasized that there are no direct data that support or refute a role for endothelial antigen presentation. Experimental observations that indirectly support a role for antigen presentation by EC will be reviewed in the next two sections of the chapter.

ANTIGEN PRESENTATION BY ENDOTHELIAL CELLS *IN VITRO*

This section of the chapter will review experimental observations that analyze the capacities of cultured EC to present antigen to T cells.

Regulation of MHC Molecule Expression on EC

Cultured human EC from a variety of tissue sources appear to behave similarly with regard to expression of class I and class II MHC molecules. The best studied system involves human umbilical vein EC (HUVEC) and the data reviewed here are derived primarily from experiments with this cell type. Under standard culture conditions HUVEC express class I molecules, (Pober and Gimbrone, 1982) and can be tissue typed for products of the A, B and C loci (Moraes and Stastny, 1977). The binding of antibody reactive with conventional class I (mouse monoclonal antibody W6/32) molecules is approximately equivalent to the level of binding of antibody reactive with β_2 microglobulin, suggesting that HUVEC to not express any significant level of unconventional class Ib molecules, but this has not been examined directly. HUVEC also express TAP-1 and TAP-2 proteins (Epperson *et al.*, 1992 and unpublished observations). The number of class I molecules per cell on HUVEC has not been rigorously calculated, but it appears (based on fluorescence intensity in comparison to other cells) to be about 25,000–50,000 molecules/cell. Two classes of proinflammatory cytokines have been shown to increase class I molecule expression: TNF/LT and IFN (both type 1 and type 2) (Lapierre *et al.*, 1988) HUVEC do not increase class I molecule expression in response to IL-1, GM-CSF, IL-4, IL-10 or any other cytokine that has been tested. Some signals other than cytokines, such as hydrogen peroxide can also increase class I expression (Bradley *et al.*, 1993), but this effect is smaller than that seen with cytokines.

Treatment with optimal concentrations of TNF or LT typically double the level of surface expression of class I molecules on HUVEC within 24 hrs and can increase expression five to ten-fold by 7 days (Collins *et al.*, 1986). TNF actions are primarily mediated through the 55kD TNF receptor which is expressed at low levels on HUVEC (Slowik *et al.*, 1993). All of the TNF effect on class I molecule expression appears to be due to increased transcription (Johnson and Pober, 1990) and, by promoter analysis of the human HLA-B7 gene, is mediated largely through a single cis regulatory site in the class I gene 5′ regulatory region, sometimes called enhancer A (Johnson and Pober, 1994). This site binds NF-κB. TNF induces the translocation from the cytosol into the nucleus of the p50p65 heterodimeric form of NF-κB, which activates transcription. In the nucleus, p50p65 heterodimers displace a constitutively expressed p50 homodimeric form of NF-κB, which is a poor activator of transcription. Other TNF actions, as yet undescribed, may also be relevant because (a) TNF translocation of p50p65 NF-κB occurs within 15 min whereas TNF-induced increases in class I synthesis exhibit a lag of 3–4 hrs; and (b) TNF activation of p50p65 NF-κB is independent of new protein synthesis whereas

TNF-induced increases in class I mRNA transcription appear to require new protein synthesis (Collins, *et al.*, 1986).

Treatment of HUVEC with optimal concentrations of type 1 or type 2 IFN cause about a five-to-ten fold increase in the level of class I expression by 24 hrs and an increase expression over twenty-fold by 7 days (Lapierre, *et al.*, 1988). All of the IFN effect on class I expression appears to be due to increased transcription (Johnson and Pober, 1990) and, by promoter analysis, is mediated in large part through an interferon concensus sequence (ICS) located 20 bp downstream of the TNF-responsive NF-κB binding site (Johnson and Pober, 1994). IFN-γ (and perhaps IFN-α/β) induces the binding of interferon response factor (IRF)-1 (also called interferon stimulated gene factor-2) to this ICS. The ICS element of the class I gene lacks the flanking sequences typically required for binding of certain other IFN-induced transcription factors such as interferon stimulated gene factor (ISGF)-3. IRF-1 binding to the ICS is probably not be the only mechanism of IFN-mediated increases of class I transcription since class I expression can be increased in response to IFN in IRF-1 knockout mice (Matsuyama, *et al.*, 1993). The likely explanation is that other IFN-responsive elements appear to map ouside the 5' regulatory region of human class I gene (Ganguly, Vasayada, and Weissman, 1989). The IFN response, like the TNF response, exhibits a lag of 3–4 hrs before new synthesis starts. The IFN effect, unlike the TNF effect, appears, to be independent of new protein synthesis (Collins, *et al.*, 1986), further implicating an IRFI independent mechanism.

Combinations of TNF or LT with type I or type 2 IFN lead to multiplicative increases in the transcriptional rate of class I genes, commonly referred to as "synergy" (Lapierre, *et al.*, 1988; Johnson and Pober, 1990). There are as yet no evidence that the factors binding to the NF-κB site and to the adjacent ICS site can directly interact, but it seems likely that the 40bp regulatory element containing both sites will act as a transcriptional enhancing unit. In other promoters, the interaction of NF-κB with other elements is facilitated by a bending of the DNA caused by binding of high mobility group (HMG)-1Y proteins to the minor groove of the DNA opposite the NF-κB binding site (Du, *et al.*, 1993).

Although TNF and IFN intend to increase the magnitude of the transcription response, the onset of new synthesis is still delayed by 3–4 hrs (Epperson, *et al.*, 1992). The basis of this lag is not understood. However, the cell is not inactive during this period: new TAP proteins are made. TAP-1 appears to be regulated by exactly the same cytokines as class I structural genes. Consequently, cytokine-treated HUVEC exhibit increased TAP expression before increased rates of class I synthesis commence (Epperson, *et al.*, 1992).

Once expressed, class I proteins are very stable (half life over 24 hrs) on HUVEC (Collins, *et al.*, 1984). Cytokine-induced increases in class I persists for days after cytokine is withdrawn, although mRNA levels decline to basal levels more rapidly. It is not known if the peptides that are bound to class I molecules can change during this period. If not, then the EC will continue to display the peptides available during the period of cytokine-induced increased synthesis.

Under standard culture conditions, HUVEC do not display any detectable class II MHC molecules (Collins, *et al.*, 1984). Upon treatment of HUVEC with optimal concentrations of IFN-γ, class II transcription and mRNA levels rise after a delay of 6–12 hrs; class II surface expression is usually not detectable before 12 hrs and reaches maximal levels of about 100,000 to 500,000 copies per cell by 7 days. Products of all three human class II loci are inducible on HUVEC, but HLA-DR and -DP are expressed at much higher levels than HLADQ molecules. Most published studies have exclusively examined HLA-DR as a surrogate for all these loci, and should be extrapolated with caution. This relative pattern to HLA-DQ expression class II loci expresion is similar to monocytes but differs from B cells which express high levels of DQ but not DP. The invariant chain is induced in parallel with class II molecules in HUVEC. Once induced, class II molecules, like class I molecules, are stable and persist for up to 4 weeks after withdrawal of cytokine. It is not known if the peptides bound to class II change during this period.

Cytokines that do not induce class II molecules on HUVEC include TNF/LT, IFN-α/β, IL-1, IL-4 or GM-CSF. Certain leukocytes, especially NK cells, may induce class II molecules by a contact-dependent pathway not involving IFN-γ (Pardi, *et al.*, 1987). TNF/LT and type 1 IFN inhibit IFN-γ mediated induction of class II molecules, but do not promote clearance of molecules already expressed (Lapierre, *et al.*, 1988). It has been reported (but not confirmed) that TNF may selectively augment HLA-DP (Wedgewood, *et al.*, 1988). IL-10 does not appear effective as an inhibitor of expression of class II molecules on HUVEC (unpublished observations Bradley and Pober).

In general, all of the preceding statements about regulation of class II molecules could equally well apply to fibroblasts, smooth muscle cells or epithelial cells. However, EC do appear exceptional in that some EC in situ appear normally to express class II molecules whereas fibroblasts, smooth muscle and epithelial cells do not. Moreover in skin organ culture, EC are exceptionally responsive to IFN-γ compared to other tissue cell types (Messadi, *et al.*, 1988). Indeed, in skin organ culture, the only cell type that appears as responsive to IFN-γ as EC is the epidermal Langerhans cells, the precursor of the lymphoid dendritic cell. The unique responsiveness of the EC appears to occur throughout this microvascular bed, including arterial, capillary and venular EC.

Formation of Antigen-MHC Molecule Complexes by Endothelial Cells

In normal situations, cells express MHC molecules occupied by peptides (as opposed to empty MHC molecules). Occupied MHC molecules can be detected biochemically (eg. by isolation followed by quantitation of peptides released under denaturating conditions) or immunologically (i.e. by cell surface recognition on the APC by a population of mono-specific T cells), but not immunocytochemically (i.e. there are no antibodies that can be used to identify empty MHC molecules). Biochemical characterization has not yet been reported for MHC molecules isolated from EC. However, immunological characterization has been performed on endothelial MHC molecules as measured by activation of mono-specific (i.e. cloned) T cells. However, even with cloned T cells, it is necessary to be certain that the specific peptide MHC complexes are in fact formed and expressed on EC rather than on a contaminating professional APC population present within the EC cultures. First, and most convincingly, monoclonal HUVEC populations have been tested as APC. This is a difficult experiment because HUVEC have only a limited replicative life span and are difficult to clone. (Clonal human EC populations should be more readily obtained in the future from immortalized EC, but this has not yet been reported. Needless to say, it will be critical in interpreting such experiments to be certain that immortalization has not conferred new capacities for antigen presentation lacking in the progenitor cell population.) However, small numbers of cloned HUVEC have been produced and found to present protein antigens to an MHC-restricted cloned allogeneic T cell population, resulting in T cell proliferation (Wagner, *et al.*, 1984). The second approach involved use of an assay that is independent of bystander effects from contaminating cells, namely cytolysis. Since cloned CTL lyse only cells that express specific peptide-MHC complexes, EC lysis by CTL cannot be explained by the presence of putative contaminating APC within EC cultures since CTL would only lyse the contaminating cells. The key observation was that cloned CTL that exhibit allogeneic recognition kill allogeneic EC expressing the appropriate foreign MHC alleles but not EC expressing irrelevant alleles (Pober, *et al.*, 1983). (To date, the experiments using CTL have depended on allogeneic recognition, but, as discussed earlier, this is a reasonable model for foreign peptide-self MHC recognition.) Both types of experiments with cloned T cells therefore support the conclusion that EC can form and express functional peptide-MHC molecule complexes.

Activation of Antigen-Specific T Cells by Endothelial Cells

Stimulation of the proliferation of cloned T cell lines and stimulation of cytolysis by cloned CTL not only established that EC can form functional peptide-MHC molecule complexes but also established that EC can activate T cell responses. However, as noted above, the responsiveness of T cells varies with history of activation, and the key question unaddressed by experiments using long term cloned T cell lines is whether EC can present antigen in a manner that results in the activation of resting, freshly isolated T cells that are more likely to represent the state of T cell circulating *in vivo*. In human experimentation, resting T cells are defined as cells isolated (generally) from peripheral blood that are not in cell cycle and do not express activation markers such as IL-2Rα chain (CD25) class II MHC molecules. As discussed in the Introduction, there are at least two different populations of resting T cells in peripheral blood. Some resting T cells have never encountered specific antigen, and thus circulate as naive T cells; other resting T cells have been altered by a previous encounter with antigen and circulate as memory T cells. Also, as discussed earlier, these cells populations differ in several respects. Naive cells generally require stronger costimulators to enter cell cycle than memory T cells. Once activated by antigen, naive CD4$^+$ T cells may proliferate more robustly but synthesize less cytokine than memory CD4$^+$ T cells. Resting memory CD4$^+$ T cells are activated as T$_H$0 helper T lymphocytes and may be further differentiated into T$_H$1 or T$_H$2-like cells. It is not known whether naive CD4$^+$ cells can also undergo such differentiation or whether they must first become memory T cells. CD8$^+$ T cells also may be divided into naive vs memory cells. It is likely that both naive and memory cells can differentiate into CTL, but most *in vitro* experiments have only analyzed CTL arising from the memory cell population.

In addition to these differences in activation requirements, resting naive and memory T cells may mediate distinct functions. For example, memory CD4$^+$ T cells better adhere to cultured endothelial cells (Damle and Doyle, 1990), better traverse endothelial cell monolayers (Pietschmann, *et al.*, 1992), and are better able to increase transendothelial leakage of macromolecules than naive CD4$^+$ T cells (Damle and Doyle, 1990). (CD8$^+$ T cells may be better at these same functions than CD4$^+$ T cells (Bender, *et al.*, 1989), but less is known about differences between the CD8$^+$ T cell naive and memory subpopulations).

These properties are consistent with the *in vivo* capacities of resting memory T cells to preferentially home to peripheral sites of inflammation whereas resting naive T cells preferentially home to secondary lymphoid organs such as lymph nodes. It is also likely that antigen presentation at peripheral sites by EC, if it occurs, will involve the activation of memory T cells. Indeed, recent experiments confirm that EC selectively activate CD45RO[+] memory T cells *in vitro*. (Epperson and Pober 1994 and unpublished observations)

T cell activation by EC (or other APC) can be assessed by a variety of assays. By definition, resting T cells are out of cell cycle (i.e. in G_0 phase), not replicating DNA, not expressing activation markers, and not synthesizing cytokines. Entry into G_1 phase of the cell cycle is evidence of activation. It can be detected using flow cytometry measuring either increased RNA content with RNA-binding dyes or an increase in cell size by light scattering. DNA replication, which occurs during S phase and increased DNA content, present in G_2 phase, can be detected using flow cytometry to measure DNA content with DNA-binding dyes. More commonly used assays to measure DNA replication quantify incorporation of tagged nucleotides, such as [^{3}H]thymidine or bromodeoxyuridine into DNA. The percentage of cells that acquire labeled nuclei during a 24 hour period constitutes a labeling index, a very accurate measure of cell replication. More simply (but less accurately reflective of cell replication) total [^{3}H]-thymidine incorporated into DNA can be measured by scintillation counting. Cell counting, which is usually the gold standard for assessing replication, is often not reliable as a measure of T cell proliferation because dividing T cells frequently die. Activation marker expression, such as IL-2Rα chain or HLA-DR, is best be quantified using flow cytometry, to measure immunofluorescence staining intensities obtained with specific antibodies. Cytokine synthesis can be measured by immunoassay (e.g. ELISA or RIA) or bioassay of conditioned medium; an alternative approach involves quantitation of mRNA (eg. by Northern blot, by nuclease protection, or most sensitively, by polymerase chain reaction-based quantitation of reverse transcribed mRNA). Cytokines commonly examined to assess T cell activation are IL-2, IL-4 and IFN-γ. Measurements of proliferation and of cytokine synthesis can be performed on very small numbers of activated T cells, permitting the use of limiting dilution analyses to determine the frequency of T cells that can be specifically activated by APC that express specific antigen MHC molecule complexes or foreign MHC molecules.

By many (if not all) of these criteria, human EC cultures can activate resting T cells specific for foreign antigen (Hirschberg, *et al.*,1980; Wagner, *et al.*, 1984; Geppert and Lipsky, 1985) or alloantigens (Hirschberg, *et al.*, 1975; Pober, *et al.*, 1983; Adams, *et al.*, 1992; Savage, *et al.*, 1993; Page, *et al.*, 1994; Westphal, *et al.*, 1994). In general, antigen-specific activation in human T cells have utilized EC and T cell populations that are allogeneic but are serologically matched at class II (HLA-DR) loci, permitting class II-restricted antigen presentation to occur. In this setting, the contribution of alloantigens cannot be fully excluded. Allogeneic differences can be avoided in experiments involving inbred animals. Mouse EC can present antigens to syngeneic mouse T cells. (McCarron, *et al.*, 1985; 1986). However, the criteria for characterizing EC cultured from mouse have often been less rigorous than those applied in human experiments, raising concerns about possible contamination of the cultures by professional APC.

The allogeneic response to human EC has been extensively studied in our laboratory (Savage, *et al.*, 1993; Epperson and Pober, 1994; Murray, Libby and Pober, 1995). Unfractionated resting blood lymphocytes at T cell:EC ratios of 20:1 proliferate and secrete IL-2 and IFN-γ when cultured with allogeneic EC. Peak proliferation typically occurs between 5 and 7 days, measured as ^{3}[H]thymidine incorporation into DNA. The time course is similar but the level of labeling is usually less than that achieved using allogeneic blood adherent cells (i.e. traditional bone marrow-derived APC) as stimulators. IL-2 and IFN-γ production is measurable in cultures with allogeneic EC by day 1 and measurable cytokine levels decline unless IL-2 utilization is prevented (eg. with IL-2R antibody). The resting EC that are placed into such co-cultures do not express class II MHC molecules; however class II molecules are induced during coculture, perhaps in response to IFN-γ-secreted by the T cells.

When the T cells are separated into CD8$^+$ and CD4$^+$ subsets, the responses of these subpopulations can be separately examined. Purified CD8$^+$ T cells proliferate in response to resting EC (peak response with T cell:EC ratios of 20–40 to 1 at 5–7 days). Human CD8$^+$ T cells stimulated by allogeneic EC secrete IL-2; IL-2 accumulate if utilization is prevented. About 10% of the CD8 cells are activated to express IL-2Rα chain. When utilization is inhibited (i.e. with antibody to IL-2Rα), proliferation is blocked, showing that CD8$^+$ T cell proliferation depends upon secreted IL-2. Purified CD8$^+$ T cells will also secrete IFN-γ and cause EC to express increased levels of class I and newly express class II MHC molecules. Pretreatment of EC with exogenous IFN-γ has little effect on the magnitude or on the time course of the CD8$^+$ T cell response. Limiting dilution analyses indicate that between 1 in 15,000 and 1 in 30,000 CD8$^+$ T cells respond to allogeneic EC by secreting IL-2.

Purified CD4$^+$ T cells will not secrete IL-2 or proliferate when cultured with resting allogeneic EC, but will do both if the EC have been pretreated with IFN-γ to induce expression of class II MHC molecules. About 10% of the CD4$^+$ T cells are activated to express IL-2Rα chain and proliferation can be blocked with antibody to IL-2Rα. Although CD4$^+$ T cells do secrete IFN-γ, they do not cause EC to express class II MHC molecules, apparently because they secrete uncharacterized soluble inhibitors of class II induction (Doukas and Pober, 1990). Limiting dilution analyses suggest that about 1 in 3,000 to 1 in 10,000 CD4$^+$ T cells respond to IFN-γ-treated EC by secreting IL-2. This frequency is clearly higher than that for CD8$^+$ T cells and the magnitude of the proliferative response is also greater, although the peak response at T cell:EC ratios of 20:1 still occurs at day 5–7.

The responses to allogeneic EC are generally similar for EC isolated from umbilical vein, aorta vein, saphenous vein and dermal microvessels. These responses should be considered in comparison to T cell responses to other allogeneic cell types. For example the adherent fraction of peripheral blood, which contains professional APC such as monocytes, B cells and dendritic cells, will generally stimulate more vigorous proliferative responses, more IL-2 production and about 5 fold higher frequencies of responders in limiting dilution assays. Some of this increased response may result from increased numbers of different peptides that can be found in association with MHC molecules on freshly isolated cell populations compared to long term cultured cell populations. However, most of the difference appears attributable to expression of stronger costimulators. In our experience, human EC, unlike bone-marrow-derived APC, do not express ligands that interact with T cell CD28 (Murray *et al*, 1994), although contrary results have been reported (Damle, *et al*., 1993). On the other hand, most tissue cell types, such as smooth muscle cells or fibroblasts, do not cause resting T cells to proliferate nor do they cause significant cytokine production. Much of the observed deficiency of tissue cells as APC can be attributed to ineffective provision of costimulation. Thus costimulation provided by EC falls between that of highly effective, professional bone marrow-derived APC and that of highly ineffective tissue cells. It should be noted that recently activated T cells, which are already in cell cycle, are effectively restimulated by all of these cell types. This is expected since requirements for costimulators are most evident for the activation of resting T cells.

Our experience with the human T cell response to allogeneic cultured EC can also be contrasted with the response to xenogeneic cultured porcine EC. In some xenogeneic species combinations (eg. mouse anti-pig); the T cell response to even professional APC is weak because direct recognition of foreign MHC molecules is lost, ie. the xenogeneic MHC molecules are too different from self MHC to invoke cross-reactions. We (Murray, *et al.*, 1994) and others (Rollins, *et al.*, 1994) have observed direct recognition of pig MHC molecules by cross-reactive human T cell receptors. In some species combinations, xenogeneic responses may also be weak because species variations in costimulator molecules and their T cell counterreceptors or adhesive interactions (eg. between T cell integrins and their counterreceptors) are too great to permit effective interactions. Again, human anti-pig interactions appear conserved (Murray, *et al.*, 1994; Rollins, *et al.*, 1994). Indeed, the most striking feature of the human T cell-porcine EC response is that by every criteria examined, it is stronger than the human allogeneic anti-EC responses. We find that pig EC, unlike human EC, express costimulators that can interact with human CD28 (Murray *et al.*, 1994). The magnitude and frequency of the human T cell anti-pig EC response thus more closely resembles that of the human T cell allogeneic response to professional APC.

Endothelial Activation of Effector T Cells

The ability of EC to present antigen and activate resting T cells raises the issue of whether T cells activated by EC acquire specific effector functions. It has been found that human microvascular EC, acquired from neonatal foreskins, are able to cause some allogeneic CD8 T cells to differentiate into alloantigen (i.e. peptide plus foreign MHC)-specific CTL if the cultures are supplemented with IL-2 (Pardi and Bender, 1991). We have found that human umbilical vein EC can cause some allogeneic CD8$^+$ T cells to synthesize perforin without exogenous IL-2. (It is not yet known whether the perforin-expressing cells are specific for the alloantigens expressed by the EC or have cytolytic ability.) As noted above CD4$^+$ T cells activated by allogeneic IFN-γ-pretreated human umbilical vein EC synthesize IL-2 and IFN-γ. IL-4 is not detectable in such cultures; however, it should be noted that immunoassays and bioassays for this human cytokine are not as sensitive as those for IL-2 and IFN-γ, and negative results must be interpreted cautiously. Nevertheless, these observations do suggest that the CD4$^+$ cells activated by EC are not T_H2-like. It is not known whether CD4$^+$ T cells repetitively activated will acquire T_H1 or T_H2 differentiation patterns if EC are used as the APC. Interestingly, mouse brain-derived EC appear to preferentially activate syngeneic T_H2 clones whereas perivascular cell populations derived from the same animals preferentially activate syngeneic T_H1 clones (Fabry *et al.*, 1993). The basis for this difference is not known. The same mouse brain EC populations are better stimulators of resting allogeneic T cells but less good at activating syngeneic T cells with peptide self MHC molecule complexes than perivascular cells (Fabry *et al.*, 1990); the basis of this difference is not clear since the kind of T cells that proliferate are probably the same in both responses.

Costimulator Functions of Endothelial Cells

The observations that EC can stimulate resting T cells to secrete IL-2 whereas other tissue cell types (e.g. fibroblasts, smooth muscle cells) cannot was attributed in the preceeding discussing to the fact that EC have stronger antigen-independent (i.e. costimulator) effects on IL-2 synthesis. Such costimulator activity have been directly tested in a number of assays. For example, one approach measures the effect of EC or other APC on IL-2 production by T cells activated with antigen-mimetic signals such as antibodies to CD3 proteins or with mitogenic lectins, such as PHA. Allogeneic human EC are very effective at increasing IL-2 synthesis in such assays at all activator concentrations (Guinan, *et al.*, 1989; Teitel, *et al.*, 1989; Hughes, *et al.*, 1990). EC can even increase IL-2 produced in response to maximal concentrations of PHA (a strong activator) by 5 to 10-fold. This capacity is shared by professional APC, such as B cells, but not by monocytes and not by most other tissue cells. (Monocytes may be required for the responses to EC when soluble antibodies are used as activators because EC do not express receptors for the Fc portion of antibodies and cannot cross-link the antibodies.) Theoretically, the allogeneic combination of APC and responder T cells used in these experiments may confound the results by superimposing allogeneic stimulation. Such cell combinations are routinely used in such assays for a practical reason: it is difficult to obtain autologous human EC and T cells. Such paired isolations have recently been accomplished using cadaveric organ donors, and it has been found that gonadal vein EC do provide costimulation to autologous T cells in such assays (Huang, *et al.*, 1994). A second recently developed approach to demonstrate costimulation, is to transiently transfect the T cells with an IL-2 promoter-reporter construct so that effects of costimulators on IL-2 transcription can be assessed more directly (Hughes and Pober, 1996). (EC and other cells with costimulators do increase endogenous IL-2 gene transcription, as detected by nuclear run off assays (Hughes and Pober, 1993), but this approach is not very sensitive and is difficult to perform on peripheral blood lymphocytes that make little IL-2.) EC are better than monocytes and nearly as good as B lymphoblastoid cells at providing transcriptional costimulation in such transfection experiments.

Data from our laboratory has shown that EC-mediated costimulation requires that the T cells be in direct contact with the EC (i.e. costimulation cannot be mediated across porous membranes) and that lightly fixed EC are as good or nearly as good at providing costimulation as living EC (Hughes, *et al.*, 1990; Savage, *et al.*, 1991). These observations point to cell surface proteins as the most important form of costimulation provided by EC. The use of polyclonal activators bypasses any role for CD4 and CD8 as costimulators in these experiments and antibodies reactive with these molecules are not inhibitory. In contrast, antibody blocking experiments have identified the CD2 signaling pathway as responsible for about one half of the EC-derived signals (Hughes, *et al.*, 1990; Savage, *et al.*, 1991). Ligands that contribute to this effect are LFA-3 (CD58), CD59, CD44 and CD2 but not CD48. LFA-3 on the EC and CD2 on T cells appear to be central to this process. CD59 and CD44, which are expressed on both cells, appear to function as augmenters of LFA-3 interaction with T cell CD2. We detect no effect on EC costimulator function by blocking that utilize the CD28 pathway on HUVEC or saphenous vein EC (Murray, *et al.*, 1994). It remains to be determined if other human EC types can utilize this pathway of costimulation. There appear to be only limited effects of pathways involving selectins, $\beta 2$ integrins (such as LFA-1 and its EC ligands ICAM-1 and ICAM-2), or $\beta 1$ integrins (such as VLA-4 and VLA-5 and their EC ligands such as fibronectin and VCAM-1) (Savage, *et al.*, 1991). As noted earlier, it has recently been appreciated that cytokines and cytokine-like molecules can interact as membrane ligand pairs. IL-1, which is expressed on EC membranes as IL-1α (Kurt-Jones, *et al.*, 1987), does not appear to be involved (Hughes, *et al.*, 1990). IL-6 also plays only a marginal role. Examination of the role of members of the TNF family expressed on T cells, such as TNF, LTα_1 β_2, CD40 ligand, and fas ligand, have not been reported in the literature.

The monoclonal antibodies that inhibit costimulation of IL-2 also inhibit proliferation of T cells to allogeneic EC, implicating a major role for the CD2 but not the CD28 costimulator pathway (Epperson and Pober, 1994; Hughes, *et al.*, 1990; Savage, *et al.*, 1993). Furthermore, the same molecules appear to be involved in the CD4$^+$ T cell response and the CD8$^+$ T cell response (Epperson and Pober, 1994; Savage, *et al.*, 1993). In addition, the proliferative responses of purified T cells to allogeneic EC also may be inhibited with antibodies that interfere with CD4 (for CD4$^+$ T cells) or CD8 (for CD8$^+$ T cells) as well as with antibodies to relevant MHC molecules. Another difference is that antibodies to β_2 or β_1 integrins are also inhibitory of allogeneic responses, suggesting that tight adhesion is more important in this setting than in costimulation assays.

The primary effect of the EC interaction mediated through the CD2 pathway is to increase IL-2 transcription (Hughes and Pober, 1996). Professional APC, such as B cells, which have ligands that engage both CD2 and CD28, utilize CD2 primarily to augment transcription and primarily utilize CD28 primarily to increase IL-2 synthesis posttranscriptionally, probably through mRNA stabilization. Interestingly, other tissue cells such as vascular smooth muscle, display equivalent levels of LFA-3, CD59 and CD44 as EC, but fail to effectively engage the CD2 pathway (Murray, Libby and Pober, 1995). The basis for this difference is not known.

Analysis of IL-2 promoter-reporter genes by site-specific mutagenesis suggests that EC costimulation of IL-2 transcription involves the same combination of cis-regulatory promoter elements as primary activation (e.g by anti-CD3 antibody or by PHA) and the same combination of cis regulatory promoter elements as B cell-mediated costimulation, (Hughes and Pober, 1996). This observation leads to the hypothesis that the primary mechanism of costimulation involves altering the composition or transcriptional activating capacity of the DNA-binding proteins that adhere to these cis-regulatory elements. Initial data from analysis of nuclear DNA binding proteins from peripheral blood T cells supports this notion (Hughes and Pober, 1993). Specifically, resting blood T cells contain c-jun homodimers that bind to the proximal AP-1 site of the IL-2 promoter. The quantity of nuclear proteins that bind to this site is not changed upon activation as assessed by quantititative electrophoratic mobility shift assays. However, upon activation with PHA, T cells synthesize c-fos and displace 5 to 10% of the c-jun homodimers with c-jun/c-fos heterodimers that are more potent at transcriptional activation. If EC are present, about 5-fold more c-fos is made and about 5 times more of the AP-1 binding complexes formed contain c-fos. Interestingly the effect on c-fos does not appear to be mediated through CD2. The question of whether similar changes may occur in the proteins that bind to other cis-regulatory elements is under investigation.

EC costimulator functions can be further analyzed by examining the effects of certain immunosuppressive drugs (Crabtree and Clipstone, 1994). Cyclosporin A and FK506 (as well as the parent compound of FK506, ascomycin) bind to related small cytoplasmic enzymes called immunophilins. When these drugs are bound, the immunophilins can interact with calcineurin, inhibiting calcineurin enzymatic activity. As noted in the Introduction section, calcineurin is phosphatase activity is required to activate certain transcription factors, such as NFAT, that are important for IL-2 synthesis. By inhibiting calcineurin, these drugs inhibit IL-2 synthesis. Living EC can render peripheral blood T cells resistant to cyclosporin A or ascomycin, requiring as much as 30 to 100-fold higher concentrations of drug to inhibit IL-2 synthesis by 50% (Karmann, *et al.*, 1994). EC are much better at this than monocytes, but the combination of monocytes plus EC appear to act cooperatively, providing resistance of 1000 fold or more. Resistance to cyclosporin A requires T cell-EC contact and develops over 6 hours. The cell surface proteins responsible for conferring resistance to cyclosporin A have not been identified. T cells cultured with EC develop pathways for cytosolic exchange of small molecule labels or dyes, consistent with gap junction communication (Guinan, *et al.*, 1988); it is possible that such pathways also contribute to the development of resistance to cyclosporin A.

ENDOTHELIAL ANTIGEN PRESENTATION *IN VIVO*

As discussed in the previous section, cultured human endothelial cells have the capacity to activate some resting peripheral blood T cells most likely a subset of memory T cells. If EC display the same capacities *in vivo*, EC could contribute to accelerated and more efficient recognition of antigen in secondary immune reactions, such as the recall response of delayed hypersensitivity. EC initiated responses are also likely to come into play when lymphocytes are confronted with a foreign vasculature, eg. after transplantation of a vascularized allograft or after transfer of lymphocytes into a foreign host. The most direct functional test of the antigen presenting capacity of EC would be to determine whether there are immunological consequences in an animal whose circulating lymphocytes could not contact endothelial cells. This experiment cannot be performed in a straight-forward way for the obvious reason that blood circulation is dependent upon an endothelial-lined system. An alternative approach may be to eliminate certain endothelial cell functions critical for antigen presentation (eg. MHC molecule expression) through genetic manipulation of a graft. This has not yet been accomplished, but may be feasible in the near future as methods for tissue-specific gene repression or gene targeting become more developed. Rats may provide an experiment of nature that confirms such expectations. Laboratory rat EC have a diminished capacity to express class II MHC molecules (Mason and Barclay, 1984) compared to other species. Of note, it is very difficult (if not impossible) to elicit recall delayed hypersensitivity in the rat. In addition, rat organs are much more readily transplanted across allogeneic barriers than organs in other mammalian species, including humans (Fabre, 1982). However, it is not clear that the EC "defect" and the immunological "defects" of rats are causally related.

Interestingly, rat EC can be induced to express class II MHC molecules when treated with IFN-γ *in vitro* (Male, *et al.*, 1987). Rat organs that have been accepted by an allogeneic host can be induced to undergo rejection if a competent APC, such a dendritic cell of the same MHC type as the organ graft (Lechler and Batchelor, 1982), is injected into the host. This and similar experiments form the basis of the "passenger leukocyte hypothesis: which states that professional APC (i.e. leukocytes) carried in the organ graft are required to initiate an immune response through direct presentation of allogeneic MHC molecules. Remarkably, injection of IFN-γ-treated rat EC (that express class II MHC molecules), but not untreated EC (which do not), can also cause rejection of a stable allograft (Ferry, *et al.*, 1987). (It is worth noting that the untreated EC do express rat class I MHC molecules, but rat CD8$^+$ T cells, unlike human CD8$^+$ T cell, cannot be activated unless CD4$^+$ T cells are also activated to provide "help" probably in the form of IL-2). Thus IFN-γ-treated EC appear to function as professional APC in this *in vivo* model.

A different functional approach to study the APC function of EC involves elimination of conventional bone-marrow derived APC to determine what APC function is left. This can be achieved experimentally by replacing the bone marrow of a first generation mouse resulting from the cross of two inbred strains (that expresses two different MHC types) with the bone marrow of one of the two parental strains (Gao, *et al.*, 1991; Kosaka, *et al.*, 1992). Such a mouse is called a bone marrow chimera. New T cells that develop in this mouse are selected to be tolerant to the MHC molecules encoded by the genes of the other parental strain. In contrast, mature T cells that isolated from animals of the parental strain used as the bone marrow donor will respond to these "foreign" MHC molecules. If introduced into a normal first generation cross bred mouse, by adoptive transfer, such parental T cells will initiate graft-vs-host disease. (It is assumed that the transferred T cells are primarily stimulated by host professional APC expressing the MHC molecules of the other parent.) However, if naive parental T cells from the same strain as the bone marrow are introduced into the bone marrow chimeric mouse, they can only directly recognize the other MHC molecules of the other parental strain on non-bone marrow-derived cells since all of the bone marrow-derived APC express only parental MHC molecules. In this setting both CD4$^+$ and CD8$^+$ T cells can be sensitized with high frequency (i.e. by direct recognition) and cause graft vs. host reactions (Gao, *et al.*, 1991; Kosaka, *et al.*, 1992). Thus non-bone marrow-derived APC are implicated as initiating the immune reaction. The only cell populations that expressed detectable levels of the "foreign" MHC" molecules (i.e. those of the other parent) in these animals are vascular EC and lymph node follicular dendritic cells (which are distinct from antigen-presenting lymphoid dendritic cells).

Another functional approach is to analyze the predicted consequences of antigen presentation by EC. Antigen presentation by EC would be expected to favor early recruitment of antigen specific T cells whereas non-specific recruitment through inflammation would be expected to show less selectivity. Careful analysis of early responses does suggest that many early infiltrating T cells appear specific for antigen (Spangrude and Daynes, 1985). Collectively, these experiments support but do not prove the hypothesis that EC can present antigen *in vivo*.

Additional support for endothelial APC function has been inferred from histological observations. For example, in acute T cell-mediated responses, in experimental animals, such as recall delayed hypersensitivity. T cell blasts have been observed within the local microvasculature in contact with the luminal surface of the EC (Dvorak, *et al.*, 1976). This pattern suggests, but does not prove that antigen recognition has occurred on the endothelial surface, Other data have come from human transplant studies. For example, most current recipients of organ transplants avoid acute rejection by treatment regimens based on cyclosporin A. However, about 30% of heart transplant recipients (and probably equal numbers of kidney transplant recipients) develop a chronic immune-mediated lesion in the graft arteries. In affected vessels, activated T cells accumulate and persist subjacent to the luminal EC (Salomon, *et al.*, 1991), This pattern of response suggests that the basis of this lesion is a host T cell chronic delayed hypersensitiviy response to graft arterial EC. However, it remains to be established that these T cells are directly responding to graft alloantigens, let alone alloantigens presented by graft EC.

CONCLUSION

The goals of this chapter were to define more precisely how T cells recognize antigen and whether EC could participate in this process by presenting antigens to resting T cells in the circulation. Our current state of knowledge permits four statements to be made about the role of endothelium as an antigen presenting cell capable of activating resting T cells. First, there is a logical reason for EC to present antigens to resting memory T cells, namely accelerated development of secondary recall responses in peripheral tissues, leading to more rapid containment of infections. Second, there are compelling data establishing the capacities of cultured human EC to act as an APC for resting memory T cells. Third, there are indirect functional and histological data consistent with the function of EC as initiators of antigen-specific responses *in vivo*. And fourth, there is as yet no direct confirmation that this can occur. The availability of new tools for genetic manipulation of animals may provide the means to test critically these ideas, answering once and for all whether (and in what circumstances) EC can present antigen to circulating T cells, thereby initiating protective immunity.

References

Adams, P.W., Lee, H.S., Waldman, W.J., Sedmak, D.D., Morgan, C.J., Ward, J.S. and Orosz, C.G. (1992). Alloantigenicity of human endothelial cells. 1. frequency and phenotype of human helper T lymphocytes that can react to allogeneic endothelial cells. *J. Immunol.*, 148:3753–3760.

Bender, J.R., Pardi, R., Kosek, J. and Engelman, E.G. (1989). Evidence that cytotoxic lymphocytes alter and traverse allogeneic endothelial cell monolayers. *Transplantation*, 47:1047–1053.

Berke, G. (1994). The binding and lysis of target cells by cytotoxic lymphocytes: molecular and cellular aspects. *Ann. Rev. Immunol.*, 12:735–773.

Bierer, B.E., Sleckman, B.P., Ratnofsky, S.E. and Burakoff, S.J. (1989). The biologic roles of CD2, CD4 and CD8 in T cell activation. *Ann. Rev. Immunol.*, 7:579–599.

Bjorkman, P.J. and Parham, P. (1990). Structure, function, and diversity of class I major histocompatibility complex molecules. *Ann. Rev. Biochem.*, 59:253–288.

Bradley, J.R., Johnson, D.R. and Pober, J.S. (1993). Endothelial activation by hydrogen peroxide:selective increases of intercellular adhesion molecule-1 and MHC class I. *Am. J. Path.*, 142:1598–1609.

Collins, T., Korman, A.J., Wake, C.T., Boss, J.M., Kappes, D.J., Fiers, W., Ault, K.A., Gimbrone, M.A., Jr., Strominger, J.L. and Pober, J.S. (1984). Immune interferon activates multiple class II major histocompatibility complex genes and the associated invariant chain gene in human endothelial cells and dermal fibroblasts. *Proc. Natl. Acad. Sci. USA*, **81**:4917–4921.

Collins, T., Lapierre, L.A., Fiers, W., Strominger, J.L. and Pober, J.S. (1986). Recombinant human tumor necrosis factor increases mRNA levels and surface expression of HLA-A,B antigens in vascular endothelial cells and dermal fibroblasts *in vitro*. *Proc. Natl. Acad. Sci. USA*, **83**:446–450.

Crabtree, G.R. and Clipstone, N.A. (1994). Signal transduction between the plasma membrane and nucleus of T lymphocytes. *Ann. Rev. Biochem.*, **63**:1045–1083.

Cresswell, P. (1994). Assembly, transport, and functionof MHC class II molecules. *Ann. Rev. Immunol.*, **12**:259–293.

Damle, N.K. and Doyle, L.V. (1990). Ability of human T lymphocytes to adhere to vascular endothelial cells and to augment endothelial permeability to macromolecules is linked to their state of post-thymic maturation. *J. Immunol.*, **144**:1233–1240.

Damle, N.K., Klussman, K., Leytze, G. and Linsley, P.S. (1993). Proliferation of human T lymphocytes induced with superantigens is not dependent on costimulation by the CD28 counter-receptor B7. *J. Immunol.*, **150**:726–735.

Doukas, J. and Pober, J.S. (1990). Lymphocyte-mediated activation of cultured endothelial cells (EC): CD4+ T cells inhibit class II MHC antigen expression despite secreting IFN-γ and increasing EC class I MHC and ICAM-1 antigen expression. *J. Immunol.*, **145**:1088–1098.

Du, W., Thanos, D. and Maniatis, T. (1993). Mechanisms of transcriptional synergism between distinct virus-inducible enhancer elements. *Cell*, **74**:887–898.

Dumonde, D.C., Pulley, M.S., Paradinas, F.J., Southcott, B.M., O'Connell, D., Robinson, M.R.G., Den Hollander, F. and Schuurs, A.H. (1982). Histological features of skin reactions to human lymphoid cell line lymphokine in patients with advanced cancer. *J. Pathol.*, **138**:289–308.

Dvorak, A.M., Mihm, M.C. and Dvorak, H.F. (1976). Morphology of delayed hypersensitivity reactions in man. II. Ultrastructural alterations affecting the microvasculature and the tissue mast cells. *Lab. Invest.*, **34**:179–189.

Epperson, D.E., Arnold, D., Spies, T., Cresswell, P., Pober, J.S. and Johnson, D.R. (1992). Cytokines increase transporter in antigen processing-1 (TAP-1) expression more rapidly than HLA Class I expression in endothelial cells. *J. Immunol.*, **149**:3297–3301.

Epperson, D.E. and Pober, J.S. (1994). Antigen presenting function of human endothelial cells: direct activation of resting CD8 T cells. *J. Immunol.*, **153**:5402–5412.

Fabre, J.W. (1982). Rat kidney allograft model: was it all too good to be true? *Transplantation*, **34**:223–225.

Fabry, Z., Waldschmidt, M.M., Moore, S.A., Hart, M.N. (1990). Antigen presentation by brain microvessel smooth muscle and endothelium. *J. Neuroimmunol.*, **28**:63–71.

Fabry, Z., Sandor, M., Gajewski, T.F., Herlein, J.A., Waldschmidt, M.M., Lynch, R.G., Hart, M.N. (1993). Differential activation of Th1 and Th2 CD4+ cells by murine brain microvessel endothelial cells and smooth muscle pericytes. *J. Immunol.*, **151**:38–47.

Ferry, B., Haltutunen, J., Leszczynski, D., Shellekens, H., van der Medie, P.H. and Hayry, P. (1987). Impact of class II major histocompatibility complex antigen expression on the immunogenic potential of isolated rat vascular endothelial cells. *Transplantation*, **44**:499–503.

Fitch, F.W., McKisie, M.D., Lancki, D.W. and Gajewski, T.F. (1993). Differential regulation of murine T lymphocyte subsets. *Ann. Rev. Immunol.*, **11**:29–48.

Ganguly, S., Vasayada, H.A. and Weissman, S.M. (1989). Multiple enhancerlike sequences in the HLA-B7 gene. *Proc. Natl. Acad. Sci. USA*, **86**:5247–5251.

Gao, E., Kosaka, H., Surh, C.D. and Sprent, J. (1991). T cell contact with Ia antigens on nonhemopoietic cells *in vivo* can lead to immunity rather than tolerance. *J. Exp. Med.*, **174**:435–446.

Geppert, T.D. and Lipsky, P.E. (1985). Antigen presentation by interferontreated endothelial cells and fibroblasts: differential ability to function as antigen-presenting cells despite comparable Ia expression. *J. Immunol.*, **135**:3750–3762.

Germain, R.H. and Margulies, D.H. (1993). The biochemistry and cell biology of antigen processing and presentation. *Ann. Rev. Immunol.*, **11**:403–450.

Gray, D. (1993). Immunological memory. *Ann. Rev. Immunol.*, **11**:49–77.

Guinan, E.C., Smith, B.R., Davies, P.F. and Pober, J.S. (1988). Cytoplasmic transfer between endothelium and lymphocytes: quantitation by flow cytometry. *Am. J. Pathol.*, **132**:406–409.

Guinan, E.C., Smith, B.R., Doukas, J.T., Miller, R.A. and Pober, J.S. (1989). Vascular endothelial cells enhance T cell responses by markedly augmenting IL2 concentrations. *Cell Immunol.*, **118**:166–177.

Halloran, P.F. and Madrenas, J. (1990). Regulation of MHC transcription. *Transplantation*, **50**:725–738.

Hirschberg, H., Bergh, O.J. and Thorsby, G. (1980). Antigen-presenting properties of human vascular endothelial cells. *J. Exp. Med.*, **152**:249s–255s.

Hirschberg, H., Evensen, S.A., Henriksen, T. and Thorsby, E. (1975). The human mixed lymphocyte-endothelium culture interaction. *Transplantation*, **19**:495–504.

Huang, E.H., Morgan, C.J., Sedmak, D.D., Ferguson, R.M. and Orosz, C.G. (1994). Alloantigenicity of human endothelial cells. IV. derivation, characterization, and utilization of gonadal vein endothelia to control endothelial alloantigenicity during lymphocyte-endothelial interactins. *Transplantation*, 57:703–711.

Hughes, C.C.W. and Pober, J.S. (1993). Costimulation of peripheral blood T cell activation by human endothelial cells:enhanced IL-2 transcription correlates with increased c-fos synthesis and increased Fos content of AP-1. *J. Immunol.*, 150:3148–3160.

Hughes, C.C.W., Savage, C.O.S. and Pober, J.S. (1990). Endothelial cells augment T cell IL-2 production by a contact-dependent mechanism involving CD2:LFA-3 interaction. *J. Exp. Med.*, 171:1453–1467.

Hughes, C.C.W. and Pober, J.S. (1996). Transcriptional regulation of the IL-2 gene in normal human peripheral blood T cells: convergence of co-stimulatory signals and differences from transformed T cells. *J. Biol. Chem.* (in press).

Janeway, C.A.J. (1992). The T-cell receptor as a multicomponent signalling machine:CD4/CD8 coreceptors and CD45 in T-cell activation. *Ann. Rev. Immunol.*, 10:645–674.

Johnson, D.R. and Pober, J.S. (1990). Tumor necrosis factor and immune interferon synergistically increase transcription of HLA class I heavy and light chain genes in vascular endothelium. *Proc. Natl. Acad. Sci. USA*, 87:5183–5187.

Johnson, D.R. and Pober, J.S. (1994). HLA class I heavy chain gene promoter elements mediating synergy between tumor necrosis factor and interferons. *Molec. Cell Biol.*, 14:1322–1332.

Jorgensen, J.L., Reay, P.A., Ehrich, E.W. and Davis, M. (1992). Molecular components of T cell recognition. *Ann. Rev. Immunol.*, 10:835–873.

Karmann, K., Pober, J.S. and Hughes, C.C.W. (1994). Endothelial cellinduced resistance to cyclosporin A in human peripheral blood T cells requires contact-dependent interactions involving CD2 but not CD28. *J. Immunol.*, 153:3929–3937.

Kosaka, H., Surh, C.D. and Sprent, J. (1992). Stimulation of active unprimed CD8+ T cells by semiprofessional antigen-presenting cells *in vivo. J. Exp. Med.*, 176:1291–1302.

Kurt-Jones, E.A., Fiers, W. and Pober, J.S. (1987). Membrane IL-1 induction on human endothelial cells and dermal fibroblasts. *J. Immunol.*, 139:2317–2324.

Lapierre, L.A., Fiers, W. and Pober, J.S. (1988). Three distinct classes of regulatory cytokines control endothelial cell MHC antigen expression: interactions with immune (γ) interferon differentiate the effects of tumor necrosis factor and lymphotoxin from those of leukocyte (α) and fibroblast (β) interferons. *J. Exp. Med.*, 167:794–804.

Lechler, R.I. and Batchelor, J.R. (1982). Restoration of immunogenicity to passenger cell-depleted kidney allografts by the addition of donor strain dendritic cells. *J. Exp. Med.*, 155:31–41.

Linsley, P.S., Ledbetter, J.A. and Parker, D.C. (1993). The role of the CD28 receptor during T cell responses to antigen. *Ann. Rev. Immunol.*, 11:191–211.

Male, D.K., Pryce, G. and Hughes, C.C.W. (1987). Antigen presentation in brain: MHC induction on brain endothelium and astrocytes compared. *Immunology*, 60:453–459.

Mason, D.W. and Barclay, A.N. (1984). Constitutive and inducible expression of Ia antigens. *Immunobiology*, 168:167–171.

Matsuyama, T., Kimura, T., Kitagawa, M., Watanabe, N., Kundig, T.M., Amakawa, R., Kishihara, K., Wakeham, A., Potter, J., Furlonger, C.L., Narendran, A., Suzuki, H., Ohashi, P.S., Paige, C.J., Taniguchi, T. and Mak, T.W. (1993). Targeted disruption of IRF-1 or IRF-2 results in abnormal type I IFN gene induction and aberrant lymphocyte development. *Cell*, 75:83–97.

McCarron, R.M., Kempski, O., Spatz, M. and McFarlin, D.E. (1985). Presentation of myelin basic protein by murine cerebral vascular endothelial cells. *J. Immunol.*, 134:3100–3103.

McCarron, R.M., Spatz, M., Kempski, O., Hogan, R.N., Muehl, L. and McFarlin, D.E. (1986). Interaction between myelin basic protein-sensitized T lymphocytes and murine cerebral vascular endothelial cells. *J. Immunol.*, 137:3428–3435.

Messadi, D.V., Pober, J.S. and Murphy, G.F. (1988). Effects of recombinant gamma interferon on HLA-DR and DQ expression by skin cells in short term organ culture. *Lab. Invest.*, 58:61–67.

Minami, Y., Kono, T., Miyazaki, T. and Taniguchi, T. (1993). The IL-2 receptor complex: its structure, function, and target genes. *Ann. Rev. Immunol.*, 11:245–267.

Moraes, J.R. and Stastny, P. (1977). A new antigen system expressed in human endothelial cells. *J. Clin. Invest.*, 60:449–454.

Munro, J.M., Pober, J.S. and Cotran, R.S. (1989). Tumor necrosis factor and interferon-γ induce distinct patterns of endothelial activation and associated leukocyte accumulation in skin of *Papio anubis. Am. J. Pathol.*, 135:121–133.

Murray, A.G., Khodadoust, M.M., Pober, J.S. and Bothwell, A.L.M. (1994). Porcine aortic endothelial cells strongly activate human T cells:direct presentation of swine MHC antigens and effective costimulation by swine ligands for human CD2 and CD28. *Immunity*, 1:57–63.

Murray, A.G., Libby, P. and Pober, J.S. (1995). Human vascular smooth muscle cells poorly costimulate and actively inhibit allogeneic CD4+ T cell proliferation *in vitro*. *J. Immunol.*, **154**:151–161.

Page, C.S., Holloway, N., Smith, H., Yacoub, M. and Rose, M.L. (1994). Alloproliferative responses of purified CD4+ and CD8+ T cells to endothelial cells in the absence of contaminating accessory cells. *Transplantation*, **57**:1628–1637.

Pardi, R., Bender, J. and Engelman, E. (1987). Lymphocyte subsets differentially induce class II human leukocyte antigens on allogeneic microvascular endothelial cells. *J. Immunol.*, **139**:2585–2592.

Pardi, R. and Bender, J.R. (1991). Signal requirements for the generation of CD4+ and CD8+ T-cell responses to human allogeneic microvascular endothelium. *Circ. Res.*, **69**:1269–1279.

Pietschmann, P., Cush, J.J., Lipsky, P.E. and Oppenheimer-Marks, N. (1992). Identification of subsets of human T cells capable of enhanced transendothelial migration. *J. Immunol.*, **149**:1170–1178.

Pober, J.S., Collins, T., Gimbrone, M.A., Jr., Cotran, R.S., Gitlin, J.D., Fiers, W., Clayberger, C., Krensky, A.M., Burakoff, S.J. and Reiss, C.S. (1983). Lymphocytes recognize human vascular endothelial and dermal fibroblast Ia antigens induced by recombinant immune interferon. *Nature*, **305**:726–729.

Pober, J.S. and Gimbrone, M.A.J. (1982). Expression of Ia-like antigens by human vascular endothelial cells is inducible *in vitro*. Demonstration by monoclonal antibody binding and immunoprecipitation. *Proc. Natl. Acad. Sci. (USA)*, **79**:6641–6645.

Reth, M. (1992). Antigen receptors on B lymphocytes. *Ann. Rev. Immunol.*, **10**:97–121.

Rollins, S.A., Kennedy, S.P., Chodera, A.J., Elliott, E.A., Zavoico, G.B. and Matis, L.A. (1994). Evidence that activation of human T cells by porcine endothelium involves direct recognition of porcine SLA and costimulation by porcine ligands for LFA-1 and CD2. *Transplantation*, **57**:1709–1716.

Salomon, R.N., Hughes, C.C.W., Schoen, F.J., Payne, D.D., Pober, J.S. and Libby, P. (1991). Human coronary transplantation-associated arteriosclerosis: evidence for a chronic immune reaction to activated graft endothelial cells. *Am. J. Pathol.*, **138**:791–798.

Savage, C.O.S., Hughes, C.C.W., McIntyre, B.W., Picard, J.K. and Pober, J.S. (1993). Human CD4+ T cells proliferate to HLA-DR+ allogeneic vascular endothelium:identification of accessory interactions. *Transplantation*, **56**:128–134.

Savage, C.O.S., Hughes, C.C.W., Pepinsky, R.S., Wallner, B.P., Freedman, A. S. and Pober, J.S. (1991). Endothelial cell lymphocyte function-associated antigen-3 and an unidentified ligand act in concert to provide costimulation to human peripheral blood CD4+ T cells. *Cell Immunol.*, **137**:150–163.

Sherman, L.A. and Chattopadhyay, S. (1993). The molecular basis of allorecognition. *Ann. Rev. Immunol.*, **11**:385–402.

Slowik, M.R., DeLuca, L.G., Fiers, W. and Pober, J.S. (1993). Tumor necrosis factor (TNF) activates human endothelial cells through the P55 TNF receptor but the P75 receptor contributes to activation at low TNF concentration. *Am. J. Pathol.*, **134**:1724–1730.

Spangrude, G.J., B.A., A. and Daynes, R.A. (1985). Site-selective homing of antigen-primed lymphocyte populations can play a critical role in the efferent limb of cell-mediated immune responses *in vivo*. *J. Immunol.*, **134**:2900–2907.

Springer, T.A. (1990). Adhesion receptors of the immune system. *Nature*, **346**:425–434.

Teitel, J.M., Shore, A., McBarron, J. and Schiavone, A. (1989). Enhanced T-cell activation due to combined stimulation by both endothelial cell sand monocytes. *Scand. J. Immunol.*, **29**:165–173.

Trowbridge, I.S. and Thomas, M.L. (1994). CD45: An emerging role as a protein tyrosine phosphatase required for lymphocyte activation and development. *Ann. Rev. Immunol.*, **12**:85–116.

Wagner, C.R., Vetto, R.M. and Burger, D.R. (1984). The mechanism of antigen presentation by endothelial cells. *Immunobiology*, **168**:453–469.

Wedgewood, J.F., Hatan, L. and Bonagura, V.R. (1988). Effect of interferon- and tumor necrosis factor on the expression of class I and class II major histocompatibility molecules by cultured human umbilical vein endothelial cells. *Cell Immunol.*, **111**:1–9.

Westphal, J.R., Williams, H.W., Tax, W.J.M., Koene, R.A.P., Ruiter, D.J. and deWaal, R.M.W. (1994). The proliferative response of human T cells to allogeneic IFN-γ treated endothelial cells is mediated via both CD2/LFA-3 and LFA-1/ICAM-1 and -2 adhesion pathways. *Transplant. Immunol.*, **1**:183–191.

2 Antigen Presentation by Brain Microvascular Smooth Muscle

Zsuzsanna Fabry, Ph.D. and Michael N. Hart, M.D.

Department of Pathology (Division of Neuropathology), University of Iowa College of Medicine, Iowa City, Iowa 52242

INTRODUCTION

Following the demonstration that endothelium, astrocytes, thyroid epithelium, and other somatic cells expressed major histocompatibility complex (MHC) class II antigens, it became more widely appreciated that many of these cells possessed at least facultative immune properties. Later studies by numerous laboratories established that many somatic cells expressing MHC class II could also activate T-lymphocytes (T-cells) with antigen-specificity. However, the *in vivo* significance of this phenomenon is not known for most of these cells. This chapter will start with a cursory review of some of the immune properties of large vessel smooth muscle followed by a treatise of our laboratory's work devoted to defining the properties of brain microvessel smooth muscle that verifies its potential as an important immunological constituent of the central nervous system.

IMMUNE PROPERTIES OF LARGE VESSEL SMOOTH MUSCLE

Vascular smooth muscle participates in various aspects of acute and chronic inflammation as evidenced by adhesion molecule expression, cytokine production, MHC class II expression and interaction with leukocytes. These properties auger smooth muscle as a potential "card-carrying" member of the immunological system and are thoroughly reported in other chapters of this book.

Most importantly, large vessel smooth muscle has been reported to express MHC class II antigens *in vivo* and *in vitro* and class II can be upregulated with gamma interferon (IFN-γ) (Warner *et al.*, 1988; Stemme *et al.*, 1990; 1992; Salomon *et al.*, 1993). Smooth muscle also produces interleukin-1 (IL-1) (Moyer and Reinisch, 1984; Libby *et al.*, 1986). Interactions of leukocytes with large vessel smooth muscle have also been explored and it is well known that IFN-γ produced by activated T-cells has an inhibitory effect on smooth muscle proliferation *in vitro* and *in vivo* (Hansson *et al.*, 1989; 1991; Nunokawa and Tanaka, 1992) (described in Chapter 8). Activation and proliferation of vascular smooth muscle cells at the site of vascular injury has also been described (Ross *et al.*, 1977), but the effect of the activated smooth muscle cells on vascular reactions and their interactions with leukocytes are not well understood. On the other hand, documentation of smooth muscle cell effects on lymphocytes has been more elusive, with at least two reported failures of smooth muscle cells to allostimulate T-cells (Pober *et al.*, 1986; Theobald *et al.*, 1993). However, monocyte activation by smooth muscle cell matrix has been reported (Kaufmann *et al.*, 1990).

Most of the immune and inflammatory regulating properties described for vascular smooth muscle *in vitro* and *in vivo* relate to large vessels. These cells express intercellular adhesion molecule-1 (ICAM-1) and vascular cell adhesion molecule-1 (VCAM-1), but not E-selectin in atherosclerotic plaques and in cultured cells. These adhesion molecules are regulated by proinflammatory cytokines, such as IL-1α, TNF-α, and monocyte chemoattractant protein-1 (Stemme *et al.*, 1992; Couffinhal *et al.*, 1993; 1994; Ikeda *et al.*, 1993; Li *et al.*, 1993; O'Brien *et al.*, 1993). The expression of adhesion molecules on large vessel SM cells suggests that these cells are participating in the focal accumulation of mononuclear cells in human atherosclerotic lesions and possibly in vasculitic states.

IMMUNE PROPERTIES OF MICROVESSEL-DERIVED SMOOTH MUSCLE CELLS

In contrast to large vessel smooth muscle, studies of inflammatory and immune properties of microvessel smooth muscle have been scant — especially in regard to the brain. Our laboratory has long been interested in the immune properties of both brain microvessel endothelium (En) and smooth muscle or pericytes (SM/P). We consider pericytes to be modified smooth muscle that are separated from En by basal lamina in the smaller microvessels in the brain. Smooth muscle is also separated from En by basal lamina, but located in postcapillary venules and larger vessels. Pericytes are distinguished at the light microscopic level by their presence at microvessel branches and at the ultrastructural level by location and by paucity of certain smooth muscle characteristics — although the latter distinction is arguable. Because we cannot be certain whether the cells we culture are pericytes, smooth muscle, or a combination of the two, we refer to them as SM/P. Most importantly, SM/P can be distinguished in culture from all other central nervous system cell types by their α-actin expression. (Figure 1).

One empirical pretext for studying the immune and inflammatory-regulating properties of SM/P lies in the fact that these cells, particularly smooth muscle, are present in postcapillary venules where the main events of the vascular phase of inflammation take place, especially leukocyte migration into the brain parenchyma. Paradoxically, vascular inflammatory events do not take place at nearly the same degree in brain capillaries (as in other organs) where it would appear that the singular barrier of En would facilitate leukocyte migration.

Our laboratory became interested in SM/P as an immune cell after discovering that mouse lymphocytes in co-culture with syngeneic brain derived SM/P became activated (proliferated and became blastic in appearance) after 6–7 days. Passive transfer of the

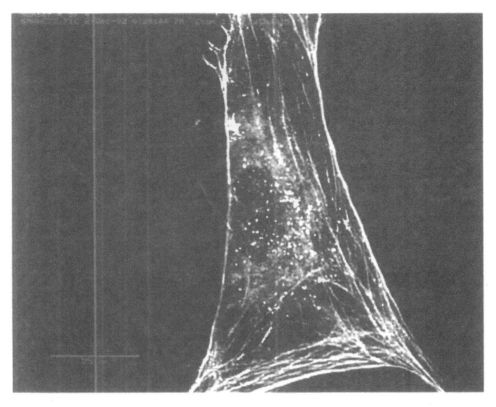

Figure 1 Analysis of α-actin expression in BALB/c brain microvessel SM/P cells by confocal microscopy. SM/P were positively identified by immunohistochemistry using a muscle-specific anti-α-actin.

SM/P activated lymphocytes into syngeneic hosts resulted in vasculitis of lungs, liver, and various other organs, albeit never in the CNS (Hart *et al.*, 1985).

Questions regarding the specificity of the lymphocyte activation were subsequently addressed. First, it was determined by flow cytometry with anti-class II antibodies that approximately 30–35% of cultured SM/P cells expressed MHC class II constitutively in contrast to En cells which showed only 5–10% constitutive expression (Hart *et al.*, 1987). MHC class II can be upregulated in both cell types by IFN-γ. Maximum upregulation is achieved with 200 U/ml, very similar to that seen in other cell types.

In many of our studies of the immune properties of SM/P we have compared BALB/c derived cells with SJL/j derived cells because the BALB/c mouse is considered a normal strain, whereas the SJL/j is autoimmune-prone and often used as a murine model for experimental allergic encephalitis. When the ability of BALB/c SM/P to activate spleen cells was compared to that of SJL/j spleen cells in syngeneic systems, the percentage of activated spleen cells was always approximately 20% greater in the BALB/c system.

It was further shown that SM/P activated T-cells preferentially in a syngeneic system — in contrast to En which activated T-cells much better when the two cell types were allo-geneic. To determine the subsets of lymphoid cells present after activation, spleen cells co-cultured for 7 days with SM/P cells were stained with different monoclonal antibodies

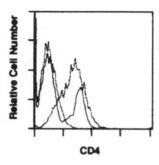 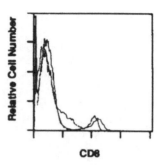

Figure 2 Flow cytometry analysis of the phenotypes of spleen cells co-cultured in the presence of syngeneic irradiated SM cells. Viable cells were isolated after the co-culture and distributed for fluorescence staining. Tracings show heavy preponderance of CD4⁺ cells with only minimal CD8⁺ cells.

directed against cell surface markers. As seen in Figure 2, after 7 days of co-culture the fraction of CD4⁺ cells present is markedly increased (~60–65%), showing a strong CD4⁺ cell activation while the percentage of CD8⁺ cells is not significantly changed (~15%) (Fabry *et al.*, 1990b). We recently demonstrated that these activated CD4⁺ T-cells produce IFN-γ, which in turn inhibits SM/P cell proliferation in the syngeneic SM/P-lymphocyte co-cultures. The evidence for this conclusion is drawn from our observations that 1) recombinant murine IFN-γ itself inhibits the proliferation of SM/P cells; 2) the supernatant from SM/P cell-activated splenic lymphocytes inhibits the proliferation of IFN-γ-sensitive WEHI 279 cells; 3) this supernatant induces the expression of class II MHC antigen of WEHI 3B cells which are also IFN-γ-sensitive; 4) the same supernatant has been found in our laboratory to be positive in an IFN-γ-sensitive ELISA. In addition to SM/P inhibition by IFN-γ, it is likely that other factors or cytokines also contribute to the inhibition as evidenced by the fact that anti-IFN-γ antibody fails to completely inhibit the effect of supernatant (unpublished observations). These other factors could be: transforming growth factor-β, glycosaminoglycans (heparin), or IL-1. The effect of IL-1 is rather controversial because it enhances the proliferation of smooth muscle cells but it can also induce the synthesis of inhibitory prostaglandins.

ANTIGEN-PRESENTING PROPERTIES OF BRAIN-DERIVED MICROVESSEL SM/P AND EN

In order to further credential SM/P as a somatic cell with immune functions, antigen presentation experiments were performed. During antigen presentation, antigen-specific T-cells are activated. α/β T-cells recognize free antigen very rarely, and their antigen recognition involves an interaction of the T-cell receptor (TCR) with fragments of antigen bound to either class I or class II MHC molecules on the surface of an antigen-presenting cell (APC) (Unanue, 1984; Townsend and Bodmer, 1989; Brodsky and Guagliardi, 1991; Kourilsky and Claverie, 1989). Class I MHC-restricted T-cells are almost exclusively CD8⁺ (cytotoxic/suppressor) phenotypes, whereas class II-restricted T-cells are CD4⁺ phenotype. The TCR is a disulfide-linked heterodimer made up of two chains, with either α and β chains on the α/β T-cells or γ and δ chain on the γ/δ T-cells (Allison and Lanier,

1987; Raulet, 1989; Allison and Havran, 1991). The TCR repertoire is formed during thymic development using different gene segments — the variable (V), diversity (D), joining (J), and constant (C) regions (Wilson *et al.*, 1988). The gene segments are randomly rearranged and, following positive and negative selection, the individual mature T-cells have single specificity when they leave the thymus. This specificity is determined by the variable regions of the α/β TCR α and β chains which form a combining site that has contact residues for both the MHC-bound peptide and the MHC molecule (Kappler *et al.*, 1987; Fowlkes and Pardoll, 1989; Schwartz, 1989a; von Boehmer *et al.*, 1989; Van Ewijk, 1991). Several data support the concept that secondary signals are generated as a result of the TCR-antigen/MHC interaction and are transmitted through CD3, a multimolecular complex expressed in a noncovalent association with the TCR on the surface of all mature T-cells. An example of a secondary signal is phosphoinositide-specific phospholipase C, which mediates breakdown of inositol phospholipids, in turn giving rise to two second messengers, namely inositol phosphate and diacylglycerol. The resulting increase in intracellular Ca^{2+} concentration and translocation of protein kinase C to the plasma membrane are thought to initiate the cascade of biochemical events leading to activation of T-cells effector functions and clonal expansion (Imboden and Stobo, 1985). In addition, tyrosine kinase activity is increased, resulting in phosphorylation of multiple substrates on tyrosine residues. At least two tyrosine kinases, p59fyn and p56lck, have been implicated in T-cells signalling and tyrosine kinase activity appears to be necessary for IL-2 production (Samelson *et al.*, 1990; Watts *et al.*, 1992). These signalling events lead to the eventual transcription of lymphokine genes and activation of other cellular functions. A T-cell encounter with specific antigens in the absence of sufficient IL-2 to complete the cell cycle will result in long-lived cellular anergy (cell unresponsiveness) or cell death (Lamb and Feldman, 1984; Schwartz, 1990). Insufficient IL-2 production is a result of the absence of adequate co-stimulation during TCR engagement.

In our experiments, ovalbumin (OVA) was given to SM/P and En as exogenous antigen for OVA-specific H2^d-restricted A2.2E10, a T-cell hybridoma (Glimcher and Shevach, 1982). Spleen cells were used as positive controls. A2.2E10 cells are known to proliferate and produce IL-2 after stimulation with OVA presented in the context of H2^d MHC (Glimcher and Shevach, 1982). Proliferation of the cells and IL-2 production from the supernatants was tested using an IL-2-dependent CTLL cell line, diagrammed in Figure 3. Figure 4 shows that unstimulated brain SM/P cells are able to present antigen to A2.2E10 cells. Whole OVA and digested OVA are presented by SM/P cells equally well. We compared the antigen-presenting capacity of SM/P cells to En cells and found that brain En cells presented OVA and digested OVA to these T-cells at a much lower level than SM/P. Other exogenous antigens, such as KLH were also tested in order to determine whether SM/P cell antigen presentation was limited to OVA. SM/P cells can present KLH antigen to the HDK-1 Th1 cell clone, detected by the increased proliferation of the HDK-1 T-cells. The antigen-presenting capacity of En cells in the HDK-1 KLH assay is also much lower than that of spleen or SM/P cells. (Fabry *et al.*, 1990a).

Class II Restriction of Antigen Specific Activation

Figure 5 shows that BALB/c brain SM/P cells are, able to present antigen to the H2^d-restricted T-cells but not to an OVA-specific H2^k-restricted T-cell demonstrating that they

ANTIGEN PRESENTATION

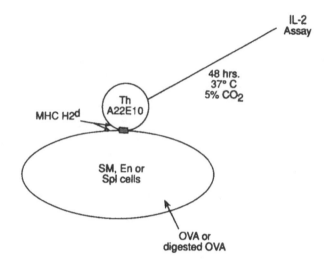

Figure 3   Antigen presentation assay schematically represented.

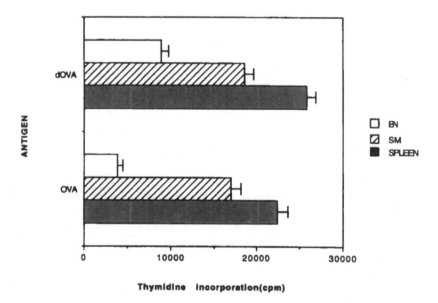

Thymidine   incorporation(cpm)

Figure 4   OVA antigen presentation by cultured brain SM cells. Irradiated spleen cells, brain SM/P or En cells were incubated with OVA-specific T-cells (1:1 ratio) in the presence of whole of digested OVA (dOVA) as an antigen. IL-2 production of T-cells was checked after 2 days' incubation using the CTLL IL-2-dependent cell line. [^{3}H] Thymidine incorporation of the CTLL cell line in the presence of culture supernatant is shown. The results represent mean cpm ± SD of triplicates in three experiments and show that SM/P presents antigen almost as well as spleen cells and much better than En in this system.

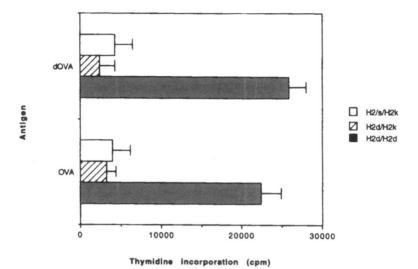

Figure 5 MHC restriction of antigen presentation. Irradiated SM/P cells were incubated for 2 days of triplicates in three experiments. The black columns represent that antigen presentation of H2^d (BALB/c) SM/P cells to H2^d-resrticted OVA antigen-specfic T-cells. Cross-hatched columns represent H2^d SM/P antigen presentation to H2^k-restricted OVA antigen-specific T-cells. Clear columns represent H2^s SM/P (SJL/j) antigen presentation to H2^d-restricted OVA-specific T-cells. The results show that antigen is presented only in the syngeneic system.

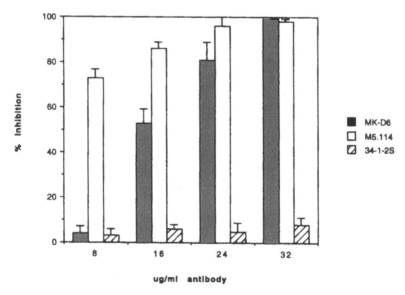

Figure 6 Effect of anti-MHC class II monoclonal antibody on antigen presentation by brain SM/P cells. Irradiated brain SM/P cells were incubated with OVA antigen and OVA antigen-specfic T-cells (1:1 ratio) in the presence of varying concentrations of anti-I-A^d (MKD6), anti-I-A^{bdq}, I-E^{dk}, (M5.114), or anti-class I (34-1-2S) monoclonal antibodies. After 2 days, IL-2 production of OVA specific T-cells was measured and compared to control cultures (antigen presentation by SM/P cells without anti-MHC monoclonal antibodies) (L mean ± SD, n = 3). More complete blockage at lower concentrations by M5.114 indicate involvement of both the IA and IE components of MHC class II.

present OVA and digested OVA in an $H2^d$-restricted fashion. In addition, SM/P of the $H2^s$ haplotype are not able to present either OVA or digested OVA to the $H2^d$-restricted cells (Fabry *et al.*, 1990a).

Blockage of Antigen-Specific Activation with Anti-MHC Class II Antibodies

The importance of MHC class II in antigen presentation by SM/P was further emphasized by co-culturing the OVA-specific T-hybridoma cells (A2.2E10) with irradiated SM/P cells ($H2^d$) with or without antigen in the presence of increasing amounts of monoclonal anti-Ia antibodies. M5.114 antibody, reacting with both I-A and I-E determinants of MHC class II, causes nearly 100% inhibition of the antigen presentation capacity of the brain cells even at the lowest concentration used (Figure 6). However, MK-D6, a monoclonal antibody reacting with the I-A determinant only, significantly inhibits the antigen presentation only in higher concentrations suggesting major antigen-presenting roles for both I-A and I-E class II MHC determinants in this system. Moreover, neither anti-MHC class I mono-clonal antibody nor anti-I-A antibody specific for the $H2^s$ haplotype influenced the antigen presentation capacity of SM/P cells (data not shown). (Fabry *et al.*, 1990a).

In summary, microvessel-derived SM/P cells are able to present antigen to an OVA specific T-cell hybridoma and to a KLH specific T-cell clone in MHC class II restricted fashion. Both class II expression on the SM/P and antigen presentation is augmented by treatment with IFN-γ. In contrast, En cells present antigen poorly, possibly because they do not process it as well as SM/P.

Antigen Specific Activation of Different Subsets of T-Helper Cells by SM/P and En

In order to help establish a possible *in vivo* function for T-cells activated by brain microvessel SM/P and En, experiments were undertaken to determine whether these somatic cells presented antigen to specific subsets of CD4+ (T-helper) cells.

T-helper (Th) (CD4+) cell subsets are identified either on the basis of the cytokines they secrete or on the basis of their relative stage of development. Two distinct subsets of T-cells have been identified among long term, cloned T-cell lines (Mosmann *et al.*, 1986; Coffman and Mosmann, 1990; Abbas *et al.*, 1991). Th1 clones secrete IFN-γ, IL-2, and lymphotoxin and promote delayed type hypersensitivity reactions. In contrast, Th2 clones produce IL-4, IL-5, IL-6, and IL-10 and promote B cell activation and antibody pro-duction (Coffman and Mosmann, 1990). Th1 and Th2 clones may also differ in their requirements for antigen presentation, since B cells preferentially stimulate Th2 clones, whereas adherent cells (macrophages/dendritic cells) preferentially stimulate Th1 clones (Gajewski *et al.*, 1991).

In order to test the hypothesis that different Th subsets might require different co-stimulatory signals for their optimal activation, four CD4+Th cell clones were selected and examined using splenocytes as APC. Some of the characteristics of these clones are listed in Table 1.

Importantly, all four clones share the same restriction elements (H-2^d); both pairs having the same antigen specificity, but differing in the cytokine pattern they produce. The OVA-specific clones (pGL2, pL3) recognize the same epitope-peptide 323–339. This peptide has been reported to be immunodominant in the H-2^d haplotype and does not

Table 1 Characteristics of Th Cell Clones Used in These Experiments

	Restriction Elements	Th Type	Antigen Specificity
pGL2	H-2^d	Th1	OVA 323–339
pL3	H-2^d	Th2	OVA 323–339
D1.1	H-2^d	Th1	Rabbit Ig
CDC35	H-2^d	Th2	Rabbit Ig

require further processing to stimulate I-A^d-restricted T-lymphocytes (Shimonkevitz *et al.*, 1984; Grey and Chesnut, 1985). These clones are maintained by weekly restimulation with irradiated syngeneic spleen cells, which also served as an APC control for subsequent experiments. Splenocytes presented antigen to both Th1 and Th2 clones, however, Th1 clones responded slightly better to splenocytes as APC in the presence of their respective antigen. (Data not presented). (Fabry *et al.*, 1993).

Antigen-Specific Activation of CD4+ Th Clones by Brain Microvessel SM/P

IFN-γ activated murine brain microvessel SM/P cells were co-cultured for 48 h with the various Th clones in the presence of their respective antigen, and the degree of the stimulation of the Th clones was determined by measuring the incorporation of [^{3}H]-TdR. Figure 7

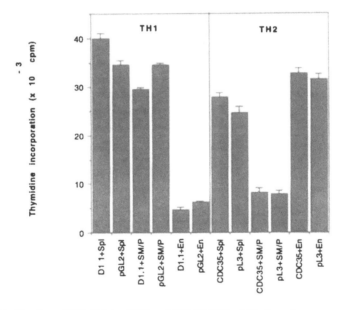

Figure 7 Proliferation of Th1 (D1.1, pGL2) and Th2 (CDC35, pL3) clones in response to splenocytes, or brain microvascular En and SM/P cells. Cloned T-cells were cultured with syngeneic splenocytes, brain microvessel En or SM/P cells (2000 rad at 1:1 ratio) in the presence of antigen. ^{3}H-TdR incorporation was measured during the last 6 hr of a 48 hr incubation. ^{3}H-thymidine incorporation without APC was < 500 cpm for all clones. The results represent mean value of triplicate cultures ± SD of four experiments, showing activation of Th1 cells by SM/P and Th2 cells by En.

shows that Th1 clones (D1.1; pGL2) respond better than Th2 clones (CDC35; pL3) when brain microvessel SM/P is used as the APC. The pGL2 Th1 clone prefers SM/P as an APC compared even to splenocytes, inasmuch as their half maximum response can be detected at a lower antigen concentration. The differential activation of these Th clones is detected not only by their proliferation, but also by their lymphokine production. The supernatant of co-cultures of SM/P with CDC35 or D1.1 clones was tested for the presence of IL-2 and IL-4. The CDC35 cells produce a very low amount of IL-4 when cultured with SM/P, whereas D1.1 secrete a significant amount of IL-2 as a result of co-culture with antigen-pulsed SM/P. Furthermore, IFN-γ-activated brain microvessel En cells were also co-cultured for 48 h with the same set of Th clones. Th1 clones (pGL2 and D1.1) do not proliferate at a wide range of antigen concentration when En cells are used as APC, however, Th2 clones do. (Fabry *et al.*, 1993)

Role of Co-Stimulatory Molecules in Differential Activation of Th1 vs. Th2 Cells

Although necessary, TCR occupancy and its associated biochemical consequences are not sufficient to induce lymphokine secretion or proliferation of Th cells; a second non-specific co-stimulatory signal is required (Mueller *et al.*, 1989). (Figure 8). Evidence

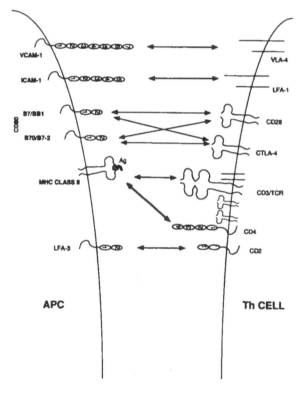

Figure 8 Adhesion molecules might mediate interactions between activated CD4⁺ T-cells and APC. TCR of the Th cells interact with MHC class II-bound peptides on the APC. This interaction is aided by several other molecules. Immunoglobulin superfamily domain structures are indicated. Molecules which have been found to be expressed by brain microvessel cells are marked in bold.

suggests that co-stimulatory signals are provided more by APC-Th cell interaction than by soluble mediators (Jenkins and Miller, 1992). The presence or absence of co-stimulatory molecules on APC will strongly influence the outcome of T-cell antigen recognition. If co-stimulators are present, antigen presentation results in cytokine gene expression and T-cell proliferation. The activated T-cells are then capable of responding to subsequent antigen exposure. In the absence of co-stimulatory molecules, there is suboptimal or no IL-2 gene expression and the T-cells do not proliferate. Subsequent activation of these T-cells may indicate that these cells are in a long-lived anergic stage. Once anergized, helper Th1 lymphocytes produce no detectable IL-2 and reduced levels of IL-3 and IFN-γ in response to stimulation via the TCR complex and yet continue to proliferate in response to exogenous IL-2. This phenomenon of clonal anergy has largely been studied using murine Th1 clones together with APC that are chemically fixed (Mueller *et al.*, 1989; Schwartz *et al.*, 1989b; Schwartz, 1990; 1992). At least five distinct adhesion molecules present on APC, B7/1, B7/2, ICAM-1 (CD54), LFA-3 (CD58), and VCAM-1 (CD106), have been individually shown to co-stimulate T-cell activation (Springer, 1990; Van Seventer *et al.*, 1990; Damle and Aruffo, 1991; Steinman and Young, 1991; Damle *et al.*, 1992a; Damle *et al.*, 1992b; Linsley and Ledbetter, 1993).

In order to determine whether adhesion or co-stimulator molecules are involved in the differential antigen-specific activation of Th1 and Th2 cells by SM/P and En, respectively, we studied the expression of a number of such molecules on En, SM/P and lymphocytes. We showed that En expressed ICAM-1 and it can be upregulated by pro-inflammatory cytokines. (Hart *et al.*, 1990; Fabry *et al.*, 1992). Although SM/P expressed virtually no ICAM-1, it is not likely that this molecule serves as the determinant of Th1 versus Th2 activation between these two APC because antibodies directed against leukocyte function molecule-1 (LFA-1), the counter receptor for ICAM-1 on lymphocytes, equally inhibits lymphocyte proliferation in co-culture with both En and SM/P. We have also studied the expression of VCAM-1 (CD106) and B7 family (CD80) on brain microvessel cells. These co-stimulatory counter-receptors function by interacting with their receptor expressed on the surface of T-cells. Thus, B7/1 and B7/2 interact with the CD28 (Linsley and Ledbetter, 1993) and CTLA-4 molecules and VCAM-1 interacts predominantly with the CD49d/CD29 (VLA-4/β1 integrin) (Damle *et al.*, 1992b). We have shown that the VCAM-1 molecule is expressed by brain microvessel En and its expression can be regulated by IFN-γ and TNF-α cytokines. However, it has not been determined as yet whether our SM/P express VCAM-1.

We have also detected B7/1 (CD80) molecule mRNA in nonstimulated and IL-1-, TNF-α and LPS-activated SM/P cells (Figure 9). Only TNF-α-stimulated En cells showed detectable amounts of B7/1 mRNA using the polymerase chain reaction (PCR) method (manuscript in preparation). However, anti CD28 mAb did not influence CD4+Th2 cell interaction with brain microvessel En cells, suggesting that B7-CD28 interaction may not be a major factor in the differential activation of Th1 and Th2 by SM/P and En, respectively.

The expression of LFA-1, CD2 and CD4 adhesion molecules was also studied on the selected Th1 and Th2 clones. Although some variation existed between individual clones in terms of expression of the particular molecules, levels of expression did not correlate with a Th1 or Th2 subset (data not shown). Although our data are not definitive yet, we favor

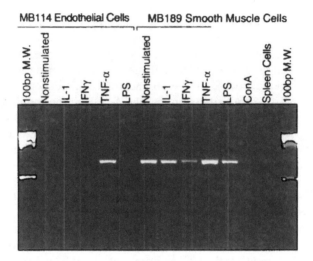

Figure 9 B7/1 gene expression in brain microvessel cells. B7/1 gene expression was determined by RT-PCR analysis of mRNA isolated from brain micorvessel cells. The predicted size of the amplified B7/1 cDNA is 840 bp. Each increment in the control DNA ladder is 100 bp.

the interpretation that the differential APC function of SM/P and En cells is best accounted for by differences in antigen presentation at the level of the co-stimulatory signal. Besides the factors which have been listed above, there could be multiple other possibilities accounting for differences between SM/P and En cells. Characterization of these factors will greatly help our understanding of inflammatory reactions at the vessel wall.

SUMMARY AND CONCLUSIONS

In this chapter we have re-capitulated experiments in our laboratory that validate brain-derived microvessel smooth muscle/pericytes having immune properties. We have shown that SM/P activate T-helper lymphocytes (CD4+) preferentially in a syngeneic system, express MHC class II antigen constitutively — which can be upregulated with IFN-γ — and presents specific antigen to CD4+ cells in an MHC class II restricted fashion. Moreover, SM/P presents antigen preferentially to Th1 lymphocytes in contrast to brain-derived En which presents to Th2 lymphocytes, suggesting different and even contrasting immune roles for these two somatic cells located at the blood-brain barrier.

Thus, a possible scenario occurring in the central nervous system during inflammatory and immune conditions would be for SM/P to both activate lymphocytes and/or confer anergy upon them. SM/P would likely do this in concert with other cells at the blood-brain barrier, such as En and astrocytes. Lymphocytes in turn, might modulate SM/P function, such as inhibiting proliferation by way of IFN-γ secretion and modulating the expression of SM/P produced cytokines, adhesion and other molecules.

References

Abbas, A.K., Williams, M.E., Burstein, H.J., Chang, T-L., Bossu, P. and Lichtman, A.H. (1991). Activation and functions of CD4[+] T-cell subsets. *Immunological Reviews*, **123**:5.

Allison, J.P. and Havran, W.L. (1991). The immunobiology of T-cells with invariant gd antigen receptors. *Annual Review Immunology*, **9**:679–705.

Allison, J.P. and Lanier, L.L. (1987). Structure, function, and serology of the T-cell antigen receptor complex. *Annual Review in Immunology*, **5**:503–40.

Brodsky, F.M. and Guagliardi, L.E. (1991). The cell biology of antigen processing and presentation. *Annual Review of Immunology*, **9**:707–44.

Coffman, R.L. and Mosmann, T.R. (1990). CD4+ T-cell subsets: regulation of differentiation and function. *Research in Immunology*, **141**:1.

Couffinhal, T., Duplaa, C., Labat, L., Lamaziere, J.M., Moreau, C., Printseva, O. and Bonnet, J. (1993). Tumor necrosis factor-alpha stimulates ICAM-1 expression in human vascular smooth muscle cells. *Arteriosclerosis and Thrombosis*, **13**:407–414.

Couffinhal, T., Duplaa, C., Moreau, C., Lamaziee, J.M. and Bonnet, J. (1994). Regulation of vascular cell adhesion molecule-1 and intercellular adhesion molecule-1 in human vascular smooth muscle cells. *Circulation Research*, **74**:225–234.

Damle, N.K. and Aruffo, A. (1991). Vascular cell adhesion molecule-1 induces T-cell antigen receptor-dependent activation of human CD4+ T-lymphocytes. *Proceedings of the National Academy of Science USA*, **88**:6403–6407.

Damle, N.K., Klussman, K. and Aruffo, A. (1992a). ICAM-2, a second ligand for CD11a/CD18 (LFA-1), provides a co-stimulatory signal for T-cell receptor-initiated activation of human T-cells. *Journal of Immunology*, **148**:665–671.

Damle, N.K., Klussman, K., Linsley, P. and Aruffo, A. (1992b). Differential co-stimulatory effects of adhesion molecules B7, ICAM-1, LFA-1, LFA-3 and VCAM-1 on resting and antigen primed CD4[+] T-lymphocytes. *Journal of Immunology*, **148**:1985–1992.

Fabry, Z., Sandor, M., Gajewski, T.F., Herlein, J.A., Waldschmidt, M.M., Lynch, R.G. and Hart, M.N. (1993). Differential activation of Th1 and Th2 CD4[+] cells by murine brain microvessel endothelial cells and smooth muscle/pericytes[1]. *Journal of Immunology*, **151**:38–47.

Fabry, Z., Waldschmidt, M.M., Hendrickson, D., Keiner, J., Love-Homan, L., Takei, F. and Hart, M.N. (1992). Adhesion molecules on murine brain microvascular endothelial cells: expression and regulation of ICAM-1 and Lgp 55. *Journal of Neuroimmunology*, **36**:1–11.

Fabry, Z., Waldschmidt, M.M., Moore, S.A. and Hart, M.N. (1990a). Antigen presentation by brain microvessel smooth muscle and endothelium. *Journal of Neuroimmunology*, **28**:63–71.

Fabry, Z., Waldschmidt, M.M., Van Dyk, L., Moore, S.A. and Hart, M.N. (1990b). Activation of CD4[+] lymphocytes by syngeneic brain microvascular smooth muscle cells. *J. Immunol.*, **145**:1099–1104.

Fowlkes, B.J. and Pardoll, D.M. (1989). Molecular and cellular events of T-cell development. *Advances in Immunology*, **44**:207–67.

Gajewski, T.F., Phinnas, M., Wong, T. and Fitch, F.W. (1991). Murine Th1 and Th2 clones proliferate optimally in response to distinct antigen-presenting cell populations. *Journal of Immunology*, **146**:1750–1758.

Glimcher, L.H. and Shevach, E.M. (1982). Production of autoreactive I region restricted T-cell hybridomas. *Journal of Experimental Medicine*, **156**:640–645.

Grey, H.M., Chesnut, R.W., Shimonkevitz, R., Marrack, P. and Kappler, J. (1984). Mechanisms of antigen processing and presentation. *Immunobiology*, **168**:202–212.

Hansson, G.K., Hellstrand, M., Rymo, L., Rubbia, L. and Gabbiani, G. (1989). Interferon-γ inhibits both proliferation and expression of differentiation-specific α-smooth muscle actin in arterial smooth muscle cells. *Journal of Experimental Medicine*, **170**:1595–1608.

Hansson, G.K., Holm, J., Holm, S., Fotev, Z., Hedrich, H.J. and Fingerle, J. (1991). T-Lymphocytes inhibit the vascular response to injury. *Proceedings of the National Academy of Sciences USA*, **88**(23), 10530–10534.

Hart, M.N., Fabry, Z., Waldschmidt, M. and Sandor, M. (1990). Lymphocyte interacting adhesion molecules on brain microvascular cells. *Molecular Immunology*, **27**:1355–1359.

Hart, M.N., Tassell, S.K., Sadewasser, K.L., Schelper, R.L. and Moore, S.A. (1985). Autoimmune vasculitis resulting from *in vitro* immunization of lymphocytes to smooth muscle. *American Journal of Pathology*, **119**:448–455.

Hart, M.N., Waldschmidt, M.M., Hanley-Hyde, J.M., Moore, S.A., Kemp, J.D. and Schelper, R.L. (1987). Brain microvascular smooth muscle expresses class II antigens[1]. *Journal of Immunology*, **138**:2960–2963.

Ikeda, U., Ikeda, M., Seino, Y., Takahashi, M., Kasahara, T., Kano, S. and Shimada, K. (1993). Expression of intercellular adhesion molecule-1 on rat vascular smooth muscle cells by pro-inflammatory cytokines. *Atherosclerosis*, **104**(1–2), 61–68.

Imboden, J.B. and Stobo, J.D. (1985). Transmembrane signalling by the T-cell antigen receptor. *Journal of Experimental Medicine*, 161:446–456.I.

Jenkins, M.K. and Miller, R.A. (1992). Memory and anergy: challenges to traditional models of T-lymphocyte differentiation. *FASEB Journal*, 6:2428.

Kappler, J.W., Wade, T. and White, J. (1987). A T-cell receptor Vb segment that imparts reactivity to a class II major histocompatibility complex product. *Cell*, 49:263–71.

Kaufmann, J., Jorgensen, R.W., Martin, B.M. and Franzblau, C. (1990). Monocyte activation by smooth muscle cell-derived matrices. *Atherosclerosis*, 85:113–125.

Kourilsky, P. and Claverie, J-M. (1989). MHC-antigen interaction: what does the T-cell receptor see? In: Dixon F., ed. *Advances in Immunology*, 45:107–94. San Diego: Academic Press.

Lamb, J.R. and Feldmann, M. (1984). Essential requirement for major histocompatibility complex recognition in T-cell tolerance induction. *Nature*, 308:72–74.

Li, H., Cybulsky, M.I., Gimbrone, M.A. Jr. and Libby, P. (1993). Inducible expression of vascular cell adhesion molecule-a by vascular smooth muscle cells *in vitro* and within rabbit atheroma. *American Journal of Pathology*, 143:1551–1559.

Libby, P., Ordovas, J.M., Birinyi, L.K., Auger, K.R. and Dinarello, C.A. (1986). Inducible interleukin-1 gene expression in human vascular smooth muscle cells. *Journal of Clinical Investigation*, 78:1432.

Linsley, P.S. and Ledbetter, J.A. (1993). The role of the CD28 receptor during T-cell responses to antigen. *Annual Review in Immunology*, 11:191.

Mosmann, T.R., Cherwinski, H., Bond, M.W., Giedlin, M.A. and Coffman, R.L. (1986). Two types of murine helper T-cell clone. I. Definition according to profiles of lymphokine activities and secreted proteins *Journal of Immunology*, 136:2348.

Moyer, C.F. and Reinisch, C.L. (1984). The role of vascular smooth muscle cells in experimental autoimmune vasculitis. *American Journal of Pathology*, 117:380.

Mueller, D.L., Jenkins, M.K. and Schwartz, R.H. (1989). Clonal expansion versus functional clonal inactivation: a co-stimulatory signalling pathway determines the outcome of T-cell antigen receptor occupancy. *Annual Review of Immunology*, 7:445–480.

Nunokawa, Y. and Tanaka, S. (1992). Interferon-gamma inhibits proliferation of rat vascular smooth muscle cells by nitric oxide generation. *Biochemical and Biophysical Research Communications*, 188:409–415.

O'Brien, K.D., Allen, M.D., McDonald, T.O., Chait, A., Harlan, J.M., Fishbein, D., McCarty, J., Ferguson, M., Hudkins, K., Benjamin, C.D., *et al.* (1993). Vascular cell adhesion molecule-1 is expressed in human coronary atherosclerotic plaques. Implications for the mode of progression of advanced coronary atherosclerosis. *Journal of Clinical Investigation*, 92:945–951.

Pober, J.S., Collins, T., Gimbrone, M.A. Jr., Libby, P. and Reiss, C.S. (1986). Inducible expression of class II major histocompatibility complex antigens and the immunogenicity of vascular endothelium. *Transplantation*, 41:141–146.

Raulet, D.H. (1989). The structure, function, and molecular genetics of the gd T-cell receptor. *Annual Review of Immunology*, 7:175–207.

Ross, R.J., Glomset, J. and Harker, L. (1977). Response to injury and atherogenesis. *American Journal of Pathology*, 86:675–684.

Salomon, R.N., Friedman, G.B., Callow, A.D., Payne, D.D. and Libby, P. (1993). Cryopreserved aortic homografts contain viable smooth muscle cells capable of expressing transplantation antigens. *Journal of Thoracic and Cardiovascular Surgery*, 106:1173–1180.

Samelson, L.E., Phillips, A.F., Luong, E.T. and Klausner, R.D. (1990). Association of the fyn protein-tyrosine kinase with the T-cell antigen receptor. *Proceedings of the National Academy Science USA*, 87:4358–4362.

Schwartz, R.H. (1989a). Acquisition of immunologic self tolerance. *Cell*, 57:1073–81.

Schwartz, R.H., Mueller, D.L., Jenkins, M.K. and Quill, H. (1989b). T-cell clonal anergy. *Cold Spring Harbor Symposium Quant., Biol.*, 2:605.

Schwartz, R.H. (1990). A Cell culture model for T-lymphocyte clonal anergy. *Science*, 248:1349–1356.

Schwartz, R.H. (1992). Co-stimulation of T-lymphocytes: the role of CD28, CTLA-4 and B7/BB1 in interleukin-2 production and immunotherapy. *Cell*, 71:1065–1068.

Shimonkevitz, R., Colon, S., Kappler, J.W., Marrack, P. and Grey, H.M. (1984). Antigen recognition by H-2-restricted T-cells. A cryptic ovalbumin peptide that substitutes for processed antigen. *Journal of Immunology*, 133:2067–2074.

Springer, T.A. (1990). Adhesion receptors of the immune system. *Nature*, 346:425–434.

Steinman, R.M. and Young, J.W. (1991). Signals arising from antigen presenting cells. *Current Opinion in Immunology*, 3:361–372.

Stemme, S., Fager, G. and Hansson, G.K. (1990). MHC class II antigen expression in human vascular smooth muscle cells is induced by interferon-gamma and modulated by tumor necrosis factor and lymphotoxin. *Immunology*, 69:243–249.

Stemme, S., Patarroyo, M. and Hansson, G.K. (1992). Adhesion of activated T-lymphocytes to vascular smooth muscle cells and dermal fibroblasts is mediated by beta 1- and beta 2-integrins. *Scandinavian Journal of Immunology*, **36**:233–242.

Theobald, V.A., Lauer, J.D., Kaplan, F.A., Baker, K.B. and Rosenberg, M. (1993). "Neutral allografts" — lack of allogeneic stimulation by cultured human cells expressing MHC class I and class II antigens. *Transplantation*, **55**:128–133.

Townsend, A. and Bodmer, H. (1989). Antigen recognition by class I-restricted T-lymphocytes. *Annual Review of Immunology*, **7**:601–24.

Unanue, E.R. (1984). Antigen-presenting function of the macrophage. *Annual Review of Immunology*, **2**:395–428.

Van Ewijk, W. (1991). T-cell differentiation is influenced by thymic micro-environments. *Annual Review of Immunology*, **9**:591–615.

Van Seventer, G.A., Shimizu, Y., Horgan, K.J. and Shaw, S. (1990). The LFA-1 ligand ICAM-1 provides an important co-stimulatory signal for T-cell receptor-mediated activation of resting T-cells. *Journal of Immunology*, **144**:4579–4586.

von Boehmer, H., The, H.S. and Kisielow, P. (1989). The thymus selects the useful and destroys the harmful. *Immunology Today*, **10**:57–61.

Warner, S.J., Friedman, G.B. and Libby, P. (1988). Regulation of major histocompatibility gene expression in human vascular smooth muscle cells. *Arteriosclerosis*, **9**:279–288.

Watts, J.D., Wilson, G.M., Ettenhadieh, E., Clark-Lewis, I., Kubanek, C.A., Astell, C.R., Marth, J.D. and Aebersold, R. (1992). Purification and initial characterization of the lymphocyte-specific protein-tyrosyl kinase p56lck from a baculovirus expression system. *Journal of Biological Chemistry*, **267**:901–907.

Wilson, R.K., Lai, E., Concannon, R., Barth, R.K. and Hood, L.E. (1988). Structure, organization and polymorphism of murine and human T-cell receptor α and β chain gene families. *Immunological Reviews*, **101**:149–172.

3 Vascular Cells Produce and Respond to Cytokines

Peter Libby, M.D.

Vascular Medicine and Atherosclerosis Unit, Cardiovascular Division,
Department of Medicine, Brigham and Women's Hospital, and Harvard Medical School,
Boston, Massachusetts

INTRODUCTION

From the last decade's ferment in vascular biology has emerged a central theme: inducible functions of the cells of the vessel wall. In the quest for the signals that switch the programs of vascular cell gene expression, the cytokines recur as common refrain. Conveniently defined as protein mediators of inflammation and immunity, the cytokines do not however include immunoglobulins and proteins of the complement cascade. Furthermore, cytokines should convey signals between cells acting at hormone-like rather than pharmacologic concentrations.

One can classify cytokines sensibly into several broad categories although not without overlap. One category includes cytokines involved particularly in non-antigen specific responses, often produced by a wide variety of cells. The mononuclear phagocytes provided the first source for many of the cytokines in this first category, hence the designation monokines (Dinarello, 1989; Oppenheim, 1985). Some of these cytokines share conserved spacing of cysteine residues, comprising a growing family known as the chemokines (Charo, 1992; Oppenheim *et al.*, 1990). Another category of cytokine mediates antigen specific immune responses, particularly those involving T-lymphocytes. The lymphokines IL-2 and interferon-gamma (IFN-γ), produced by a restricted range of cell types, T lymphocytes or Natural Killer (NK) cells, fall into this second category, the lymphokines. Finally, many cytokines have important roles in hematopoiesis. This class of cytokines includes the colony stimulating factors (CSFs), more or less selective for various lineages of blood cells, such as macrophage colony stimulating factor (M-CSF), granulocyte-macrophage colony stimulating factor (GM-CSF) or granulocyte colony stimulating factor (G-CSF). Interleukin-3 also falls into this latter category of cytokines involved in hematopoiesis.

Many cytokines bear the name "Interleukin" indicating the original concept that the cytokines mediated exchange of signals among leukocytes. As knowledge of the biology of cytokines has increased, this original concept has broadened considerably. We now know that many non-leukocytic cell types can produce as well as respond to cytokines. In fact, cytokines currently seem nearly universal as messengers of intercellular communication in many species.

In the context of vascular biology, cytokines have assumed a particularly prominent place because they regulate many vascular functions involved in homeostasis, defenses against injury, and in pathobiology of vascular diseases. The effects of cytokines on blood vessels has implications that reach beyond a narrow interpretation of vascular biology. Indeed, blood vessels play a prominent role in inflammation in general. Three classical cardinal signs of inflammation result primarily from alterations in blood vessel function. The redness (rubor) characteristic of inflammation results from increased local blood flow due to vasodilatation. The swelling (tumor) of inflamed tissues results from increased vascular permeability leading to extravasation of protein followed by fluid. The warmth (calor) follows upon the increased blood flow due to regional vasodilatation.

Another fundamental characteristic of the host-response during inflammation regards leukocyte recruitment to the inflamed zone. We now understand that alterations in vascular endothelial function contribute fundamentally to recruitment of leukocytes at sites of tissue inflammation, infection or injury (see below for details) (Gimbrone *et al.*, 1990; Bevilacqua, 1993). Metastasis of tumors by vascular routes likewise involves adhesive interactions of malignant cells with endothelial adhesion molecules subject to cytokine regulation. These examples illustrate the central role of cytokine-induce alterations in vascular biology *per se*, in generalized and local host defenses, in inflammatory responses, and in pathology in the broadest sense.

Immunologists in particular have generally regarded the vascular systems as a mere conduit for lymphocytes. However, more thoughtful practitioners of immunology recognize a more fundamental role for blood vessels in the immune response (Pober *et al.*, 1986; Butcher, 1986). Obviously, lymphocyte recruitment to areas of antigen-specific immune responses constitutes a special case of leukocyte recruitment via the vasculature as described above. However, lymphocyte recirculation occurs continuously as a homeostatic process as recognized since the time of Gowans and as elaborated by the contemporary work of Weissman, Butcher and colleagues (Butcher, 1986; Butcher *et al.*, 1986). Thus, lymphocytes interact with specialized endothelial cells on the venules of peripheral lymph nodes or Peyer's patches, where they can enter the lymphoid tissue. The lymphocyte circulatory system constitutes an important facet of lymphocyte physiology and immune surveillance.

Another broad area of interface between immunology and vascular biology concerns transplant rejection. A variety of reactions of the host to allografted organs or tissues involve blood vessels as primary targets. For example, hyperacute rejection results from a humoral immune response mediated by preformed natural alloantibodies reactive with vascular antigens in the allografted organ (For an extensive treatment of this topic see Chapter 7). This hyperacute process produces sudden vascular thrombosis, graft ischemia, and immediate failure.

Acute parenchymal rejection also involves blood vessels. As pointed out by Pober and colleagues, the host immune system first encounters the allogeneic tissue of the graft at the endothelial interface (Pober *et al.*, 1984). This graft endothelium bears the first wave of attack of cytolytic T-cells during an allogeneic response. The pathology of acute allograft rejection shows prominent perivascular "cuffing" due to mononuclear infiltrates, a further indication for the importance of blood vessels in this particular type of immune reaction.

Table 1 Selected Examples of Cytokine Actions in Vascular Pathophysiology

Interleukin-1	IL-1	● Induces adhesion molecule expression by endothelium ● Augments prostaglandin production by smooth muscle and endothelial cells ● Stimulates growth factor production by smooth muscle cells ● Increases expression of nitric oxide synthases (with other cytokines)
Tumor necrosis factor-α	TNF-α	● similar to IL-1
Macrophage chemo-attractant protein-1	MCP-1 (MCAF)	● Activates macrophage chemotaxis and activation
Macrophage-colony stimulating factor	M-CSF (CSF-1)	● Co-mitogenic for macrophages ● Simulates apolipoprotein E and scavenger receptor expression by macrophages
Gamma interferon	IFN-γ	● Induces class II major histocompatibility antigens on endothelial and smooth muscle cells as well as macrophages and T and B lymphocytes ● Cytostatic for endothelial and smooth muscle cells ● Inhibits collagen gene expression by smooth muscle cells ● Activates macrophages ● Increases expression of nitric oxide synthases (with other cytokines)
Interleukin-6	IL-6	● Activates B lymphocytes
Interleukin-2	IL-2	● Mitogenic for T lymphocytes
Interleukin-8	IL-8	● Chemoattractant and activator for granulocytes ● Inhibits granulocyte adhesion to endothelium under some circumstances

Table 2 Selected Sources of Cytokines Relevant in Vascular Pathophysiology

Cytokine		*Endothelium*	*Smooth Muscle*	*T-cells*	*Macrophages*
Interleukin-1	IL-1	+	+	+	++++
Tumor necrosis factor-α	TNF-α	−	+	+	++++
Macrophage chemoattractant protein-1	MCP-1 (MCAF)	+	++	?	+++
Macrophage-colony stimulating factor	M-CSF (CSF-1)	+	+	?	?
Interleukin-6	IL-6	+	+++	+	++
Interleukin-2	IL-2	−	−	+++	−
Gamma interferon	IFN-γ	−	−	+++	−
Interleukin-8	IL-8	+	+	+	?

Finally, in the context of transplantation biology, we and others have hypothesized an important role for a cellular immune reaction in pathogenesis of allograft vascular disease (Libby *et al.*, 1989; Salomon *et al.*, 1991). This form of "chronic" rejection involves a fibro-proliferative response of the vessels of the allograft leading eventually to chronic graft ischemia and failure. These examples illustrate vascular involvement in all phases of allograft rejection. For all of these reasons, understanding of many aspects of immunology requires an appreciation of vascular biology. As cytokines regulate many of the very functions of blood vessels important in immune and inflammatory responses (Table 1), cytokines elaborated by cells of the immune system convey many of the signals that alter functions of blood vessels during such responses (Table 2). These considerations then provide the background for consideration of cytokines in the context of vascular immunology.

Vascular Cells Produce a Variety of Cytokines

Interleukin-1

Interleukin-1, the prototypic cytokine, possesses many biological actions (Dinarello, 1994). Recognized early on as an endogenous pyrogen, biochemical studies suggested the identity of interleukin-1 with an independently characterized "lymphocyte activating factor" (Dinarello, 1981; Rosenwasser and Dinarello, 1981). The molecular characterization of IL-1 led to the recognition that many biological activities studied in laboratories across the globe were actually due to IL-1 (Auron *et al.*, 1984; March *et al.*, 1985). The astonishing range of IL-1's cellular targets run a gamut from osteoclasts to neuroglia. Interleukin-1 exists as two isoforms, interleukin-1 α and β, which share limited sequence similarities (26%) at the amino acid level but resemble each other at the three dimensional structural level quite closely (Zhang *et al.*, 1991). Although IL-1 was originally characterized as a soluble mediator, neither isoform of IL-1 contains a recognizable signal sequence as expected for a protein secreted through the usual pathways. The cDNAs encoding IL-1 α and β were first cloned from monocytes.

Both endothelial cells and smooth muscle cells elaborate thymocyte co-stimulatory activity characteristic for IL-1 (Libby *et al.*, 1986a; 1986b). The availability of cDNA reagents made it possible to test whether vascular cells could actually transcribe the newly defined IL-1 α and β genes. Indeed, when stimulated with bacterial endotoxin or other appropriate stimuli, human vascular endothelial and smooth muscle cells accumulated mRNA encoding both isoforms of IL-1 (Libby *et al.*, 1986a; 1986b). Moreover, both of these cell types elaborated thymocyte co-stimulatory activity that could be neutralized by the polyclonal antisera then available raised against biochemically purified interleukin-1.

As mentioned above, IL-1 does not appear to utilize the traditional secretory pathway as both isoforms lack the characteristic sequences signaling export from the cell. This paradox became even more perplexing when supernatants of appropriately activated human vascular cells were assayed for interleukin-1 biological activity using more selective reporter cell lines as they became available. Although the mRNA encoding IL-1 could readily be induced in vascular cells, media conditioned by these cells did not appear to contain substantial IL-1 activity as assessed by the more refined assays (Loppnow and Libby, 1992). Subsequent work has helped resolve these apparent paradoxes.

In the case of interleukin-1β, the original translation product lacks biological activity. Proteolytic cleavage by a highly specific cysteine protease, interleukin-1 beta converting enzyme, produces the biologically active species of this cytokine (Thornberry *et al.*, 1992). Thus, the accumulation of interleukin-1 beta mRNA or immunoreactive protein do not by themselves necessarily indicate the presence of biologically active material. Also, we now know that the IL-1 family contains an additional member. The IL-1 receptor antagonist bears substantial sequence similarity with IL-1 but does contain a legitimate signal sequence (Arend *et al.*, 1990; Dinarello and Thompson, 1991; Hannum *et al.*, 1990; Matsushime *et al.*, 1991). Vascular cells can elaborate the receptor antagonist in response to some of the same stimuli that cause IL-1 mRNA accumulation. Thus simultaneous release of the inhibitory isoform of IL-1 may mask its biological activity in conditioned media.

More importantly, although vascular cells can transcribe the IL-1 gene, they may not secrete biologically active materials, as neither the alpha nor beta isoform of IL-1 contain a recognizable signal sequence. Rather, vascular cells may accumulate the IL-1 precursors destined for release only under special circumstances, by a pathway as yet incompletely defined. Furthermore, vascular smooth muscle cells appear to exhibit surface-associated IL-1 activity serologically identified as the alpha isoform. Thus vascular smooth muscle cells appear not to elaborate soluble IL-1, but express IL-1 activity only with cells that contact their surface (Loppnow and Libby, 1992). The next section will discuss the probable nature of the soluble thymocyte co-stimulatory activity secreted by vascular cells after stimulation.

Interleukin-6

Like IL-1, interleukin-6 was originally described in many laboratories investigating a diverse variety of phenomena. The molecular characterization of IL-6 led to the coalescence of a number of such activities including B cell stimulatory factor, hybridoma growth factor, and beta2 interferon among others as due to this molecular entity (Aarden *et al.*, 1985; 1987; Hirano *et al.*, 1986; Zuberstein *et al.*, 1986; May *et al.*, 1986). In contrast to interleukin-1, IL-6 has a traditional signal sequence. Vascular endothelial and smooth muscle cells stimulated by bacterial endotoxin, interleukin-1, and other stimuli, transcribe the IL-6 gene (Loppnow and Libby, 1989a; 1989b). Furthermore, they translate this mRNA and appear to secrete the protein product virtually co-translationally. Vascular cells, particularly vascular smooth muscle cells, can elaborate astonishing quantities of IL-6. We have documented the production of picograms of IL-6 protein per smooth muscle cells following stimulation with IL-1 (Loppnow and Libby, 1990). Moreover, exposure to growth factors, such as platelet-derived growth factor (PDGF), will also stimulate IL-6 gene expression by vascular smooth muscle cells (Loppnow and Libby, 1990).

The broad spectrum of biological actions of IL-6 include the ability to participate in T-cell activation. Although IL-6 has relatively weak thymocyte co-stimulatory activity compared to IL-1, vascular smooth muscle cells elaborate IL-6 in such prodigious quantity that we believe that much of the thymocyte co-stimulatory activity elaborated by these cells is actually due to IL-6. Early experiments showed inhibition of much of the thymocyte co-stimulatory activity derived from activated vascular smooth muscle cells by anti-sera raised against IL-1. However, this reagent, prepared before the discovery of IL-6, and raised against biochemically purified IL-1, probably contained antibodies that neutralized IL-6 as well as IL-1 (Libby *et al.*, 1986b).

Although IL-6 may weakly promote mitogenesis of rat smooth muscle cells (Ikeda *et al.*, 1991), we find negligible effect of IL-6 on the proliferation of human smooth muscle cells. Indeed, our laboratory has not documented any action of IL-6 on vascular cells. These findings suggest to us the following model. Interleukin-1, which has manifold effects on intrinsic vascular wall cells does not appear to be secreted under usual circumstances. Vascular smooth muscle cells appear to require close cellular contact in order to elicit IL-1-induced signaling. This tight control of IL-1 biological activity appears to restrict its potent actions and resist an accelerated propagation of IL-1-induced signaling within an inflamed blood vessel. IL-6 in contrast appears to lack substantial effects on intrinsic vascular cells. IL-6's major targets include T- and B-lymphocytes. As these lymphocytes do not reside within the normal vessel but must be recruited, it is teleologically appealing to consider that IL-6, readily secreted in a soluble form that can act at a distance, and participate in recruitment and activation of B and T lymphocytes. IL-6 might in this manner be an important mediator in certain particular vascular inflammatory responses, such as angiocentric vasculidities including lymphocytic granulomatosis. In addition to T lymphocytes, atheroma contain cells likely derived from B lymphocytes, thus IL-6 may play a role in this aspect of atherogenesis as well.

Interleukin-8

Interleukin-8 exhibits more restricted biological activity than IL-1 or IL-6. It appears to function primarily as a stimulator of granulocyte function. Interestingly, IL-8 production by endothelial cells was first documented by a circuitous route. Interleukin-1-treated endothelial cells elaborate an inhibitor of leukocyte adhesion in static assays (Wheeler *et al.*, 1988). The biochemical purification of this leukocyte adhesion inhibitory activity showed that it resided in a truncated form of the previously described cytokine IL-8 (Gimbrone *et al.*, 1989). Thus, IL-1 stimulated endothelial cells can secrete this activator of polymorphonuclear leukocytes. IL-8 appears capable of exerting both pro inflammatory and anti-inflammatory actions depending on the assay. Smooth muscle cells may also transcribe IL-8 gene (Wang *et al.*, 1991). Local IL-8 production by vascular cells might participate in granulocyte recruitment in acute "leukoclastic" vasculitides such as the Arthus reaction or other forms of vasculitis associated with infiltrates rich in polymorphonuclear leukocytes (see Chapter 5).

Monocyte Chemoattractant Protein-1

This cytokine exemplifies a member of the chemokine family of particular potential significance in chronic vascular diseases. As usual in the cytokine field, the molecular characterization of a particular entity leads to the recognition that a variety of biological activities studied in different laboratories converge on a given molecule. The case of monocyte chemoattractant protein-1 (MCP-1) illustrates this principle. MCP-1 is also known as monocyte activating and chemoattractant factor (MCAF) (Furutani *et al.*, 1989; Larsen *et al.*, 1989; Matsushima *et al.*, 1988; Matsushima and Oppenheim, 1989; Matsushima *et al.*, 1989). Mouse fibroblasts treated with PDGF transcribe an originally anonymous gene, denoted JE, as a prominent early response. The JE gene turned out to encode the murine homologue of human MCP-1. Both vascular endothelial and smooth muscle cells can produce and elaborate MCP-1 (Wang *et al.*, 1991; Sica *et al.*, 1990; Rollins *et al.*, 1990; Cushing *et al.*, 1990). In particular, vascular smooth muscle cells were known to secrete a chemoattractant for mononuclear phagocytes (Valente *et al.*, 1984). MCP-1 accounts for this activity which may be important in the pathogenesis of vascular diseases including atherosclerosis, characterized by infiltration of the blood vessel by mononuclear phagocytes (Nelken *et al.*, 1991).

Tumor Necrosis Factor-α

Tumor necrosis factor shares many of IL-1's biological actions, despite its distinct primary structure (Nera *et al.*, 1992). The laboratories of Old and Cerami discovered tumor necrosis factor independently in the Old sought the identity of a factor that led to necrosis of transplantable tumors in mice previously treated with endotoxin (Old, 1985). Cerami sought a factor which mediated cachexia in animals with parasitic infections, hence the name "cachectin" originally proposed by their group (Beutler and Cerami, 1986). The cloning of TNF revealed that these two activities resided in a single entity now commonly known as tumor necrosis factor-α (Tracey and Cerami, 1994). Furthermore, a T-cell-derived mediator denoted lymphotoxin exhibited substantial sequence similarity with TNF-α and was dubbed by some tumor necrosis factor-β (Gray et al., 1984). In contrast to the other cytokines mentioned above, we are unaware of definitive evidence that vascular endothelial cells transcribe TNF genes.

However, vascular smooth muscle cells can transcribe TNF-α (Warner and Libby, 1989). Our original experiments utilized "superinduction" conditions to elicit substantial TNF-α mRNA accumulation by vascular smooth muscle cells. We initially doubted the biological significance of this observation which required treatment with a protein synthesis inhibitor together with the inducing stimulus such as bacterial endotoxin (Warner and Libby, 1989). Despite our concerns that we were dealing with a cell culture artifact, TNF production by smooth muscle cells appears to occur more readily *in vivo* than *in vitro*. Human smooth muscle cells in atherosclerotic lesions express TNF-α (Barath et al., 1990a; 1990b). Smooth muscle cells produce TNF-α in a variety of experimentally-produced vascular lesions in rabbits (Tanaka et al., 1994; Clausell et al., 1994). Administration of soluble TNF receptors to hearts allografted in rabbits can inhibit the development of graft coronary disease (Clausell et al., 1994). Thus, despite our initial reservations, vascular cell-derived TNF-α appears pathophysiologically significant.

Granulocyte-Macrophage Colony Stimulating Factor

Within the micro-environment of the bone marrow, leukopoiesis occurs in close proximity to microvessels. Bagby and colleagues showed early on that interleukin-1 treatment induced the expression of granulocyte-monocyte colony stimulating factor (GM-CSF) in cultured vascular endothelial cells (Bagby et al., 1986). This result was the first demonstration of expression of a hematopoietic growth factor by a vascular cell. This finding raised the possibility that local paracrine influences derived from the microvasculature of the bone marrow may contribute to the regulation of leukopoiesis.

Macrophage-Colony Stimulating Factor

Macrophages figure prominently in the pathogenesis of certain chronic vascular diseases including atherosclerosis. Accordingly, the possibility that intrinsic vascular wall cells can also produce macrophage-colony stimulating factor (M-CSF) has intrigued several groups. As opposed to other colony stimulating factors, M-CSF circulates at measurable levels, and mononuclear phagocytes absolutely require M-CSF for survival.

In addition to promoting proliferation and differentiation of mononuclear phagocytes during leukopoiesis, M-CSF exerts a number of specific effects on macrophages of considerable interest in vascular biology. For example, M-CSF can induce the expression of scavenger receptors from modified low density lipoprotein on the surface of mononuclear phagocytes (Clinton et al., 1992). This effect may enhance the ability of macrophages to undergo transformation into foam cells by imbibing lipid. Furthermore, M-CSF can induce the expression of apolipoprotein E by macrophages. This apolipoprotein binds to the low density lipoprotein receptor with high affinity (Mahley, 1988). Local production of apolipoprotein E by macrophages within atherosclerotic lesions may participate in choles-terol removal by enhancing the peripheral catabolism of high density lipoprotein particles involved in cholesterol removal (Mahley, 1988; Brown and Goldstein, 1983; Basu *et al.*, 1981; Mahley *et al.*, 1989). Thus, the observation that vascular endothelial and smooth muscle cells can express the M-CSF gene and elaborate M-CSF protein has important implications for the pathogenesis and regression or stabilization of atherosclerotic lesions (Clinton *et al.*, 1992; Rajavashisth *et al.*, 1990). The finding that modified low-density lipoprotein can stimulate M-CSF expression by vascular cells provides an important link between dyslipidemia and cytokine gene regulation of immense potential significance in understanding atherogenesis (Clinton *et al.*, 1992; Rajavashisth *et al.*, 1990).

Overview of Cytokine Production by Vascular Cells

The above discussion does not aim to present an encyclopedic listing of all possible cytokines produced by vascular cells. Rather we have concentrated on a few well-studied examples which illustrate various general features of this phenomenon (Table 2). The more we learn about the range of cells that can produce cytokines, the wider that gamut appears. Ultimately, cells that do not express various cytokines may prove the exceptions rather than the rule. Vascular endothelial and smooth muscle cells can be induced to accumulate the mRNAs that encode a wide variety of cytokines. However, the examples mentioned above indicate why one cannot necessarily conclude that the elaboration of biologically active cytokines automatically ensues following increases in mRNA. For example, in the case of interleukin-1, vascular cells appear to secrete biologically active IL-1 only under unusual circumstances. In contrast, tumor necrosis factor, which we would have predicted not to be produced by vascular smooth muscle cells under physiologic conditions based on our *in vitro* experiments, does appear to be readily expressed *in vivo*.

Even when well established, the ability of vascular cells to elaborate particular cytokines does not itself justify conclusions regarding the biological significance of these findings. Rather, carefully designed *in vivo* experiments should allow more rigorous delineation of the biological significance of vascular cell-derived cytokines in various vascular responses and pathological conditions.

Cytokines Regulate Key Functions of Vascular Endothelial and Smooth Muscle Cells

Cytokines Regulate Hemocompatability of Vascular Endothelium

The normal vascular endothelium possesses a remarkable ability to maintain blood in a liquid state during prolonged contact. Few other materials, either synthetic or natural, exhibit such remarkable hemocompatibility. The mechanisms which underlie the throm-boresistance of normal endothelium have become increasingly clear over the last decade. Initially, the elaboration of arachidonic acid derivatives such as prostacyclin were thought to confer upon endothelium the ability to inhibit the aggregation and release reactions of platelets (Weksler *et al.*, 1977; Gimbrone, 1986). Subsequently, heparan sulfate proteoglycans capable of binding anti-thrombin III and thus inhibiting the action of thrombin were localized to the endothelial surface (Marcum and Rosenberg, 1985). Endothelial cells also bear on their surface thrombomodulin, a protein that can inhibit blood coagulation by activating the protein C system (Esmon, 1987a; 1987b).

If a stray blood clot should begin to form in the vicinity of an endothelial cell, endogenous fibrinolytic mechanisms may speed up lysis further assuring the thromboresistance of this important endovascular lining cell (Collen *et al.*, 1989). Endothelial cells can express the gene that encodes tissue-type plasminogen activator (tPA). In addition, endothelial cells can express urokinase type plasminogen activator (uPA) and bear the receptor for binding this fibrinolytic enzyme as well (Levin and Loskutoff, 1982; Barnathan *et al.*, 1990). In summary, the surface of endothelial cells exhibits a number of molecular strategies to impede plaque formation and destabilize clots should they form. These mechanisms explain the physiologic hemocompatibility of the normal endothelium.

However, in some instances intravascular thrombosis may prove adaptive and desirable. For example, hemostasis following injury can stem blood loss. Accordingly, the endothelial cell possesses pro-coagulant mechanisms, many of which require induction by inflammatory or injurious stimuli for their expression. Cytokines play such a regulatory role. The pro-coagulant molecules expressed by endothelial cells include tissue factor and von Willebrand factor (vWF) (Jaffe *et al.*, 1976). The inactivator of plasminogen activator known as PAI-1 constitutes a major secretory product of vascular endothelial cells (Loskutoff *et al.*, 1983).

Tissue factor, a cell surface membrane glycoprotein, activates blood coagulation via factors VII and X. Expressed at low levels on normal endothelium, cytokines such as interleukin-1 or TNF readily induce expression of tissue factor activity by endothelial cells (Bevilacqua *et al.*, 1984; Stern *et al.*, 1985a; 1985b). The observation that treatment with interleukin-1 induces pro-coagulant activity on endothelial cells antidates the cloning of tissue factor (Morrissey *et al.*, 1987; Spicer *et al.*, 1987). Cytokine treatment can tip the fibrinolytic balance of the endothelial surface toward clot stabilization by enhancing the expression of PAI-1. Thus, cytokines exert a concerted action on endothelial cells to promote blood coagulation and inhibit fibrinolysis.

The consumption coagulopathy that accompanies septic shock illustrates the functional importance of this cytokine-induced shift in endothelial hemocompatibility. Gram negative sepsis provides an instructive example. Bacterial cell wall lipopolysaccharides induce expression of cytokines such as IL-1 or TNF from phagocytic cells. Circulating levels of these cytokines rise early on during sepsis. The full-blown syndrome of septic shock characteristically includes disseminated intravascular coagulation. Many of the dreaded consequences of Gram-negative sepsis involve intravascular coagulation in various specific organ beds. For example, the adult respiratory distress syndrome often involves microvascular thrombosis, as well as cytokine-induced capillary leak. Acute renal cortical necrosis also involves coagulation within the kidney's microvessels. The acute adrenal failure seem in Waterhouse-Friderichsen syndrome involves intraadrenal hemorrhage and thrombosis as well. The cutaneous manifestation of bacterial sepsis including purpura fulminans involves microthrombi in the vasculature of the skin as well. This extreme example underscores the importance of the hemostatic balance of the endothelial cells as regulated by cytokines.

Cytokines Regulate the Expression of Leukocyte Adhesion Molecules by Vascular Endothelium

As noted in the introduction to this Chapter, the endothelium serves as the gatekeeper for leukocyte trafficking physiologically and in pathologic states. The expression on the endothelial surface of leukocyte adhesion molecules governs the adhesive interactions of white cells with this cell type. Two major classes of endothelial-leukocyte adhesion molecule exist. Members of the immunoglobulin superfamily exemplified by intercellular adhesion molecule-1 (ICAM-1) or vascular cell adhesion molecule-1 (VCAM-1) interact with integrin molecules on the surface of leukocytes and mediate tight adhesive interactions (Springer, 1990; Carlos and Harlan, 1994). Members of the selectin family include E-selectin (formerly known as ELAM-1) and P-selectin (previously known as GMP-140 or PADGEM) (Bevilacqua *et al.*, 1991; Bevilacqua and Nelson, 1993). The third known member of the selectin family, L-selectin, is expressed by the leukocyte rather than the endothelial cell.

As a rule, vascular cells do not express such adhesion receptors at high levels in the basal state (resting endothelial cells do express low levels of ICAM-1 or in some cases of VCAM-1) (Dustin *et al.*, 1986). Cytokines consistently augment the expression of members of both classes of adhesion molecules. For example, IL-1 and TNF rapidly induce the expression of E-selectin by endothelial cells which normally do not express this molecule (maximal at 4 hours of stimulation) (Bevilacqua *et al.*, 1985, 1987). Exposure of endothelial cells to the same cytokines or to γ-interferon will augment the expression of ICAM-1, constitutively expressed at low levels by these cells (Dustin *et al.*, 1986). Increased ICAM-1 expression induced by cytokines occurs more slowly than E-selectin induction and continues for up to several days of stimulation. Specific leukocyte adhesion molecules tend to exhibit some selective affinity for various leukocyte subclasses. For example, E-selectin interacts preferentially with cells of the polymorphonuclear leukocyte series, although it can also bind mononuclear phagocytes (DiCorleto and de la Motte, 1985; Shankar *et al.*, 1994). ICAM-1 in contrast exhibits considerable promiscuity, interacting with many leukocyte subclasses which bear the LFA-1 member of the CD-11/CD-18 integrin family (Springer, 1990). VCAM-1 interacts more selectively with cells of the mononuclear lineages, including lymphocytes and monocyte macrophages (Osborn *et al.*, 1989). VCAM-1 binds to these mononuclear cells via its cognate ligand, the VLA-4 integrin (Elices *et al.*, 1990). Cytokines regulate the expression of VCAM-1, on the surfaces of both vascular endothelial and smooth muscle cells (Carlos *et al.*, 1990; Li *et al.*, 1993).

Cell culture experiments led to the identification and molecular characterization of endothelial-leukocyte adhesion molecules. *In vitro* studies also provided the basis for their function in leukocyte adhesion. The results of current studies of genetically modified mice that lack the ability to express one or another adhesion molecule verify in many cases the functional predictions that emerge from cell culture studies. For example, animals deficient in P-selectin or E-selectin exhibit impaired abilities to mount a leukocytic infiltrated response to peritoneal irritation (Mayadas *et al.*, 1993). There appears to be considerable overlap in the function of P- and E-selectin in this regard. More complete abrogation of the polymorphonuclear infiltrated response in such animals requires concurrent administration of antibody directed against the remaining endothelial selectin.

Similar use of antibody neutralizing strategies alone or in conjunction with genetically modified mice will continue to shed new light on the pathophysiologic importance of endothelial-leukocyte adhesion molecules. However, sufficient evidence exists to validate the initial model proposed by Gimbrone some years ago of the critical importance of these surface ligands for leukocytes in leukocyte recruitment during inflammatory responses. Thus, cytokine-inducible leukocyte adhesion molecules play a central role in this important aspect of inflammation.

Cytokines Induce the Expression of Growth Factors and Further Cytokines in Vascular Smooth Muscle and Endothelial Cells

The ability of cytokines to induce further cytokine production and expression of genes encoding other mediators including peptide growth factors has proven a consistent feature. Vascular cells share this characteristic of cytokine action. Early reports of interleukin-1 gene expression in human vascular endothelial cells indicated that in addition to bacterial endotoxin, TNF-α stimulated the expression of IL-1 α and β genes (Libby *et al.*, 1986a; Nawroth *et al.*, 1986). Tumor necrosis factor also elicits IL-1 α and β gene expression in human smooth muscle cells (Warner and Libby, 1989).

Perhaps more remarkably, interleukin-1 induces its own gene expression. This phenomenon, originally described in vascular smooth muscle cells, has proven widely applicable (Warner *et al.*, 1987). IL-1 induces gene expression in other cell types and *in vivo* as well. This property of IL-1 to induce its own gene expression suggests the presence of a positive feedback loop which could yield runaway expression of this mediator. Two points mitigate this disquieting scenario. First, as explained at length in the previous section, vascular cells probably do not secrete IL-1 in a soluble form under usual circumstances. Second, IL-1 induces the expression of its own inhibitor, the interleukin-1 receptor antagonist, as well as prostanoids (see below) which can in many instances counteract some of the pro-inflammatory or growth promoting effects of IL-1 (Rossi *et al.*, 1985; Libby *et al.*, 1988).

IL-1 not only induces expression of its own gene but of a wide variety of cytokines and growth factors. For example, IL-1 induces TNF gene expression in vascular smooth muscle cells (Warner and Libby, 1989). As already mentioned, IL-1 potently induces IL-6 and IL-8 gene expression. IL-1 also augments the expression of certain hematopoietic growth factors such as GM-CSF and M-CSF in vascular cells (Bagby *et al.*, 1986; Clinton *et al.*, 1992). IL-1 thus appears to serve as a master regulator of cytokine gene expression orchestrating many aspects of the cytokine cascade during inflammatory responses.

IL-1 and/or TNF can also induce the expression of genes encoding peptide growth factors for mesenchymal cells. TNF treatment of human vascular endothelial cells elicits the secretion of platelet-derived growth factor (PDGF) and heparin-binding epidermal growth factor (Hajjar *et al.*, 1987; Yoshizumi *et al.*, 1992). Treatment of human smooth muscle cells with IL-1 leads to production of PDGF AA homodimer and the expression of basic fibroblast growth factor (bFGF) (Raines *et al.*, 1989; Gay and Winkles, 1990; 1991). IL-1 can also induce expression of the endothelin gene in vascular endothelial cells (Yoshizumi *et al.*, 1989). Endothelin may stimulate the proliferation of smooth muscle cells under some conditions (Hirata *et al.*, 1989; Nakaki *et al.*, 1989).

The ability of cytokines such as IL-1 or TNF to induce secondary growth factors has important implications in the pathogenesis of vascular diseases. The response of the artery to various types of injury including atherogenic stimuli induce a fibroproliferative response characterized by smooth muscle cell migration and replication. Peptide mitogens and chemoattractants such as PDGF or bFGF may mediate aspects of this fibroproliferative response. In this manner, the cytokines may participate in this important biological response of arterial wall cells.

Cytokines Regulate the Production of Vasoactive Molecules by Vascular Wall Cells

For many years, cytokines such as IL-1 have been known to augment the production of products of the cyclooxygenase pathway in various cells. Human endothelial cells exposed to IL-1 elaborate prostacyclin (Rossi *et al.*, 1985; Breviario *et al.*, 1990). Human smooth muscle cells exposed to IL-1 or TNF release prostaglandin E2, as well as lesser amounts of prostacyclin, as desribed above. In addition to the anti-aggregatory properties of prostacyclin for platelets previously mentioned, prostaglandin potently dilates many types of vessels. Prostaglandin E2 can also regulate vascular tone. Cytokines such as IL-1 regulate the expression of the enzymes (cyclooxygenases I and II) that catalyze the rate limiting step in prostaglandin synthesis from arachidonic acid (Maier *et al.*, 1990; Hla *et al.*, 1993).

Much recent attention has focused on nitric oxide (NO), another small molecule regulator of vascular tone elaborated by endothelial cells, nitric oxide (NO) (Knowles and Moncada, 1994; Michel and Smith, 1993; Morris and Billiar, 1994). Both endothelial and smooth muscle cells can produce NO, originally characterized as an endothelial-dependent vasodilator. Nitric oxide arises from the guanidino group of L-arginine by the action of a family of enzymes known as nitric oxide synthases (NOS). Endothelial cells express one form of NOS constitutively although TNF-α may augment the activity of this enzyme. Smooth muscle cells (at least in rodents) express a cytokine-inducible form of NOS that produces relatively large amounts of NO (Nakayama *et al.*, 1992; Nunokawa *et al.*, 1993; Geng *et al.*, 1994). The isoform expressed in smooth muscle cells resembles the NOS inducible in macrophages. Production of NO by macrophages probably represents an important cytotoxic mechanism used in defense against intracellular microorganisms (Nathan and Hibbs, 1991). By controlling the expression of NOS, cytokines such as TNF, interferon-γ, or IL-1 may influence vascular tone. In addition, NO can regulate aspects of thrombosis (by inhibiting platelet aggregation) and leukocyte interaction with endothelial cells (by inhibiting leukocyte adhesion). The extent to which cytokine-inducible NOS contributes to vascular homeostasis for inflammatory states in humans remains uncertain. If so, cytokines would be expected to regulate vascular tone in this manner as well as by modulating prostanoid metabolism.

Cytokines Regulate Synthesis and Degradation of the Vascular Extracellular Matrix

Much of the volume of normal human vessels and a majority of hyperplastic arterial lesions consist of a complex extracellular matrix. A variety of macromolecules contribute to the formation of this matrix. Interstitial collagen molecules (principally types I and III) make up a substantial portion of the extracellular matrix of the tunica media and the adventitia of blood vessels and of atherosclerotic intimal lesions as well (Wagner, 1990). Nonfibrillar collagens (e.g., types IV and V) localize in the basement membrane underlying endothelial cells in the vascular intima. Proteoglycans of all three major classes also contribute to the vascular extracellular matrix (Wight, 1989). Other molecules such as elastin also contribute importantly to the matrix of the tunica media of arteries. Adhesive glycoproteins such as fibronectin and thrombospondin occur in the vascular matrix in addition and may play a regulatory as well as structural role. Cytokines can modulate the biosynthesis of many of these macromolecules. For example, IL-1 and TNF weakly stimulate synthesis of the genes that encode procollagens I and III (Amento *et al.*, 1991). More impressively, the lymphokine interferon-γ potently inhibits this process (Amento *et al.*, 1991). Even vascular smooth muscle cells stimulated with transforming growth factor-β, the most potent stimulus for interstitial collagen gene expression known, exhibit markedly reduced levels of RNA and biosynthesis for the interstitial procollagens when exposed simultaneously to interferon-γ. IL-1 can also modulate the expression of the core protein decorin, an essential constituent of the arterial proteoglycans (Edwards *et al.*, 1991).

The degradation of vascular extracellular matrix components also appear subject to regulation by cytokines. A family of speccialized enzymes known as matrix metalloproteinases (MMP) participate in a concerted pathway leading to degradation of many components of the extracellular matrix. Interleukin-1 can induce the expression by vascular smooth muscle cells of interstitial collagenase, a metalloproteinase required for the initial proteolytic cleavage of fibrillar collagens in their native tightly coiled triple helix (Yanagi *et al.*, 1991; Galis *et al.*, 1994). IL-1 and TNF can also induce the expression of a gelatinolytic and elastinolytic enzyme known variously as 92-kD gelatinase or gelatinase B (Galis *et al.*, 1994; Southgate *et al.*, 1992). IL-1 and TNF further induce the expression of the metalloproteinase stromelysin, an enzyme with a broad substrate specificity for various constituents of the vascular extracellular matrix (Galis *et al.*, 1994).

This aspect of cytokine influences on vascular function has considerable clinical interest. The regulation of matrix metabolism by cytokines may contribute decisively to the evolution of the final stages of the atherosclerotic plaque. We now understand the majority of acute thrombotic events complicating advanced atherosclerotic lesions follow upon rupture or fissure of the plaque (Davies and Thomas, 1985; Fuster, 1994). The propensity of an atheroma to such physical destabilization depends in great measure on the integrity of the extracellular matrix. T-lymphocytes in atherosclerotic plaques exhibit markers of chronic activation and elaborate the cytokine interferon-γ (Hansson *et al.*, 1989; Stemme *et al.*, 1992). As noted above, we have shown that this lymphokine potently inhibits the expression of interstitial collagen genes by vascular smooth muscle cells, the major source of these matrix constituents in atheroma (Amento *et al.*, 1991). Therefore, areas within plaques infiltrated by chronically activated T-cells should exhibit impaired ability to maintain the integrity of the matrix. At the same time, IL-1 and TNF-α can augment expression of a broad panel of matrix metalloproteinases by both smooth muscle cells and macrophages. These metalloproteinases, acting coordinately, can further destabilize the matrix of the atheroma by breakdown of various matrix constituents. This weakened matrix at sites of chronic inflammation and cytokine action probably render the atheroma susceptible to physical disruption such as might be precipitated by a hypertensive crisis or some other source of mechanical stress on the atherosclerotic plaque (Richardson *et al.*, 1989; Cheng *et al.*, 1993).

CONCLUSION

The studies described above establish the existence of a local cytokine network potentially contributing to the pathobiology of arterial diseases and acting locally within the
vessel wall. Virtually all cell types found in normal and diseased vessels can synthesize
various cytokines. These mediators can in turn elicit a coordinated program of pro-
inflammatory responses from both vascular endothelial and smooth muscle cells. Such
responses doubtless prove highly adaptive and beneficial in terms of host defenses
against pathogenic microorganisms and responses to injury.

However, when expressed inappropriately, the local cytokine cascade and consequent
alterations in vascular functions can hasten the development of various vascular diseases.
We have discussed the dramatic example of the vascular responses to Gram-negative
sepsis. In this situation, the host's defense mechanism overshoots and becomes maladap-
tive. With respect to vascular pathology, cytokines are likely to contribute to a variety of
chronic vasculitic processes (including but not exclusively the angiocentric vasculidites).
Locally produced cytokines may even signal deranged endothelial cell growth in
Kaposi's sarcoma (Salahuddin *et al.*, 1988). A spectrum of acute and chronic forms of
transplantation rejection most likely involves the vascular responses to cytokines.
Atherosclerosis provides an example of a chronic inflammatory process that includes
cytokine signaling as well. These examples illustrate how the ability of the blood vessel
to produce and respond to various cytokines takes on considerable significance in view of
the panoply of vascular diseases in which these mediators may participate.

As mentioned above, many questions remain regarding cytokine actions within blood
vessels. One must always bear in mind the difficulties in extrapolating from *in vitro*
experiments and inviting intellectual constructs to conclusions about the *in vivo* roles of
various mediators. This caveat certainly applies to the understanding the roles of
cytokines. We have discussed how the advent of genetically modified animals and vascular gene transfer technologies may permit experimental verification of many of the
hypotheses of cytokines functions in vascular pathophysiology generated by *in vitro*
work.

In terms of vascular immune responses, cytokines no doubt contribute to lymphocyte
recirculation, recruitment to sites of cellular immune responses, and in the vascular complications of transplantation previously discussed. Vascular endothelial cells may also be
important targets in autoimmune diseases and immunopathologic reactions that involve
humoral responses as well. Other Chapters in this volume consider the role of vascular
endothelial and smooth muscle cells in antigen presentation (see Chapter X).

The cytokine network seems so complex, multidimensional, and redundant that it
would seem to defy therapeutic interruption (in addition to stretching the memory of
casual students). However, as noted above, simultaneous induction of inhibitory pathways may limit positive feedback and help to keep the action of renegade cytokines in
check. The spectre of the redundancy of cytokine networks in vascular inflammation
does suggest that simple approaches to antagonizing cytokines may prove difficult.
Various strategies for neutralizing specific cytokines, such as therapeutic administration
of IL-1 receptor antagonist or soluble TNF receptors in septic shock have proven disap-
pointing in clinical trials. The prospect of local neutralization of cytokines during
chronic vascular inflammatory processes could prove even more difficult. Despite these

potential frustrations to therapeutic intervention in vascular cytokine signaling pathways, only by further study of this fascinating network will we achieve mastery over the biology of vascular diseases.

ACKNOWLEDGEMENTS

Work from our laboratory reported in this chapter was supported by grants from the U.S. National Heart Lung and Blood Institute (HL 34636, HL-43364, and HL 48743) and the American Heart Association.

References

Aarden, L.A., Lansdorp, P.M. and De Groot, E.R. (1985). A growth factor for B cell hybridomas produced by human monocytes. *Lymphokines*, 10:175–185.

Aarden, L.A., De Groot, E.R., Schaap, O.L. and Lansdorp, P.M. (1987). Production of hybridoma growth factor by human monocytes. *Eur. J. Immunol.*, 17:1411–1416.

Amento, E.P., Ehsani, N., Palmer, H. and Libby, P. (1991). Cytokines positively and negatively regulate intersitial collagen gene expression in human vascular smooth muscle cells. *Arteriosclerosis*, 11:1223–1230.

Arend, W.P., Welgus, H.G., Thompson, R.C. and Eisenberg, S.P. (1990). Biological properties of recombinant human monocyte-derived interleukin 1 receptor antagonist. *J. Clin. Invest.*, 85:1694–7.

Auron, P.E., Webb., A.C., Rosenwasser, L.J., Mucci, S.F., Rich, A., Wolff, S.M. and Dinarello., C.A. (1984). Nucleotide sequence of human monocyte interleukin-1 precursor cDNA. *Proc. Natl. Acad. Sci. USA*, 81:7907–7911.

Bagby, G.C J., Dinarello, C.A., Wallace, P., Wagner, C., Hefeneider, S. and McCall, E. (1986). Interleukin 1 stimulates granulocyte macrophage colony-stimulating activity release by vascular endothelial cells. *J. Clin. Invest.*, 78:1316–1323.

Barath, P., Fishbein, M.C., Cao, J., Berenson, J., Helfant, R.H. and Forrester, J.S. (1990a). Detection and localization of tumor necrosis factor in human atheroma. *Am. J. of Cardiology*, 65:297–302.

Barath, P., Fishbein, J.O., Berenson, J., Helfant, R.H. and Forrester, J.S. (1990b). Tumor necrosis factor gene expression in human vascular intimal smooth muscle cells detected by in situ hybridization. *Am. J. Pathol.*, 137:503–509.

Barnathan, E.S., Kuo, A., Kariko, K., Rosenfeld, L., Murray, S.C., Behrendt, N., Ronne, E., Weiner, D., Henkin, J. and Cines, D.B. (1990). Characterization of human endothelial cell urokinase-type plasminogen activator receptor protein and messenger RNA. *Blood*, 76:1795–806.

Basu, S.K., Brown, M.S., Ho, Y.K., Havel, R.J. and Goldstein, J.L. (1981). Mouse macrophages synthesize and secrete a protein resembling apolipoprotein E. *Proc. Natl. Acad. Sci. USA*, 78:7545–9.

Beutler, B. and Cerami, A. (1986). Cachectin and tumour necrosis factor as two sides of the same biological coin. *Nature*, 320:584–588.

Bevilacqua, M.P., Pober, J.S., Majeau, G.R., Cotran, R.S. and Gimbrone, M.A., Jr. (1984). Interleukin-1 (IL-1) induces biosynthesis and cell surface expression of procoagulant activity in human vascular endothelial cells. *J. Exp. Med.*, 160:618–623.

Bevilacqua, M.P., Pober, J.S., Majeau, G.R., Cotran, R.S. and Gimbrone, M.A., Jr. (1985). Interleukin-1 acts on cultured human vascular endothelium to increase the adhesion of polymorphonuclear leukocytes, monocytes and related leukocyte cell lines. *J. Clin. Invest.*, 76:2003–2011.

Bevilacqua, M.P., Pober, J.S., Mendrick, D.L., Cotran, R.S. and Gimbrone Jr., M.A. (1987). Identification of an inducible endothelial-leukocyte adhesion molecule. *Proc. Natl. Acad. Sci. USA*, 84:9238–9242.

Bevilacqua, M., Butcher, E., Furie, B., Furie, B., Gallatin, M., Gimbrone, M., Harlan, J., Kishimoto, K., Lasky, L., McEver, R., et al. (1991). Selectins: a family of adhesion receptors. *Cell*, 67:233.

Bevilacqua, M.P. (1993). Endothelial-leukocyte adhesion molecules. *Ann. Rev. Immunol.*, 11:767–804.

Bevilacqua, M.P. and Nelson, R.M. (1993). Selectins. *J. Clin. Invest.* 91:379–87.

Breviario, F., Proserpio, P., Bertocchi, F., Lampugnani, M.G., Mantovani, A. and Dejana, E. (1990). Interleukin-1 stimulates prostacyclin production by cultured human endothelial cells by increasing arachidonic acid mobilization and conversion. *Arteriosclerosis*, 10:129–34.

Brown, M.S. and Goldstein, J.L. (1983). Lipoprotein metabolism in the macrophage: implications for cholesterol deposition in atherosclerosis. *Ann. Review Biochem.*, 52:223–261.

Butcher, E.C. (1986). The regulation of lymphocyte traffic. *Curr. Top. Microbiol. Immunol.*, 128:85–122.

Butcher, E.C., Lewinsohn, D., Duijvestijn, A., Bargatze, A., Wu, N. and Jalkanen, S. (1986). Interactions between endothelial cells and leukocytes. *J. Cell Biochem.*, 30:121–131.

Carlos, T.M., Schwartz, B.R., Kovach, N.L., Yee, E., Rosa, M., Osborn, L., Chi, R.G., Newman, B., Lobb, R., Rosso, M., *et al.* (1990). Vascular cell adhesion molecule-1 mediates lymphocyte adherence to cytokine-activated cultured human endothelial cells [published erratum appears in Blood 1990 Dec 1;76(11):2420]. *Blood*, 76:965–70.

Carlos, T.M. and Harlan, J.M. (1994). Leukocyte-endothelial adhesion molecules. *Blood*, 84:2068–101.

Charo, I. (1992). Monocyte-endothelial cell interactions. *Curr. Opinion Lipidol.*, 3:335–343.

Cheng, G.C., Loree, H.M., Kamm, R.D., Fishbein, M.C. and Lee, R.T. (1993). Distribution of circumferential stress in ruptured and stable atherosclerotic lesions: a structural analysis with histopathologic correlation. *Circulation*, 87:1179–1187.

Clausell, N., Molossi, S., Sett, S. and Rabinovitch, M. (1994). *In vivo* blockade of tumor necrosis factor-alpha in cholesterol-fed rabbits after cardiac transplant inhibits acute coronary artery neointimal formation. *Circulation*, 89:2768–79.

Clinton, S., Underwood, R., Sherman, M., Kufe, D. and Libby, P. (1992). Macrophage-colony stimulating factor gene expression in vascular cells and in experimental and human atherosclerosis. *Am. J. Path.*, 140:301–316.

Collen, D., Lijnen, H.R., Todd, P.A. and Goa, K.L. (1989). Tissue-type plasminogen activator. A review of its pharmacology and therapeutic use as a thrombolytic agent. *Drugs*, 38:346–88.

Cushing, S.D., Berliner, J.A., Valente, A.J., Territo, M.C., Navab, M., Parhami, F., Gerrity, R., Schwartz, C.J. and Fogelman, A.M. (1990). Minimally modified low density lipoprotein induces monocyte chemotactic protein 1 in human endothelial cells and smooth muscle cells. *Proc. Natl. Acad. Sci. USA*, 87:5134–8.

Davies, M.J. and Thomas, A.C. (1985). Plaque fissuring–the cause of acute myocardial infarction, sudden ischemic death, and crescendo angina. *Br. Heart J.*, 53:363–373.

DiCorleto, P.E. and de la Motte, C.A. (1985). Characterization of the adhesion of the human monocytic cell line U937 to cultured endothelial cells. *J. Clin. Invest.*, 75:1153–61.

Dinarello, C.A. (1981). Demonstration of a human pyrogen-inducing factor during mixed leukocyte reactions. *J. Exp. Med.*, 153:1215–1224.

Dinarello, C.A. (1989). Interleukin 1 and its biologically related cytokines. *Adv. Immunol.*, 44:153–205.

Dinarello, C. and Thompson, R. (1991). Blocking IL-1: interleukin 1 receptor antagonist *in vivo* and *in vitro*. *Immunol. Today*, 12:404–410.

Dinarello, C. (1994). The interleukin-1 family: 10 years of discovery. *FASEB Journal*, 8:1314–1325.

Dustin, M.L., Rothlein, R., Bhan, A.K., Dinarello, C.A. and Springer, T.A. (1986). Induction by IL-1 and interferon-gamma: tissue distribution, biochemistry, and function of a natural adherence molecule (ICAM-1). *J. Immunol.*, 137:245–254.

Edwards, I.J., Xu, H., Wright, M.J. and Wagner, W.D. (1994). Interleukin-1 upregulates decorin production by arterial smooth muscle cells. *Arteriosclerosis and Thrombosis*, 14:1032–9.

Elices, M J., Osborn, L., Takada, Y., Crouse, C., Luhowskyj, S., Hemler, M.E. and Lobb, R.R. (1990). VCAM-1 on activated endothelium interacts with the leukocyte integrin VLA-4 at a site distinct from the VLA-4/fibronectin binding site. *Cell*, 60:577–84.

Esmon, C.T. (1987a). The regulation of natural anticoagulant pathways. *Science*, 235:1348–1352.

Esmon, N.L. (1987b). Thrombomodulin. *Semin. Thromb. Hemost.*, 13:454–463.

Furutani, Y., Nomura, H., Notake, M., Oyamada, Y., Fukui, T., Yamada, M., Larsen, C.G., Oppenheim, J.J. and Matsushima, K. (1989). Cloning and sequencing of the cDNA for human monocyte chemotactic and activating factor (MCAF). *Biochem. Biophys. Res. Comm.*, 159:249–55.

Fuster, V. (1994). Lewis A. Conner Memorial Lecture. Mechanisms leading to myocardial infarction: insights from studies of vascular biology. *Circulation*, 90:2126–46.

Galis, Z., Muszynski, M., Sukhova, G., Simon-Morrisey, E., Unemori, E., Lark, M., Amento, E. and Libby, P. (1994). Cytokine-stimulated human vascular smooth muscle cells synthesize a complement of enzymes required for extracellular matrix digestion. *Circ. Res.*, 75:181–189.

Gay, C.G. and Winkles, J.A. (1990). Heparin-binding growth factor-1 stimulation of human endothelial cells induces platelet-derived growth factor A-chain gene expression. *J. Biol. Chem.*, 265:3284–92.

Gay, C.G. and Winkles, J A. (1991). Interleukin 1 regulates heparin-binding growth factor 2 gene expression in vascular smooth muscle cells. *Proc. Natl. Acad. Sci. USA*, 88:296–300.

Geng, Y.-j., Almquist, M. and Hansson, G.K. (1994). cDNA cloning and expression of imducible nitric oxide synthase from rat vascular smooth muscle cells. *Biochim. Biophys. Acta.*, 1281:421–424.

Gimbrone, M.A.J. (1986). Vascular Endothelium in Hemostasis and Thrombosis. ed.), Churchill Livingstone, Edinburgh.

Gimbrone Jr., M.A., Obin, M.S., Brock, A.F., Luis, E.A., Hass, P.E., Hébert, C.A., Yip, Y.K., Leung, D.W., Lowe, D.G., Kohr, W.J., Darbonne, W.C., Bechtol, K.B. and Baker, J.B. (1989). Endothelial interleukin-8: A novel inhibitor of leukocyte-endothelial interactions. *Science*, 246:1601–1603.

Gimbrone, M.A.J., Bevilacqua, M.P. and Cybulsky, M.I. (1990). Endothelial-dependent mechanisms of leuko-cyte adhesion in inflammation and atherosclerosis. *Ann. N. Y. Acad. Sci.*, **598**:77–85.

Gray, P.W., Aggarwal, B.B., Benton, C.V., Bringman, T.S., Henzel, W.J., Jarrett, J.A., Leung, D.W., Moffat, B., Ng, P., Svedersky, L.P., Palladino, M. A. and Nedwin, G. E. (1984). Cloning and expression of cDNA for human lymphotoxin, a lymphokine with tumour necrosis activity. *Nature*, **312**:721–724.

Hajjar, K.A., Hajjar, D.P., Silverstein, R.L. and Nachman, R.L. (1987). Tumor necrosis factor-mediated release of platelet-derived growth factor from cultured endothelial cells. *J. Exp. Med.*, **166**:235–245.

Hannum, C.H., Wilcox, C.J., Arend, W.P., Joslin, F.G., Dripps, D.J., Heimdal, P.L., Armes, L.G., Sommer, A., Eisenberg, S.P. and Thompson, R.C. (1990). Primary structure and functional expression from comple-mentary DNA of a human interleukin-1 receptor antagonist. *Nature*, **343**:341–6.

Hansson, G.K., Holm, J. and Jonasson, L. (1989). Detection of activated T lymphocytes in the human athero-sclerotic plaque. *Am. J. Pathol.*, **135**:169–175.

Hirano, T., Yasukawa, K., Harada, H., Taga, T., Watanabe, Y., Matsuda, T., Kashiwamura, S., Nakajima, K., Koyama, K., Iwamatsu, A., Tsunasawa, S., Sakiyama, F., Matsui, H., Takahara, Y., Taniguchi, T. and Kishimoto, T. (1986). Complementary DNA for a novel human interleukin (BSF-2) that induces B lym-phocytes to produce immunoglogulin. *Nature*, **324**:73–76.

Hirata, Y., Takagi, Y., Fukuda, Y. and Marumo, F. (1989). Endothelin is a potent mitogen for rat vascular smooth muscle cells. *Atherosclerosis*, **78**:225–8.

Hla, T., Ristimaki, A., Appleby, S. and Barriocanal, J.G. (1993). Cyclooxygenase gene expression in inflamma-tion and angiogenesis. *Ann. N.Y. Acad. Sci.*, **696**:197–204.

Ikeda, U., Ikeda, M., Oohara, T., Oguchi, A., Kamitani, T., Tsuruya, Y. and Kano, S. (1991). Interleukin 6 stimulates growth of vascular smooth muscle cells in a PDGF-dependent manner. *Am. J. Physiol.*, **260**:H1713–H1717.

Jaffe, E.A., Hoyer, L.W. and Nachman, R.L. (1976). Synthesis of von Willebrand factor by cultured human endothelial cells. *Proc. Natl. Acad. Sci. USA*, **71**:1906–9.

Knowles, R.G. and Moncada, S. (1994). Nitric oxide synthases in mammals. *Biochem. J.*, **298**:249–58.

Larsen, C.G., Zachariae, C.O., Oppenheim, J.J. and Matsushima, K. (1989). Production of monocyte chemotac-tic and activating factor (MCAF) by human dermal fibroblasts in response to interleukin 1 or tumor necro-sis factor. *Biochem Biophys. Res. Comm.*, **160**:1403–8.

Levin, E.G. and Loskutoff, D.J. (1982). Cultured bovine endothelial cells produce both urokinase and tissue-type plasminogen activators. *J. Cell. Biol.*, **94**:631–636.

Li, H., Cybulsky, M.I., Gimbrone Jr., M.A. and Libby, P. (1993). Inducible expression of vascular cell adhesion molecule-1 (VCAM-1) by vascular smooth muscle cells *in vitro* and within rabbit atheroma. *Am. J. Path.*, **143**:1551–1559.

Libby, P., Ordovàs, J.M., Auger, K.R., Robbins, H., Birinyi, L.K. and Dinarello, C.A. (1986a). Endotoxin and tumor necrosis factor induce interleukin-1 gene expression in adult human vascular endothelial cells. *Am. J. Path.*, **124**:179–186.

Libby, P., Ordovas, J.M., Birinyi, L.K., Auger, K.R. and Dinarello., C.A. (1986b). Inducible interleukin-1 expression in human vascular smooth muscle cells. *J. Clin. Invest.*, **78**:1432–1438.

Libby, P., Warner, S.J.C. and Friedman, G.B. (1988). Interleukin-1: a mitogen for human vascular smooth muscle cells that induces the release of growth-inhibitory prostanoids. *J. Clin. Invest.*, **88**:487–498.

Libby, P., Salomon, R.N., Payne, D.D., Schoen, F.J. and Pober, J.S. (1989). Functions of vascular wall cells related to the development of transplantation-associated coronary arteriosclerosis. *Transplantation Proc.*, **21**:3677–3684.

Loppnow, H. and Libby, P. (1989a). Adult human vascular endothelial cells express the IL6 gene differentially in response to LPS or IL1. *Cell. Immunol.*, **122**:493–503.

Loppnow, H. and Libby, P. (1989b). Comparative analysis of cytokine induction in human vascular endothelial and smooth muscle cells. *Lymphokine Res.*, **8**:293–299.

Loppnow, H. and Libby, P. (1990). Proliferating or interleukin 1-activated human vascular smooth muscle cells secrete copious interleukin 6. *J. Clin. Invest.*, **85**:731–738.

Loppnow, H. and Libby, P. (1992). Functional significance of human vascular smooth muscle cells-derived interleukin 1 in paracrine and autocrine regulation pathways. *Exp. Cell. Res.*, **198**:283–290.

Loskutoff, D.J., Van Mourik, J.A., Erickson, L.A. and Lawrence, D. (1983). Detection of an unusually stable fibrinolytic inhibitor produced by bovine endothelial cells. *Cell. Biol.*, **80**:2956–2960.

Mahley, R.W. (1988). Apolipoprotein E: cholesterol transport protein with expanding role in cell biology. *Science*, **240**:622–30.

Mahley, R.W., Weisgraber, K.H., Hussain, M.M., Greenman, B., Fisher, M., Vogel, T. and Gorecki, M. (1989). Intravenous infusion of apolipoprotein E accelerates clearance of plasma lipoproteins in rabbits. *J. Clin. Invest.*, **83**:2125–2130.

Maier, J.A., Hla, T. and Maciag, T. (1990). Cyclooxygenase is an immediate-early gene induced by interleukin-1 in human endothelial cells. *J. Biol. Chem.*, **265**:10805–8.

March, C.J., Mosley, B., Larsen, A., Cerretti, D.P., Braedt, G., Price, V., Gillis, S., Henney, C.S., Kronheim, S.R., Grabstein, K., Conlon, P.J., Hopp, T.P. and Cosman, D. (1985). Cloning, sequence and expression of two distinct human interleukin-1 complementary DNAs. Nature (Lond.), 315:641–***.

Marcum, J.A. and Rosenberg, R.D. (1985). Heparin like molecules with anticoagulant activity are synthesized by cultured endothelial cells. *Biochem. Biophys. Res. Comm.*, 126:365-372.

Matsushima, K., Morishita, K., Yoshimura, T., Lavu, S., Kobayashi, Y., Lew, W., Appella, E., Kung, H.F., Leonard, E.J. and Oppenheim, J.J. (1988). Molecular cloning of a human monocyte-derived neutrophil chemotactic factor (MDNCF) and the induction of MDNCF mRNA by interleukin 1 and tumor necrosis factor. *J. Exp. Med.*, 167:1883–93.

Matsushima, K. and Oppenheim, J.J. (1989). Interleukin 8 and MCAF: Novel inflammatory cytokines inducible by IL1 and TNF. *Cytokine*, 1:2-13.

Matsushima, K., Larsen, C.G., DuBois, G.C. and Oppenheim, J.J. (1989). Purification and characterization of a novel monocyte chemotactic and activating factor produced by a human myelomonocytic cell line. *J. Exp. Med.*, 169:1485–90.

Matsushime, H., Roussel, M.F., Matsushima, K., Hishinuma, A. and Sherr, C.J. (1991). Cloning and expression of murine interleukin-1 receptor antagonist in macrophages stimulated by colony-stimulating factor 1. *Blood*, 78:616–23.

May, L.T., Helfgott, D.C. and Sehgal, P.B. (1986). Anti-b-interferon antibodies inhibit the increased expressioin of HLA-B7 mRNA in tumor necrosis factor-treated human fibroblasts: structural studies of the β-interferon involved. *Proc. Natl. Acad. Sci. USA*, 83:8957–8961.

Mayadas, T.N., Johnson, R.C., Rayburn, H., Hynes, R.O. and Wagner, D.D. (1993). Leukocyte rolling and extravasation are severely compromised in P selectin-deficient mice. *Cell*, 74:541–54.

Michel, T. and Smith, T.W. (1993). Nitric oxide synthases and cardiovascular signaling. *Am. J. Card.*, 72:9.

Morris, S., Jr. and Billiar, T.R. (1994). New insights into the regulation of inducible nitric oxide synthesis. *Am. J. Physiol.*, 266:

Morrissey, J.H., Fakhrai, H. and Edgington, T.S. (1987). Molecular cloning of the cDNA for tissue factor, the cellular receptor for the initiation of the coagulation protease cascade. *Cell*, 50:129–35.

Nakaki, T., Nakayama, M., Yamamoto, S. and Kato, R. (1989). Endothelin-mediated stimulation of DNA synthesis in vascular smooth muscle cells. *Biochem. Biophys. Res. Comm.*, 158:880–3.

Nakayama, D.K., Geller, D.A., Lowenstein, C.J., Chern, H.D., Davies, P., Pitt, B.R., Simmons, R.L. and Billiar, T.R. (1992). Cytokines and lipopolysaccharide induce nitric oxide synthase in cultured rat pulmonary artery smooth muscle [published erratum appears in *Am. J. Respir. Cell Mol. Biol.*, 1993 9, 229]. *Am. J. Resp. Cell and Mol. Biol.* 7:471–6.

Nathan, C.F. and Hibbs, J.B.J. (1991). Role of nitric oxide synthesis in macrophage antimicrobial activity. *Curr. Opin. Immunol.*, 3:65–70.

Nawroth, P.P., Bank, I., Handley, D., Cassimeris, J., Chess, L. and Stern, D. (1986). Tumor necrosis factor/cachectin interacts with endothelial cell receptors to induce release of interleukin 1. *J. Exp. Med.*, 163:1363–1375.

Nelken, N., Coughlin, S., Gordon, D. and Wilcox, J. (1991). Monocyte chemoattractant protein-1 in human atheromatous plaques. *J. Clin. Invest.*, 88:1121–1127.

Neta, R., Sayers, T.J. and Oppenheim, J.J. (1992). Relationship of TNF to interleukins. *Immunol. Series*, 56:499–566.

Nunokawa, Y., Ishida, N. and Tanaka, S. (1993). Cloning of inducible nitric oxide synthase in rat vascular smooth muscle cells. *Biochem. Biophys. Res. Comms.*, 191:89–94.

Old, L.J. (1985). Tumor necrosis factor. *Science*, 230:630–633.

Oppenheim, J.J. (1985). Antigen nonspecific lymphokines: an overview. *Meth. Enzymol.*, 116:357–372.

Oppenheim, J.J., Zachariae, C.O., Mukaida, N. and Matsushima, K. (1991). Properties of the novel proinflammatory supergene "intercrine" cytokine family. *Ann. Rev. of Immunol.*, 9:617–48.

Osborn, L., Hession, C., Tizard, R., Vassallo, C., Luhowskyj, S., Chi-Rosso, G. and Lobb, R. (1989). Direct expression cloning of vascular cell adhesion molecule 1, a cytokine-induced endothelial protein that binds to lymphocytes. *Cell*, 59:1203–1211.

Pober, J.S., Gimbrone, M.A., Jr., Collins, T., Cotran, R.S., Ault, K.A., Fiers, W., Krensky, A.M., Clayberger, C., Reiss, C.S. and Burakoff, S.J. (1984). Interactions of T lymphocytes with human vascular endothelial cells: role of endothelial cells surface antigens. *Immunobiol.*, 168:483–494.

Pober, J.S., Collins, T., Gimbrone, M.A., Jr., Libby, P. and Reiss, C.S. (1986). Inducible expression of class II major histocompatibility complex antigens and the immunogenicity of vascular endothelium. *Transplantation*, 41:141–146.

Raines, E.W., Dower, S.K. and Ross, R. (1989). Interleukin-1 mitogenic activity for fibroblasts and smooth muscle cells is due to PDGF-AA. *Science*, 243:393–396.

Rajavashisth, T.B., Andalibi, A., Territo, M.C., Berliner, J.A., Navab, M., Fogelman, A.M. and Lusis, A.J. (1990). Induction of endothelial cell expression of granulocyte and macrophage colony-stimulating factors by modified low-density lipoproteins. *Nature*, 344:254–257.

Richardson, P.D., Davies, M.J. and Born, G.V. (1989). Influence of plaque configuration and stress distribution on fissuring of coronary atherosclerotic plaques. *Lancet*, 2:941–4.

Rollins, B.J., Yoshimura, T., Leonard, E.J. and Pober, J.S. (1990). Cytokine-activated human endothelial cells synthesize and secrete a monocyte chemoattractant, MCP-1/JE. *Am. J. Pathol.*, 136:1229–33.

Rosenwasser, L.J. and Dinarello, C.A. (1981). Ability of human leukocytic pyrogen to enhance phytohemagglutinin-induced murine thymocyte proliferation. *Cell. Immunol.*, 63:134–142.

Rossi, V., Breviario, F., Ghezzi, P., Dejana, E. and Mantovani, A. (1985). Prostacyclin synthesis induced in vascular cells by interleukin-1. *Science*, 229:174.

Salahuddin, S.Z., Nakamura, S., Biberfeld, P., Kaplan, M.H., Markham, P.D., Larsson, L. and Gallo, R.C. (1988). Angiogenic properties of Kaposi's sarcoma-derived cells after long-term culture *in vitro*. *Science*, 242:430–433.

Salomon, R.N., Hughes, C.C.W., Schoen, F.J., Payne, D.D., Pober, J.S. and Libby, P. (1991). Human coronary transplantation-associated arteriosclerosis: Evidence for a chronic immune reaction to activated graft endothelial cells. *Am. J. Path.*, 138:791–8.

Shankar, R., de la Motte, C.A., Poptic, E.J. and DiCorleto, P.E. (1994). Thrombin receptor-activating peptides differentially stimulate platelet-derived growth factor production, monocytic cell adhesion, and E-selectin expression in human umbilical vein endothelial cells. *J. Biol. Chem.*, 269:13936–13941.

Sica, A., Wang, J.M., Colotta, F., Dejana, E., Mantovani, A., Oppenheim, J.J., Larsen, C.G., Zachariae, C.O. and Matsushima, K. (1990). Monocyte chemotactic and activating factor gene expression induced in endothelial cells by IL-1 and tumor necrosis factor. *J. Immunol.* 144:3034–3038.

Southgate, K.M., Davies, M., Booth, R.F. and Newby, A.C. (1992). Involvement of extracellular-matrix-degrading metalloproteinases in rabbit aortic smooth-muscle cell proliferation. *Biochem. J.*, 288:93–9.

Spicer, E.K., Horton, R., Bloem, L., Bach, R., Williams, K.R., Guha, A., Kraus, J., Lin, T.C., Nemerson, Y. and Konigsberg, W.H. (1987). Isolation of cDNA clones coding for human tissue factor: primary structure of the protein and cDNA. *Proc. Natl. Acad. Sci. USA*, 84:5148–52.

Springer, T.A. (1990). Adhesion receptors of the immune system. *Nature*, 346:425–34.

Stemme, S., Holm, J. and Hansson, G.K. (1992). T lymphocytes in human atherosclerotic plaques are memory cells expressing CD45RO and the integrin VLA-1. *Arterioscler Thromb.*, 12:206–211.

Stern, D.M., Bank, I., Nawroth, P.P., Cassimeris, J., Kisiel, W., Fenton, J.W. 2., Dinarello, C., Chess, L. and Jaffe, E.A. (1985a). Self-regulation of procoagulant events on the endothelial cell surface. *J. Exp. Med.*, 162:1223–1235.

Stern, D., Nawroth, P., Handley, D. and Kisiel, W. (1985b). An endothelial cell-dependent pathway of coagulation. *Proc. Natl. Acad. Sci. USA*, 82:2523–2527.

Tanaka, H., Sukhova, G. and Libby, P. (1994). Interaction of the allogeneic state and hypercholesterolemia in arterial lesion formation in experimental cardiac allografts. *Arteriosclerosis and Thrombosis*, 14:734–745.

Thornberry, N.A., Bull, H.G., Calaycay, J.R., Chapman, K.T., Howard, A.D., Kostura, M.J., Miller, D.K., Molineaux, S.M., Weidner, J.R., Aunins, J.; *et al.*, (1992). A novel heterodimeric cysteine protease is required for interleukin-1 beta processing in monocytes. *Nature*, 356:768–74.

Tracey, K.J. and Cerami, A. (1994). Tumor necrosis factor: a pleiotropic cytokine and therapeutic target. *Ann. Rev. Med.*, 45:491–503.

Valente, A.J., Fowler, S.R., Sprague, E.A., Kelley, J.L., Suenram, C.A. and Schwartz, C.J. (1984). Initial characterization of a peripheral blood mononuclear cellchemoattractant derived from cultured arterial smooth muscle cells. *Am. J. Pathol.*, 117:409–417.

Wagner, W. (1990). Modification of collagen and elastin in the human atherosclerotic plaque. Editor Springer Verlag, City, State.

Wang, J., Sica, A., Peri, G., Walter, S., Martin-Padura, I., Libby, P., Ceska, M., Lindley, I., Colotta, F. and Mantovani, A. (1991). Expression of monocyte chemotactic protein and interleukin-8 by cytokine-activated human vascular smooth muscle cells. *Arteriosclerosis*, 11:1166–1174.

Warner, S.J.C. and Libby, P. (1989). Human vascular smooth muscle cells: Target for and source of tumor necrosis factor. *J. Immunol.*, 142:100–109.

Warner, S.J.C., Auger, K.R. and Libby, P. (1987). Human interleukin 1 induces interleukin 1 gene expression in human vascular smooth muscle cells. *J. Exp. Med.*, 165:1316–1331.

Weksler, B.B., Marcus, A.J. and Jaffe, E.A. (1977). Synthesis of prostaglandin I2 (prostacyclin) by cultured human and bovine endothelial cells. *Proc. Natl. Acad. Sci. USA*, 74:3922–3926.

Wheeler, M.E., Luscinskas, F.W., Bevilacqua, M.P. and Gimbrone, M.A.J. (1988). Cultured human endothelial cells stimulated with cytokines or endotoxin produce an inhibitor of leukocyte adhesion. *J. Clin. Invest.*, 82:1211–1218.

Wight, T.N. (1989). Cell biology of arterial proteoglycans. *Arteriosclerosis*, 9:1–20.

Yanagi, H., Sasaguri, Y., Sugama, K., Morimatsu, M. and Nagase, H. (1991). Production of tissue collagenase (matrix metalloproteinase 1) by human aortic smooth muscle cells in response to platelet-derived growth factor. *Atherosclerosis*, 91:207–16.

Yoshizumi, M., Kourembanas, S., Temizer, D.H., Cambria, R.P., Quertermous, T. and Lee, M.E. (1992). Tumor necrosis factor increases transcription of the heparin-binding epidermal growth factor-like growth factor gene in vascular endothelial cells. *J. Biol. Chem.*, **267**:9467–9.

Yoshizumi, M., Kurihara, H., Morita, T., Yamashita, T., Oh-hashi, Y., Sugiyama, T., Takaku, F., Yanagisawa, M., Masaki, T. and Yazaki, Y. (1989). Interleukin 1 increases the production of endothelin by cultured endothelial cells. *Circulation*, **80**:II–5.

Zhang, J.D., Cousens, L.S., Barr, P.J. and Sprang, S.R. (1991). Three-dimensional structure of human basic fibroblast growth factor, a structural homolog of interleukin 1 beta. *Proc. Natl. Acad. Sci. USA.*, **88**:3446–50.

Zilberstein, A., Ruggieri, R., Korn, J.H. and Revel, M. (1986). Structure and expression of cDNA and genes for human interferon-beta-2, a distinct species inducible by growth-stimulatory cytokines. *EMBO J.*, **5**:2529–2537.

4 Chemokines in Vascular Pathophysiology

**Alberto Mantovani, Paola Allavena, Francesco Colotta,
Silvano Sozzani**

Istituto di Ricerche Farmacologiche, Mario Negri, Via Eritrea 62, I-20157 Milano, Italy

INTRODUCTION

The recruitment of leukocytes from the blood compartment into tissues is a central event in a variety of physiological and pathological processes. Leukocyte accumulation is also a hallmark of disease processes which directly involve the vessel wall, including various forms of vasculitis, atherosclerosis and neoplastic transformation. Polymorphonuclear cells (PMN) have served as prototypic professional migrants to construct a multistep paradigm of leukocyte recruitment and lymphocyte recirculation (for recent review Springer, 1994). The "area code" model involves multiple molecules (selectins; integrins interacting with Ig superfamily counter-receptors; chemokines) acting in concert and, to some extent, in sequence in a multistep process, from rolling to extravasation. Selective or preferential accumulation of leukocyte populations (e.g. eosinophils in allergic reactions) is a hallmark of leukocyte recruitment in normal or diseased tissues. In the conceptual framework of the area code model, selectivity is the end result of multiple factors, each with relatively wide spectrum of action (Springer, 1994; Butcher, 1991). Vascular cells play an active role in leukocyte recruitment by producing the determinants of leukocyte extravasation, which include vasoactive molecules, adhesion molecules and chemoattractants (Figure 1). While the central importance of chemoattractants and adhesion molecules is widely recognized and reviewed, vasodilation may represent a forgotten classic in current versions of the multistep paradigm of recruitment (Mantovani and Dejana, 1989; Mantovani *et al.*, 1992b).

Vasodilation is an early event of inflammatory and immune reactions and some of the classic manifestations of inflammation (rubor, calor; Cornelius Celsus, 30 BC to AD 38) are direct consequences of hyperhemia. Vasodilation *per se* does not cause formation of exudate or PMN extravasation (Wedmore and Williams, 1981; Williams and Peck, 1977). However it is permissive and important for both to occur. PMN emigration caused by local application of classic leukocyte attractants (e.g. FMLP, LTB4) has long been known to be dramatically potentiated by concomitant prostaglandin (PG)-induced vasodilation

Supported by Piano Nazionale Farmaci Consorzio Nireco

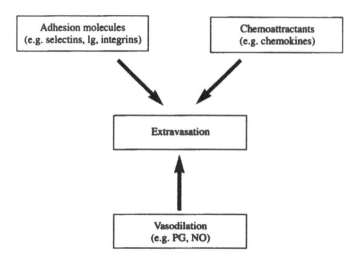

Figure 1 The concerted action of adhesion molecules, chemokines and vasodilatory mediators in recruitment in tissues.

(Issekutz, 1981; Issekutz and Bhimji, 1982; Movat *et al.*, 1984; Rampart *et al.*, 1989; Colditz, 1990). Moreover, treatment with inhibitors of production of PG, one class of vasodilatory substances at play, caused partial block of PMN recruitment at inflammatory sites (Wedmore and Williams, 1981; Issekutz, 1981; Issekutz and Bhimji, 1982; Movat *et al.*, 1984). More recently, the importance of concomitant vasodilation was also demonstrated in studies with the prototypic chemokine interleukin-8 (IL-8). Application of a vasodilatory PG dramatically augmented the potency (at least 2 logs) and/or maximum effect elicited by IL-8 *in vivo* (Colditz, 1990; Rampart *et al.*, 1989). Changes in blood rheology may also be permissive for the action of adhesion molecules (Mantovani *et al.*, 1992b; Lawrence *et al.*, 1990).

IL-1 and tumor necrosis factor (TNF), central mediators of inflammation and inducers of chemokines and adhesion molecules in endothelium, regulate production of vasoactive substances by endothelial cells (Rossi *et al.*, 1985). For instance, IL-1 and TNF induce production of PGI_2 and NO by endothelial cells by affecting expression of enzymes involved in production of these short-lived mediators (for review Mantovani *et al.*, 1992b). Thus, IL-1 and TNF cause sustained production by endothelial cells of vasodilatory mediators. Concomitantly they cause expression of adhesion molecules and, as discussed here, production of chemokines. The concerted action of permissive rehological changes, adhesion and attraction underlies recruitment.

Here we will summarize current information on how chemokines are produced by vessel wall elements *in vitro* and *vivo* and how some of them in turn act on vascular cells. Emerging information on the actual *in vivo* relevance of chemokines in vessel wall disorders, including neoplasia, will be discussed. The analysis of chemokines in vessel wall pathophysiology will be preceeded by a brief overview of the general properties and spectrum of action of members of this complex superfamily of inflammatory mediators. For a more in depth analysis of chemokines, the reader is referred to recent reviews (Oppenheim *et al.*, 1991; Baggiolini *et al.*, 1994; Mantovani, 1994).

CHEMOKINES: AN OVERVIEW

The selective recruitment of different leukocyte populations from the blood compartment into tissues has started to be better understood with the discovery of a number of chemotactic proteins now known as chemokines. Chemokines are small inducible low molecular weight (8–10 kDa) chemotactic proteins which have a marked affinity for heparin and possess four conserved cysteine residues. Two subfamilies may be distinguished according to the position of the first two cysteines, which are either separated by one amino acid (C-X-C) or adjacent (C-C) (Oppenheim *et al.*, 1991; Miller and Krangel, 1992; Baggiolini *et al.*, 1994).

C-X-C chemokines include IL-8, neutrophil-activating protein (NAP)-2, GROα, β and γ, epithelial-cell-derived neutrophil-activating protein (ENA-78) and granulocyte chemotactic protein-2 (GCP-2). All these proteins show about 25 to 45% homology with IL-8, and contain at the N-terminal domain a three amino acid sequence, Glu, Leu, Arg (ELR) that is critical for the binding to the receptors. Thus, the only two proteins that lack the ELR sequence, IP-10 and platelet factor-4, are devoid of neutrophil activating properties (Baggiolini *et al.*, 1994).

C-C chemokines include monocyte chemotactic protein (MCP)-1, MCP-2, MCP-3, RANTES, MIP-1α, MIP-1β and I-309. These proteins show 30–70% homology with MCP-1, with the highest homology among MCP-2 and MCP-3 with respect to MCP-1 (62 and 71%, respectively) and between MIP-1α and MIP-1β ($\cong$70% homology).

C-X-C and C-C chemokines, also called chemokines α and β, show a certain degree of selectivity among the leukocyte subpopulations. The former are active on neutrophilic granulocytes but not on monocytes (with the only exception of IP-10), the latter are active on monocytes but not on neutrophils (Table 1). IL-8 and MCP-1 are the best characterized proteins for the C-X-C and C-C families, respectively. Both proteins behave as classical chemotactic agonists being able to activate the oxidative burst, granule exocytosis, formation of bioactive lipids and integrin upregulation. Nevertheless, chemotaxis appears to be the most efficient biological activity induced by both C-X-C and C-C chemokines in human phagocytes.

As shown in Table 1, C-C chemokines also are potent basophil and eosinophil activators (Baggiolini and Dahinden, 1994). MCP-3, MIP-1α and RANTES are chemoattractants and secretagogue agents for both cell types. On the contrary MCP-1 is active on basophils but not on eosinophils, and is the first cytokine able to distinguish between these two cell types. MCP-1-induced histamine release is present in normal cells and enhanced after priming with GM-CSF, IL-3 and IL-5. After priming, release of leukotriene C_4 is also observed. Histamine release from basophils is also observed after RANTES and MIP-1α stimulation, with the first being a better chemoattractant than MCP-1. MIP-1α is a weaker agonist than other C-C chemokines active on these cells *in vitro*, but induces a conspicuous infiltration and activation of mast cell *in vivo*. MCP-3 appears to be the strongest agonist in human eosinophils in terms of both chemotaxis and exocytosis (Baggiolini and Dahinden, 1994).

IL-8, RANTES, MIP-1α and MIP-1β induce migration of T lymphocytes with different spectrum of action on lymphocyte subpopulations or activation state (Table 1) (Larsen *et al.*, 1989; Schall *et al.*, 1990; Taub *et al.*, 1993; Schall *et al.*, 1993). RANTES is a strong attractant of both resting and activated T cells, whereas for MIP-1α and β, chemotaxis is

Table 1   The spectrum of action of C-X-C and C-C chemokines

Family	Molecule	Neu	Eo	Ba	Mo	T Ly CD4	T Ly CD8	B Ly	Other
Cys-X-Cys	IL-8	++	±	±	−	±	±	−	melanomas, keratinocytes endothelium
	NAP-2	++	nt	±	−	nt	nt	nt	
	GROα	++	nt	nt	−	nt	nt	nt	
	IP-10	−	nt	nt	+	+	+	−	
Cys-Cys	MCP-1	−	−	++	++	−	−	−	−
	MCP-2	−	nt	nt	+	nt	nt	nt	nt
	MCP-3	−	+++	++	+	nt	nt	nt	nt
	RANTES	−	++	++	+	++§	++	+	nt
	MIP-1α	±*	+	+	+	+	++	+	hematopoietic precursors
	MIP-1β	−	−	−	+	++	±	−	−
	I309	−	nt	nt	+	?	?	nt	nt

The activity considered is migration. In general activated T cells respond better than resting cells, except for RANTES. For references, see text.
Neo, neutrophil; Eo, eosinophil; Ba, basophil; Mo, monocyte; Ly lymphocyte; nt, not tested.
§ CD4 cells with a memory phenotype may be preferentially affected. See text.

best observed with activated cells (Taub *et al.*, 1993). RANTES was selective for CD4[+] T cells with a memory phenotype in one study (Schall *et al.*, 1990) but not in another (Taub *et al.*, 1993). MIP-1α was found preferentially active on CD8[+] T cells, whereas MIP-1β was selective for CD4[+] T cells (Taub *et al.*, 1993; Schall *et al.*, 1993). In addition to inducing migration, chemokines, soluble or bound to proteoglycans, induce lympho-cyte adhesion to endothelium (Taub *et al.*, 1993; Schall *et al.*, 1993; Tanaka *et al.*, 1993).

All chemokines known, with the only exception of MCP-2 (Sozzani *et al.*, 1994), induce a rapid increase of intracellular calcium concentration evaluated in cells in sus-pension. At least for C-C chemokines, influx of calcium across membrane channels is the main mechanism responsible for the increase in intracellular calcium concentration (Sozzani *et al.*, 1993). Elevated intracellular calcium levels are required for activation of phospholipase A_2 and release of arachidonic by MCP-1, RANTES and MIP-1α (Locati *et al.*, 1994).

Information about chemokine receptors starts to be available. Two receptors which bind with high affinity IL-8, one of which also binds with high affinity NAP-2 and GROs were cloned from a cDNA library of differentiated HL-60 cells (Holmes *et al.*, 1991; Murphy and Tiffany, 1991). A promiscuous receptor for MIP-1α and RANTES also was cloned independently by two different groups from a similar cDNA library (Neote *et al.*, 1993; Gao *et al.*, 1993). More recently, two receptors for MCP-1 were cloned in MonoMac6 cells, a monocytic cell line (Charo *et al.*, 1994). All these receptors belong to the seven-transmembrane domain family of GTP-binding protein-associated receptors and show a certain degree of homology with the receptors for FMLP, PAF, C5a, others classical chemotactic agonists. It will be important to molecularly identify novel chemokine receptors (e.g. Sozzani *et al.*, 1994) and to define their expression in hematopoietic and nonhematopoietic elements including vascular cells (see later).

CHEMOKINES PRODUCED BY VASCULAR CELLS

In Vitro Studies

Endothelial Cells

EC produce various chemokines in response to signals representative of inflammatory reactions, immunity and thrombosis (Mantovani *et al.*, 1992b). Inflammatory cytokines (IL-1 and TNF) and bacterial lipopolysaccharides (LPS) induce expression and release of IL-8 and GROα (Strieter *et al.*, 1989; Schroder and Christophers, 1989; Sica *et al.*, 1990a; Dixit *et al.*, 1990; Sica *et al.*, 1990b; Rollins *et al.*, 1990; Gimbrone *et al.*, 1989; Wen *et al.*, 1989). Induction of IL-8 expression is associated with and depends on gene transcription (Sica *et al.*, 1990a). IL-4 and IL-3 are weak inducers of IL-8 expression and amplify induction by inflammatory cytokines (Rollins and Pober, 1991; Howell *et al.*, 1991; Colotta *et al.*, 1992; Korpelainen *et al.*, 1993). Hypoxia has recently been shown to induce IL-8 expression in EC, a finding potentially relevant for pathological conditions in which activation and recruitment of leukocytes may amplify tissue damage (Karakurum *et al.*, 1993). Platelets contain IL-1 and, when they interact with vascular EC, induce IL-8 gene expression (Kaplanski *et al.*, 1993).

As a result of proteolytic cleavage, IL-8 versions with a different NH_2 terminus and length can be produced (Baggiolini *et al.*, 1994). It has been suggested that EC release predominantly a 77aa version of IL-8, which is a less active species at activating leukocytes than the most common 73 residue form (Gimbrone *et al.*, 1989; Hebert *et al.*, 1990). The proteolitic conversion to smaller versions of the molecule can be catalyzed by thrombin (Hebert *et al.*, 1990).

The influence of IL-8 on the interaction of polymorphonuclear cells with vascular EC has been the object of seemingly conflicting observations, which seem now to reflect different experimental protocols and, most interestingly, different functions exerted by this cytokine under different pathophysiological conditions. IL-8 increased the adhesiveness of normal PMN for normal EC (Carveth *et al.*, 1989). In apparent contrast with these findings, EC-derived IL-8 was reported to inhibit binding of the PMN to a activated EC (Gimbrone *et al.*, 1989). Although it elicits PMN extravasation when given locally, IL-8 inhibits recruitment if administered systemically by the i.v. route (Hechtman *et al.*, 1991; Ley *et al.*, 1993). The seemingly paradoxic anti-inflammatory effects of high levels of systemic IL-8, possibly dependent upon the action of a reverse chemotactic gradient and leukocyte deactivation, may represent a feedback mechanism to control tissue damage.

The role of IL-8 produced locally by vascular cells was recently reexamined using reconstructed vessel wall models (Huber *et al.*, 1991). Unequivocal evidence was obtained for the importance of IL-8 in transendothelial migration induced by inflammatory cytokines (Huber *et al.*, 1991; Smith *et al.*, 1993).

EC of postcapillary venules bind IL-8, possibly via heparin-like molecules (Rot, 1992). Solid phase IL-8 elicits haptotactic migration (Wang *et al.*, 1990). Thus, locally produced IL-8 may be retained on the surface of EC and activate adhesive interactions and migration (Rot, 1992).

EC activated *in vitro* by inflammatory cytokines express GROα, which according to one report, could in turn act on EC (Wen *et al.*, 1989 see below).

IP10, a member of the C-X-C family but unique in that it attracts monocytes, is expressed in certain endothelia of mice exposed *in vivo* to interferonγ (IFNγ) or to LPS (Narumi *et al.*, 1992; Gómez-Chiarri *et al.*, 1993). There are no reports on *in vitro* expression of this chemokine in EC.

EC produce substantial amounts of the C-C chemokine MCP-1 (Sica *et al.*, 1990b; Rollins *et al.*, 1990). The proinflammatory signals IL-1, TNF and, to a lesser extent, LPS are potent stimuli for MCP-1 production (Sica *et al.*, 1990b; Rollins *et al.*, 1990). Under the same conditions, MCP-2 was undetectable in EC supernatants (J. Van Damme, personal communication). IL-4 and IL-13 are less active, but active, inducers of MCP-1 expression (Rollins and Pober, 1991; Howell *et al.*, 1991; Colotta *et al.*, 1992). INFγ was recently shown to induce MCP-1 in human microvascular EC (Brown *et al.*, 1994). Given the role that lipids and monocytes play in the natural history of atherosclerosis, it is of interest that minimally modified low density lypoproteins (MM-LDL) induce MCP-1 production in EC smooth cells (Cushing *et al.*, 1990). Thrombin was recently found to induce expression of MCP-1 in monocytes and, less prominently, in EC (Colotta *et al.*, 1994).

The molecular basis of stimulation of chemokine expression in EC has been studied to a limited extent. Induction by inflammatory signals and thrombin is protein synthesis independent in EC, but, interestingly, not in monocytes (Colotta *et al.*, 1994). Direct demonstration of enhanced gene transcription was obtained for MCP-1 and IL-8 by nuclear run off analysis (Sica *et al.*, 1990b; Sica *et al.*, 1990a). The 5' regulatory region of the IL-8 gene contains NFkB sequences which are involved in induction of expression in other cell types (Baggiolini *et al.*, 1994). It is of interest that IL-1 and TNF induce in EC the inhibitor of NFkB (IKB) which is likely to dampen the expression of NFkB-regulated genes including chemokines (d'Aniello *et al.*, 1993).

Smooth Muscle Cells (SMC) and Mesangial Cells

Already in early studies on MCP-1, it had been described that vascular SMC secreted a monocyte chemoattractant (Valente *et al.*, 1984; Valente *et al.*, 1988) which resembled a similar factor produced by tumor lines (Bottazzi *et al.*, 1983). The SMC-derived factor was subsequently identified as MCP-1. Indeed IL-1, TNF, and MM-LDL induce expression of MCP-1 in SMC with mechanisms and kinetics resembling those observed in EC (Wang *et al.*, 1991; Cushing *et al.*, 1990). IL-1 and TNF also stimulate expression and release of IL-8 in SMC (Wang *et al.*, 1991).

Kidney mesangial cells may have an ontogenetic relationship with SMC. They express and release MCP-1 and IL-8 in response to IL-1 and TNF (Zoja *et al.*, 1991; Rovin *et al.*, 1992; Satriano *et al.*, 1993b; Satriano *et al.*, 1993a). Of special importance in relation to pathology is induction of MCP-1 and IP10 by aggregated immunoglobulins (Satriano *et al.*, 1993b; Satriano *et al.*, 1993a). Reactive oxygen intermediates act as second messengers in induction of MCP-1 by aggregated Ig (Satriano *et al.*, 1993a). These results may have considerable relevance in kidney pathology involving mononuclear phagocyte infiltration.

In Vivo Studies

In vivo studies on chemokines in vessel wall pathology have largely been restricted to atherosclerosis. MCP-1 expression has been detected in atheromatous lesions of rabbits, primates and man (Takeya *et al.*, 1993; Yu *et al.*, 1992; Yla Herttuala *et al.*, 1991; Nelken *et al.*, 1991). Chemokine gene expression has been detected in various cellular elements, including SMC, EC and mononuclear phagocytes, with somewhat different results in different studies. In the only study with mAb (Takeya *et al.*, 1993), cell populations positive for MCP-1 were different in lesions representative of different stages of the natural history of atherosclerosis. EC staining was prominent in diffuse intimal thickening and in fatty streaks, whereas it was weak in atheromatous lesions. Subendothelial macrophages were strongly positive for MCP-1 in fatty streak lesions and in atherosclerotic plaques. In plaques, a few intima SMC stained for MCP-1. These results suggest that EC and macrophages are the major source of MCP-1 in early atherosclerotic lesions (Takeya *et al.*, 1993). Monocyte adhesion and infiltration is an early event in the natural history of atherosclerosis (Libby and Hansson, 1991; Ross, 1993). Mononuclear phagocyte infiltration is also a prominent feature of vasculitis (Fauci *et al.*, 1978). Locally produced MCP-1 may play an important role in regulating extravasation of leukocytes, of monocytes in particular, in vessel wall pathology.

EFFECTS OF CHEMOKINES ON VASCULAR ELEMENTS

By and large, the spectrum of action of chemokines is restricted to leukocytes. However, recent reports have suggested that some chemokines may affect EC function. IL-8 has recently been shown to induce migration and proliferation of EC (Koch *et al.*, 1992; Strieter *et al.*, 1992). It has also been shown to course angiogenesis *in vivo* models in rodents (Koch *et al.*, 1992; Strieter *et al.*, 1992). IL-8 was also reported to be chemotactic for SMC (Yue *et al.*, 1993). In the same vein, groα affected EC proliferation in one study (Wen *et al.*, 1989) but others failed to observe binding and activity of this chemokine on EC (Rot, 1992).

We have been unable to detect of activities of various chemokines, and in particular of MCP-1, on EC (unpublished). However the mouse C-C chemokine FIC has been shown to bind EC (Heinrich *et al.*, 1993).

Platelet factor 4 (PF4), a C-C chemokine contained in the α granules of platelets, of largely unknown function, has been reported to inhibit growth factor-induced proliferation of EC and angiogenesis *in vivo* (Maione *et al.*, 1990).

The above results point to the possibility that some chemokines may regulate the proliferation and migration of vessel wall elements. Identification of chemokine receptors on vascular cells will be important to define the nature and significance of this interaction.

CHEMOKINES IN VASCULAR TUMORS

Transformed cells frequently produce chemokines (for review Mantovani *et al.*, 1992a; Mantovani, 1994). For instance, MCP-1, 2 and 3 have been identified as tumor-derived chemoattractants. There is evidence based on studies with MCP-1 that tumor-derived chemotactic factors contribute to macrophage infiltration of neoplastic tissues. At least in certain tumors, tumor-associated macrophages (TAM) provide a microenvironment favourable to neoplastic growth and angiogenesis (Mantovani *et al.*, 1992a; Mantovani, 1994).

Neoplastic transformation can affect vessel wall elements, causing hemangiomas, hemangiosarcomas and Kaposi's sarcoma (KS). At least some mouse polyoma middle T-transformed hemangiomas lines, which cause opportunistic vascular tumors characterized by host cell recruitment and leukocyte infiltration (Williams *et al.*, 1989; Garlanda *et al.*, 1994), express the C-X-C chemokine KC (possibly the homologue of human gro) and the C-C molecule MCP-1.

KS is an opportunistic vascular tumor characterized by a conspicuous infiltrate at least in the early phases of its natural history. We recently observed that cultured KS cells express and release IL-8 and MCP-1 and that production of these molecules is amplified by IL-1 and TNF (Sciacca *et al* in preparation). More importantly, *in situ* hybridization revealed expression of MCP-1 *in vivo* in KS lesions. Infiltrating host leukocytes, and TAM in particular, can play an important role in the regulation of tumor growth and progression. TAM are potent producers of growth factors and promote angiogenesis (Mantovani *et al.*, 1992a; Mantovani, 1994). Thus production of chemokines may amplify growth and angiogenesis in these vascular tumors.

SOME OPEN QUESTIONS AND CONCLUDING REMARKS

Chemokines are an essential component of the current paradigm of leukocyte extravasation and recruitment in normal and pathological conditions. Their distinct spectrum of action provides a basis for selective or preferential accumulation of different leukocyte populations under different conditions, a long known key feature of inflammatory/immune reactions. However, the redundancy of the chemokine system, with substantial overlap among individual molecules, is intriguing. It this vein, it is puzzling that chemokines with different target leukocytes are induced concomitantly with similar kinetics by the same signals. For instance, IL-8, active mainly on PMN, and MCP-1, active mainly on mononuclear phagocytes, are produced by vessel wall elements *in vitro* in response to the same signals and we are not aware of substantial dissociations in terms of kinetics or inducers. It can be speculated that other factors, including inhibitors (Wang *et al.*, 1986) or regulation of survival in tissues, play an important role in dictating the type of leukocyte ultimately accumulating in a diseased blood vessel. While the results summarized here point to a central role of chemokines in the pathophysiology of blood vessels, little direct information is available *in vivo*. In addition to in situ analysis, antibodies to rodent molecules and gene targeting will be required to dissect the *in vivo* function of chemokines.

Table 2 Chemokine production by vascular cells

Cell type	Chemokine	Stimuli	Selected references
Endothelium	IL-8 (C-X-C)	IL-1, TNF, LPS	(Strieter *et al.*, 1989; Schroder and Christophers, 1989; Sica *et al.*, 1990a; Gimbrone *et al.*, 1989)
		IL-4	(Rollins and Pober, 1991; Colotta et al., 1992)
		IL-3	(Korpelainen *et al.*, 1993)
		platelets (via IL-1)	(Kaplanski *et al.*, 1993)
		hypoxia	(Karakurum *et al.*, 1993)
	groα (C-X-C)	TNF	(Wen *et al.*, 1989)
	IP-10 (C-X-C)	LPS	(Narumi *et al.*, 1992; Gómez-Chiarri *et al.*, 1993)
		IFNγ	(Narumi *et al.*, 1992; Gómez-Chiarri *et al.*, 1993)
	MCP-1 (C-C)	IL-1, TNF, LPS	(Sica *et al.*, 1990b; Rollins *et al.*, 1990)
		IL-4	(Colotta *et al.*, 1992)
		IFNγ	(Brown *et al.*, 1994)
		MM-LDL	(Cushing *et al.*, 1990)
		thrombin	(Colotta *et al.*, 1994)
Smooth muscle cells	IL-8 (C-X-C)	IL-1, TNF	(Wang *et al.*, 1991)
	MCP-1 (C-C)	MM-LDL	(Cushing *et al.*, 1990)
		IL-1, TNF	(Wang *et al.*, 1991; Valente *et al.*, 1984)
Mesangial cells	IL-8 (C-X-C)	IL-1, TNF	(Zoja *et al.*, 1991)
	IP-10 (C-X-C)	Aggregated IgG	(Gómez-Chiarri *et al.*, 1993)
	MCP-1 (C-C)	IL-1, TNF	(Zoja *et al.*, 1991)
		IFNγ	(Satriano *et al.*, 1993a; Satriano *et al.*, 1993b)
		Aggregated IgG	(Satriano *et al.*, 1993a)

References

Baggiolini, M. and Dahinden, C.A. (1994). CC Chemokines in Allergic Inflammation. *Immunol. Today*, **15**:127–133.

Baggiolini, M., Dewald, B. and Moser, B. (1994). Interleukin-8 and related chemotactic cytokines — CXC and CC chemokines. *Adv. Immunol.*, **55**:99–179.

Bottazzi, B., Polentarutti, N., Acero, R., Balsari, A., Boraschi, D., Ghezzi, P., Salmona, M. and Mantovani, A. (1983). Regulation of the macrophage content of neoplasms by chemoattractants. *Science*, **220**:210–212.

Brown, Z., Gerritsen, M.E., Strieter, R.M., Kunkel, S.L. and Westwick, J. (1994). Chemokine gene expression and secretion by cytokine activated human microvascular endothelial cells: differential regulation of MCP-1 and IL-8 in response to interferon-gamma. *Am. J. Pathol.*, **145**:913–921.

Butcher, E.C. (1991). Leukocyte-endothelial cell recognition: three (or more) steps to specificity and diversity. *Cell*, **67**:1033–1036.

Carveth, H.J., Bohnsack, J.F., McIntyre, T.M., Baggiolini, M., Prescott, S.M. and Zimmerman, G.A. (1989). Neutrophil activating factor (NAF) induces polymorphonuclear leukocyte adherence to endothelial cells and to subendothelial matrix proteins. *Biochem. Biophys. Res. Commun.*, **162**:387–393.

Charo, I.F., Myers, S.J., Herman, A., Franci, C., Connolly, A.J. and Coughlin, S.R. (in press). Molecular cloning and functional expression of two monocyte chemoattractant protein 1 (MCP-1) receptors reveals alternative splicing of the carboxyl-terminal tails. *Proc. Natl. Acad. Sci. USA.*, **91**:2752–2756.

Colditz, I.G. (1990). Effect of exogenous prostaglandin E2 and actinomycin D on plasma leakage induced by neutrophil-activating peptide-1/interleukin-8. *Immunol. Cell Biol.*, **68**:397–403.

Colotta, F., Sironi, M., Borre, A., Luini, W., Maddalena, F. and Mantovani, A. (1992). Interleukin 4 amplifies monocyte chemotactic protein and interleukin 6 production by endothelial cells. *Cytokine*, **4**:24–28.

Colotta, F., Sciacca, F.L., Sironi, M., Luini, W., Rabiet, J.R. and Mantovani, A. (1994). Expression of monocyte chemotactic protein-1 (MCP-1) by monocytes and endothelial cells exposed to thrombin. *Am. J. Pathol.*, **144**:975–985.

Cushing, S.D., Berliner, J.A., Valente, A.J., Territo, M.C., Navab, M., Parhami, F., Gerrity, R., Schwartz, C.J. and Fogelman, A.M. (1990). Minimally modified low density lipoprotein induces monocyte chemotactic protein 1 in human endothelial cells and smooth muscle cells. *Proc. Natl. Acad. Sci. USA.*, 87:5134–5138.

d'Aniello, E.M., Breviario, F., Martin Padura, I., Lampugnani, M.G., Dejana, E., Mantovani, A. and Introna, M. (1993). Interleukin-1 and tumor necrosis factor induce transient expression of an inhibitor of nuclear factor kB in endothelial cells. *Endothelium*, 1:161–165.

Dixit, V.M., Green, S., Sarma, V., Holzman, L.B., Wolf, F.W., O'Rourke, K., Ward, P.A., Prochownik, E.V. and Marks, R.M. (1990). Tumor necrosis factor-alpha induction of novel gene products in human endothelial cells including a macrophage-specific chemotaxin. *J. Biol. Chem.*, 265:2973–2978.

Fauci, A.S., Haynes, B.F. and Katz, P. (1978). The spectrum of vasculitis. *Ann. Intern. Med.*, 89 (Part 1): 660–676.

Gao, J.L., Kuhns, D.B., Tiffany, H.L., McDermott, D., Li, X., Francke, U. and Murphy, P.M. (1993). Structure and functional expression of the human macrophage inflammatory protein 1 alpha/RANTES receptor. *J. Exp. Med.*, 177:1421–1427.

Garlanda, C., Parravicini, C., Sironi, M., De Rossi, M., Wainstok de Calmanovici, R., Carozzi, F., Bussolino, F., Colotta, F., Mantovani, A. and Vecchi, A. (1994). Progressive growth in immunodeficient mice and host cell recruitment by mouse endothelial cells transformed by polyoma middle T: implications for the pathogenesis of opportunistic vascular tumors. *Proc. Natl. Acad. Sci. USA.*, 91:7291–7295.

Gimbrone, M.A.J., Obin, M.S., Brock, A.F., Luis, E.A., Hass, P.E., Hebert, C.A., Yip, Y.K., Leung, D.W., Lowe, D.G., Kohr, W.J. and et al, (1989). Endothelial interleukin-8: a novel inhibitor of leukocyte-endothelial interactions. *Science*, 246:1601–1603.

Gómez-Chiarri, M., Hamilton, T.A., Egido, J. and Emancipator, S.N. (1993). Expression of IP-10, a lipopolysaccharide- and interferon-gamma-inducible protein, in murine mesangial cells in culture. *Am. J. Pathol.*, 142:433–439.

Hebert, C.A., Luscinskas, F.W., Kiely, J.M., Luis, E.A., Darbonne, W.C., Bennett, G.L., Liu, C.C., Obin, M.S., Gimbrone, M.A.J. and Baker, J.B. (1990). Endothelial and leukocyte forms of IL-8. Conversion by thrombin and interactions with neutrophils. *J. Immunol.*, 145:3033–3040.

Hechtman, D.H., Cybulsky, M.I., Fuchs, H.J., Baker, J.B. and Gimbrone, M.A.J. (1991). Intravascular IL-8. Inhibitor of polymorphonuclear leukocyte accumulation at sites of acute inflammation. *J. Immunol.*, 147:883–892.

Heinrich, J.N., Ryseck, R.P., Macdonaldbravo, H. and Bravo, R. (1993). The product of a novel growth factor-activated gene, fic, Is a biologically active C-C-type cytokine. *Mol. Cell Biol.*, 13:2020–2030.

Holmes, W.E., Lee, J., Kuang, W.J., Rice, G.C. and Wood, W.I. (1991). Structure and functional expression of a human interleukin-8 receptor. *Science*, 253:1278–1280.

Howell, G., Pham, P., Taylor, D., Foxwell, B. and Feldmann, M. (1991). Interleukin 4 induces interleukin 6 production by endothelial cells: synergy with interferon- gamma. *Eur. J. Immunol.*, 21:97–101.

Huber, A.R., Kunkel, S.L., Todd, R.F. and Weiss, S.J. (1991). Regulation of transendothelial neutrophil migration by endogenous interleukin-8 . *Science*, 254:99–102.

Issekutz, A.C. (1981). Vascular responses during acute neutrophilic inflammation. Their relationship to *in vivo* neutrophil emigration. *Lab. Invest.*, 45:435–441.

Issekutz, A.C. and Bhimji, S. (1982). Effect of nonsteroidal anti-inflammatory agents on immune complex-and chemotactic factor-induced inflammation. *Immunopharmacology*, 4:253–266.

Kaplanski, G., Porat, R., Aiura, K., Erban, J.K., Gelfand, J.A. and Dinarello, C.A. (1993). Activated platelets induce endothelial secretion of interleukin-8 *in vitro* via an interleukin-1-mediated event. *Blood*, 81:2492–2495.

Karakurum, M., Shreeniwas, R., Chen, J., Pinsky, D., Yan, S.D., Anderson, M., Sunouchi, K., Major, J., Hamilton, T., Kuwabara, K., Rot, A., Nowygrod, R. and Stern, D. (1993). Hypoxic induction of interleukin-8 gene expression in human endothelial cells. *Blood*, 81:2492–2495.

Koch, A.E., Polverini, P.J., Kunkel, S.L., Harlow, L.A., DiPietro, L.A., Elner, V.M., Elner, S.G. and Strieter, R.M. (1992). Interleukin-8 as a macrophage-derived mediator of angiogenesis. *Science*, 258:1798–1801.

Korpelainen, E.I., Gamble, J.R., Smith, W.B., Goodall, G.J., Qiyu, S., Woodcock, J.M., Dottore, M., Vadas, M.A. and Lopez, A.F. (1993). The receptor for interleukin 3 is selectively induced in human endothelial cells by tumor necrosis factor alpha and potentiates interleukin 8 secretion and neutrophil transmigration. *Proc. Natl. Acad. Sci. USA.*, 90:11137–11141.

Larsen, C.G., Anderson, A.O., Appella, E., Oppenheim, J.J. and Matsushima, K. (1989). The neutrophil-activating protein (NAP-1) is also chemotactic for T lymphocytes . *Science*, 243:1464–1466.

Lawrence, M.B., Smith, C.W., Eskin, S.G. and McIntire, L.V. (1990). Effect of venous shear stress on CD18-mediated neutrophil adhesion to cultured endothelium. *Blood*, 75:227–237.

Ley, K., Baker, J.B., Cybulsky, M.I., Gimbrone, M.A. and Luscinskas, F.W. (1993). Intravenous interleukin-8 inhibits granulocyte emigration from rabbit mesenteric venules without altering L-selectin expression or leukocyte rolling. *J. Immunol.*, 151:6347–6357.

Libby, P. and Hansson, G.K. (1991). Biology of disease. Involvement of the immune system in human atherogenesis: current knowledge and unanswered questions. *Lab. Invest.*, 64:5–15.

Locati, M., Zhou, D., Luini, W., Evangelista, V., Mantovani, A. and Sozzani, S. (1994). Rapid induction of Arachidonic acid release by Monocyte Chematactic Protein-1 and related chemokines. *J. Biol. Chem.*, **269**:1–8.

Maione, T.E., Gray, G.S., Petro, J., Hunt, A.J., Donner, A.L., Bauer, S.I., Carson, H.F. and Sharpe, R.J. (1990). Inhibition of angiogenesis by recombinant human platelet factor-4 and related peptides. *Science* **247**:77–79.

Mantovani, A., Bottazzi, B., Colotta, F., Sozzani, S. and Ruco, L. (1992a). The origin and function of tumor-associated macrophages. *Immunol. Today*, **13**:265–270.

Mantovani, A., Bussolino, F. and Dejana, E. (1992b). Cytokine regulation of endothelial cell function. *FASEB. J.*, **6**:2591–2599.

Mantovani, A. (1994). Tumor-associated macrophages in neoplastic progression: a paradigm for the *in vivo* function of chemokines. *Lab. Invest.*, **71**:5–16.

Mantovani, A. and Dejana, E. (1989). Cytokines as communication signals between leukocytes and endothelial cells. *Immunol. Today*, **10**:370–375.

Miller, M.D. and Krangel, M.S. (1992). Biology and biochemistry of the chemokines: a family of chemotactic and inflammatory cytokines. *Crit. Rev. Immunol.*, **12**:17–46.

Movat, H.Z., Rettl, C., Burrowes, C.E. and Johnston, M.G. (1984). The *in vivo* effect of Leukotriene B4 on polymorphonuclear leukocytes and the microcirculation. *Am. J. Pathol.*, **115**:233–244.

Murphy, P.M. and Tiffany, H.L. (1991). Cloning of complementary DNA encoding a functional human inter-leukin-8 receptor. *Science*, **253**:1280–1283.

Narumi, S., Wyner, L.M., Stoler, M.H., Tannenbaum, C.S. and Hamilton, T.A. (1992). Tissue-specific expression of murine IP-10 mRNA following systemic treatment with interferon-gamma. *J. Leukoc. Biol.*, **52**:27–33.

Nelken, N.A., Coughlin, S.R., Gordon, D. and Wilcox, J.N. (1991). Monocyte chemoattractant protein-1 in human atheromatous plaques. *J. Clin. Invest.*, **88**:1121–1127.

Neote, K., DiGregorio, D., Mak, J.Y., Horuk, R. and Schall, T.J. (1993). Molecular cloning, functional expression and signaling characteristics of a C-C chemokine receptor. *Cell*, **72**:415–425.

Oppenheim, J.J., Zachariae, C.O., Mukaida, N. and Matsushima, K. (1991). Properties of the novel proinflammatory supergene "intercrine" cytokine family. *Annu. Rev. Immunol.*, **9**:617–648.

Rampart, M., Van Damme, J., Zonnekeyn, L. and Herman, A.G. (1989). Granulocyte chemotactic protein/interleukin-8 induces plasma leakage and neutrophil accumulation in rabbit skin. *Am. J. Pathol.*, **135**:21–25.

Rollins, B.J., Yoshimura, T., Leonard, E.J. and Pober, J.S. (1990). Cytokine-activated human endothelial cells synthesize and secrete a monocyte chemoattractant, MCP-1/JE. *Am. J. Pathol.*, **136**:1229–1233.

Rollins, B.J. and Pober, J.S. (1991). Interleukin-4 induces the synthesis and secretion of MCP-1JE by human endothelial cells. *Am. J. Pathol.*, **138**:1315–1319.

Ross, R. (1993). The pathogenesis of atherosclerosis: a perspective for the 1990s. *Nature*, **362**:801–809.

Rossi, V., Breviario, F., Ghezzi, P., Dejana, E. and Mantovani, A. (1985). Prostacyclin synthesis induced in vascular cells by interleukin-1. *Science*, **229**:174–176.

Rot, A. (1992). Endothelial cell binding of NAP-1/IL-8: role in neutrophil emigration. *Immunol. Today*, **13**:291–294.

Rovin, B.H., Yoshimura, T. and Tan, L. (1992). Cytokine-induced production of monocyte chemoattractant protein-1 by cultured human mesangial cells. *J. Immunol.*, **148**:2148–2153.

Satriano, J.A., Hora, K., Shan, Z., Stanley, E.R., Mori, T. and Schlondorff, D. (1993a). Regulation of monocyte chemoattractant protein-1 and macrophage colony-stimulating factor-1 by IFN-gamma, tumor necrosis factor-alpha, IgG aggregates and cAMP in mouse mesangial cells. *J. Immunol.*, **150**:1971–1978.

Satriano, J.A., Shuldiner, M., Hora, K., Xing, Y., Shan, Z. and Schlondorff, D. (1993b). Oxygen radicals as second messengers for expression of the monocyte chemoattractant protein, JE/MCP-1 and the monocyte colony-stimulating factor, CSF-1, in response to tumor necrosis factor-alpha and immunoglobulin-G — evidence for involvement of reduced nicotinamide adenine dinucleotide phosphate (NADPH)-dependent oxidase. *J. Clin. Invest.*, **92**:1564–1571.

Schall, T.J., Bacon, K., Toy, K.J. and Goeddel, D.V. (1990). Selective attraction of monocytes and T lymphocytes of the memory phenotype by cytokine RANTES. *Nature*, **347**:669–671.

Schall, T.J., Bacon, K., Camp, R.D., Kaspari, J.W. and Goeddel, D.V. (1993). Human macrophage inflammatory protein alpha (MIP-1 alpha) and MIP-1 beta chemokines attract distinct populations of lymphocytes. *J. Exp. Med.*, **177**:1821–1826.

Schroder, J.M. and Christophers, E. (1989). Secretion of novel and homologous neutrophil-activating peptides by LPS-stimulated human endothelial cells. *J. Immunol.*, **142**:244–251.

Sica, A., Matsushima, K., Van Damme, J., Wang, J.M., Polentarutti, N., Dejana, E., Colotta, F. and Mantovani, A. (1990a). IL-1 transcriptionally activates the neutrophil chemotactic factor/IL-8 gene in endothelial cells. *Immunology*, **69**:548–553.

Sica, A., Wang, J.M., Colotta, F., Dejana, E., Mantovani, A., Oppenheim, J.J., Larsen, C.G., Zachariae, C.O. and Matsushima, K. (1990b). Monocyte chemotactic and activating factor gene expression induced in endothelial cells by IL-1 and tumor necrosis factor. *J. Immunol.*, **144**:3034–3038.

Smith, W.B., Gamble, J.R., Clarklewis, I. and Vadas, M.A. (1993). Chemotactic desensitization of neutrophils demonstrates interleukin-8 (IL-8)-dependent and IL-8-independent mechanisms of transmigration through cytokine-activated endothelium. *Immunology*, **78**:491–497.

Sozzani, S., Molino, M., Locati, M., Luini, W., Cerletti, C., Vecchi, A. and Mantovani, A. (1993). Receptor-activated calcium influx in human monocytes exposed to monocyte chemotactic protein-1 and related cytokines. *J. Immunol.*, **150**:1544–1553.

Sozzani, S., Zhou, D., Locati, M., Rieppi, M., Proost, P., Magazin, M., Vita, N., Van Damme, J. and Mantovani, A. (1994). Receptors and transduction patways for Monocyte Chemotactic Protein-2 (MCP-2) and MCP-3: similarities and differences with MCP-1. *J. Immunol.*, **152**:3615–3622.

Springer, T.A. (1994). Traffic signal for lymphocyte recirculation and leukocyte emigration: the mutistep paradigm. *Cell*, **76**:301–314.

Strieter, R.M., Kunkel, S.L., Showell, H.J., Remick, D.G., Phan, S.H., Ward, P.A. and Marks, R.M. (1989). Endothelial cell gene expression of a neutrophil chemotactic factor by TNF-alpha, LPS and IL-1 beta. *Science*, **243**:1467–1469.

Strieter, R.M., Kunkel, S.L., Elner, V.M., Martonyi, C.L., Koch, A.E., Polverini, P.J. and Elner, S.G. (1992). Interleukin-8. A corneal factor that induces neovascularization. *Am. J. Pathol.*, **141**:1279–1284.

Takeya, M., Yoshimura, T., Leonard, E.J. and Takahashi, K. (1993). Detection of monocyte chemoattractant protein-1 in human atherosclerotic lesions by an anti-monocyte chemoattractant protein-1 monoclonal antibody. *Hum. Pathol.*, **24**:534–539.

Tanaka, Y., Adams, D.H., Hubscher, S., Hirano, H., Siebenlist, U. and Shaw, S. (1993). T-cell adhesion induced by proteoglycan-immobilized cytokine MIP-1 beta. *Nature*, **361**:79–82.

Taub, D.D., Conlon, K., Lloyd, A.R., Oppenheim, J.J. and Kelvin, D.J. (1993). Preferential migration of activated CD4+ and CD8+ T cells in response to MIP-1 alpha and MIP-1 beta. *Science*, **260**:355–358.

Valente, A.J., Fowler, S.R., Sprague, E.A., Kelley, J.L., Suenram, C.A. and Schwartz, C.J. (1984). Initial characterization of a paripheral blood mononuclear cell chemoattractant derived from cultured arterial smooth muscle cells. *Am. J. Pathol.*, **117**:409–417.

Valente, A.J., Graves, D.A., Vialle-Valentin, C.E., Delgado, R. and Schwartz, C.J. (1988). Purification of a monocyte chemotactic factor secreted by nonhuman primate vascular cells in culture. *Biochemistry*, **27**:4162–4168.

Wang, J.M., Cianciolo, G.J., Snyderman, R. and Mantovani, A. (1986). Coexistence of a chemotactic factor and a retroviral P158-related chemotaxis inhibitor in human tumor cell culture supernatant. *J. Immunol.*, **137**:2726–2732.

Wang, J.M., Taraboletti, G., Matsushima, K., Van Damme, J. and Mantovani, A. (1990). Induction of haptotactic migration of melanoma cells by neutrophil activating protein/interleukin-8. *Biochem. Biophys. Res. Commun.*, **169**:165–170.

Wang, J.M., Sica, A., Peri, G., Walter, S., Padura, I.M., Libby, P., Ceska, M., Lindley, I., Colotta, F. and Mantovani, A. (1991). Expression of monocyte chemotactic protein and interleukin-8 by cytokine-activated human vascular smooth muscle cells. *Arterioscler. Thromb.*, **11**:1166–1174.

Wedmore, C.V. and Williams, T.J. (1981). Control of vascular permeability by polymorphonuclear leukocytes in inflammation. *Nature*, **289**:646–650.

Wen, D., Rowland, A. and Derynck, R. (1989). Expression and secretion of *gro*/MGSA by stimulated human endothelial cells. *EMBO J.*, **8**:1761–1766.

Williams, R.L., Risau, W., Zerwes, H.G., Drexler, H., Aguzzi, A. and Wagner, E.F. (1989). Endothelioma cells expressing the polyoma middle T oncogene induce hemangiomas by host cell recruitment. *Cell*, **57**:1053–1063.

Williams, T.J. and Peck, M.J. (1977). Role of prostaglandin-mediated vasodilatation in inflammation. *Nature*, **270**:530–532.

Yla Herttuala, S., Lipton, B.A., Rosenfeld, M.E., Sarkioja, T., Yoshimura, T., Leonard, E.J., Witztum, J.L. and Steinberg, D. (1991). Expression of monocyte chemoattractant protein 1 in macrophage-rich areas of human and rabbit atherosclerotic lesions. *Proc. Natl. Acad. Sci. USA.*, **88**:5252–5256.

Yu, X., Dluz, S., Graves, D.T., Zhang, L., Antoniades, H.N., Hollander, W., Prusty, S., Valente, A.J., Schwartz, C.J. and Sonenshein, G.E. (1992). Elevated expression of monocyte chemoattractant protein 1 by vascular smooth muscle cells in hypercholesterolemic primates. *Proc. Natl. Acad. Sci. USA.*, **89**:6953–6957.

Yue, T.L., Mckenna, P.J., Gu, J.L. and Feuerstein, G.Z. (1993). Interleukin-8 is chemotactic for vascular smooth muscle cells. *Eur. J. Pharmacol.*, **240**:81–84.

Zoja, C., Wang, J.M., Bettoni, S., Sironi, M., Renzi, D., Chiaffarino, F., Abboud, H.E., Van Damme, J., Mantovani, A., Remuzzi, G. and *et al*, (1991). Interleukin-1 beta and tumor necrosis factor-alpha induce gene expression and production of leukocyte chemotactic factors, colony-stimulating factors and interleukin-6 in human mesangial cells. *Am. J. Pathol.*, **138**:991–1003.

5 Immunopathological Approaches to Clarify the Etiopathogenesis of Systemic Arteritis

Masahisa Kyogoku, Masato Nose, Masaaki Miyazawa, Kazuhiro Murakami, Mitsuyasu Kato, Jun-ichi Fujiyama and Junpei Itoh

Department of Pathology, Tohoku University School of Medicine

INTRODUCTION

The first example of the diseases that indicated the role of immune responses in the etiopathogenesis of systemic arteritis was serum sickness. Rich and Gregory (1943) first described a rabbit model of serum sickness and analyzed the process of immune complex mediated tissue injury. In 1958 Dixon *et al.* (1958) published the famous article in *Arch. of Pathol.* on the one-shot model of acute serum sickness. According to their observation the vasculitis appeared during its third or catabolic phase when immune complexes were detected in the circulation. The complexes of an antigen, antibodies, and complement components were deposited in the sites of glomerulonephritis, vasculitis and arthritis. During the late 60's and early 70's Cochrane *et al.* (Cochrane and Hawkins, 1968; Cochrane, 1971; Cochrane and Koffler, 1973) analysed the model in more detail. They speculated that IgE, PAF and platelet factors augmented the endothelial permeability, and that 19S immune complexes, preformed in an antigen excess condition, precipitated beneath the endothelia and formed fibrinoid deposits *in situ*.

If one repeatedly injects a small amount of antigen every day, a different type of vasculitis develops instead of the above-described acute necrotizing fibrinoid arteritis (Germuth and Heptinstall, 1957). In such a condition the kinetics and incidence of the development and histological appearance of arteritis are dependent on the schedule of sensitization, molecular characters of the antigen used, the ratio between antigen and antibody or sizes of immune complexes. Thus, a precise condition that induces vasculitis is quite difficult to establish and, therefore, the incidence of arteritis is very low in such a chronic type of serum sickness.

Nishikawa (1979) and Watanabe (1984) demonstrated that not the circulating immune complexes but immune complexes made *in situ* in the adventitia from preexisting antibodies and antigens coming through adventitial connective tissue venules were much more important to form necrotizing arteritis of the fibrinoid type. In their models the fibrinoid substances were sometimes found on the medioadventitial margins. Some adhesion molecules may work in such sites.

These early efforts using animal models established a relatively firm idea among pathologists that immune complexes played a crucial role in the pathogenesis of systemic arteritis. Demonstration of deposited immunoglobulins along with or even without complement components in vascular walls has been regarded by may as an adequate evidence to suggest the involvement of immune complexes in the pathogenesis of observed tissue injuries. However, the deposition of immunoglobulins or other macromolecules into vascular walls may sometimes be only a result of tissue damage rather than a cause of it. In this chapter, we will review previous works on the pathogenesis of systemic arteritis, and discuss about how much of vascular injuries can be explained by the immune complex-mediated mechanisms and how much cannot, mostly based upon our own research data.

AN OVERVIEW OF ANIMAL MODELS OF ARTERITIS ON AN ETIOLOGICAL POINT OF VIEW

According to our bibliographical survey, about 500 reports that dealt with animal experiments on vascular diseases had been published in the last decade. They can be classified into three categories standing upon the etiological point of view: 1) virus induced 2) bacterial or other prokaryotic or eukaryotic infection and 3) autoimmune diseases or other immunological disturbances (Table 1). The animals used were mostly mammals, and species varied from horses to mice. Most of the virally induced models were spontaneously developing, and found coincidentally. On the contrary, most of the bacterial infection- or toxin-induced models were intentionally produced using an agent that was suspected to be causing a human disease. (Kyogoku *et al.*, 1988)

Virus-Related Models of Vasculitis

The species of virus that can induce vasculitis in animals are quite diverse; herpesviridae, parvoviridae, coronaviridae, togaviridae, and retroviridae. Among these, equine arteritis virus threw the Kentucky horse farms into panic in 1984, where a number of foals suffered from systemic necrotizing arteritis. Concentrated examination revealed that the disease was caused by a toga-virus. Foals were preferentially infected, and the virus seemed to be disseminated through the semen of the carrier stallions during mating procedures. The literature also tells us that this virus was contagious to newborn horses and the histopathology of the arterial lesions was quite similar to that of Kawasaki Disease (KD) (Jones *et al.*, 1957; McCollum *et al.*, 1971; Porterfield *et al.*, 1978; Werner *et al.*, 1984; Timoney *et al.*, 1986).

As murine models of vasculitis, 3 strains are well known and widely used; MRL/Mp-*lpr/lpr* (MRL/*lpr*), SL/Ni, and (NZB × NZW)F1 (BWF1). These three models all express endogenous retroviruses, which are common in mice, and the envelope glycoprotein, gp70, of an endogenous virus seems to act as an antigen composing circulating immune complexes, which ultimately induce glomerulonephritis and occasionally systemic necrotizing vasculitis. A detailed description of the arteritis in SL/Ni and MRL/Mp-*lprl/lpr* mice will be presented later in this review.

Most of the vasculitides induced by viruses appeared on the Table 1 seem to be the direct results of lytic viral infection, but some are the results of antibody responses against viral particles of virus-infected cells as are seen in the cases of murine retroviruses. (Alexandersen *et al.*, 1987, 1989)

Table 1 Animal Models Aiming at Vasculitides — Bibliographical Survey 1980–1988

[I] Virus induced
    Equine arteritis virus (toga virus) [Timoney 1986]
    Canine vasculitis (Rabies, parvovirus)
    Feline vasculitis (Coronavirus)
    Mink Aleutian (parvovirus) [Alexandersen 1987, 1989]
    Marmosett (hepatitis A)
    Sheep (ovine progressive pneumonia virus)
    Cattle (African malignant catarrhal fever, herpes)
    Piglet (Aujeszky's disease virus)
    Chelonian (giant cell)
    Murine
      MRL/Mp-*lpr/lpr* (retrovirus) [Nose 1987, 1989a, 1989b]
      SL/Ni (ecotropic retrovirus) [Kyogoku 1977b, 1978, 1980, 1981; Shirane 1979; Kizaki 1979;
                        Matsumoto 1979; Nose 1980; Miyazawa 1987]
        NZB/WF1 (gp70 IC)
        hepatitis virus 3
        polyoma virus

[II] Bacteriae, toxin and others
    Streptococcus pyogenes proteoglycan (mouse) [Ohkuni 1987]
    Erysipelothrix rhusiopathiae neuraminidase (rat) [Nakato 1987]
    E. Coli, endotoxin, LPS (rat, rabbit) [Fujiyama 1986; Kato 1989, 1990; Jones 1957]
    Lactobacillus, cell wall (mouse) [Lehman 1985]
    Pseudomonas, with immunodeficiency [Keren & Wolman 1984]
    Propionibacterium acnes [Kato 1983]
    Staphylococcus
    Candida albicans, alkali extract (mouse) [Murata 1987]
    Mollicutes (cell wall deficient bacteria) of plant origin
    Toxoplasma

[III] Autoimmune and/or immunodeficiency
    Anti-smooth muscle, cellular or humoral [Hart 1985; Moyer 1984; Saji 1987]
    Anti-endothelial [Hart 1985]
    Excessive Ia expression [Moyer 1984; Hansson 1987; Leung 1986]
    GvH [Pals 1985]
    angry macrophage [Nose 1987, 1989a, 1989b]
    Cyclosporin A [Nield 1984]
    Nitrogen mustard, Cyclophosphamide-induced immunideficiency [Keren 1984]

    Athymic rat + hypertension [Christiansen 1983]
    Nude mouse
    Young animals are more sensitive to toxin [Nakato 1987; Fujiyama 1986]

Bacteria and Their Components

Most of the bacterial agents used for the studies of vasculitides are suspected to be an etiological agent of human diseases based on clinical and pathological observations of vasculitis
patients. The suspected bacteria or their components were injected into various experimental
animals expecting to induce histopathological lesions similar to those of humans.
Streptococci (Ohkuni *et al.*, 1987), *Propionibacteria* (Kato *et al.*, 1983), *Pseudomonas*
(Keren and Wolman, 1984), *Lactobacilli* (Lehman *et al.*, 1985) and *Erysipelothrix rhusiopathiae* (Nakato *et al.*, 1987) are all common around us and are not pathogenic to healthy
adult humans. Generally speaking, most of the vasculitides induced by injection of bacteria
or their components are of the immune-complex type. Young rats are more sensitive to
the arteritis induced with the bacteria. Preference to coronary arteries is common in these

bacteria-induced or immune complex type arteritides. The main branches of coronary arteries look like a common vulnerable portion of the vasculature in mammals.

Another experimental animal model using a mold as an inducing agent was reported. Murata *et al.* (1987) injected an alkali extract of *Candida albicans MCLS*-2 strain, which was isolated from feces of KD patients, into the mice and about 80~90% of the animals suffered from granulomatous arteritis. Its histogenetical analysis was, however, insufficient so far.

Immunodeficiency and Autoimmunity

Wolman's experiments (Karen and Wolman, 1984) about *Pseudomonas*-induced arteritis strongly suggested that in immunosuppressed conditions a small dose of common non-pathogenic bacteria could induce systemic vasculitis. Similar phenomena were described in the experiments using immunosuppressive agents such as Cyclosporin A (Neild *et al.*, 1984), nitrogen mustard, cyclophosphamide, or in those performed in thymectomized (Christiansen *et al.*, 1983), athymic nude, or younger mice. In these experiments, immunologically immature or deranged animals showed higher incidences of arteritides. The reason why younger animals are more susceptible to arteritis is still not clear, but we are convinced that without the mature defense mechanism, various toxic or infective agents can directly attack and destroy the vascular wall and can thus cause vasculitides.

Immune responses against various components of vascular walls, such as endothelial (Pals *et al.*, 1985; Leung *et al.*, 1986; Hansson, 1987) or muscle cells (Moyer and Reinisch, 1984; Hart *et al.*, 1985; Saji *et al.*, 1987), and even the responses against their cell surface molecules, such as adhesion molecules, are also suspected to cause arteritis. Some are caused by antibody-induced immunocytolysis, but most are thought to be mediated by cellular immune responses. Cellular attack is more efficient for the destruction of vascular walls. Immunocompetent cells, mostly macrophages, and probably a kind of activated macrophages as observed in MRL/*lpr* mice, have a high efficiency to attack the arterial endothelium as well as medial myocytes, which occasionally express more MHC class II antigens during the course of arteritis than in the normal state. Human endothelial cells usually express HLA-DR antigens even under the normal condition, but smooth muscle cells do not express any class II antigens when not stimulated. Therefore, class II antigen expression on the myocytes is a completely pathological manifestation, as were observed in the cases of human arteritides.

SYSTEMIC VASCULITIDES FROM A PATHOLOGICAL POINT OF VIEW

Table 2 is a classification of vasculitides proposed by Dr. Rüttner of Zürich in the International Congress of Geographical Pathology in 1975. Kawasaki Disease (KD), which will be discussed in detail in the following section, was not listed in this table, because its pathological characteristics had not yet been reported internationally. However, KD should be classified in the second or third category.

The principle of this classification is simple, "in the order of calibers of affected vessels." However, it is very interesting that some histopathological characteristics of arteritides become clearer depending on calibers of affected vessels, that is, in the arteries

Table 2   Proposed classification of vascular diseases (International Society of Geographical Pathology 12th Conference, Zürich (Switzerland) 15th–18th September, 1975)

Classification of Inflammatory Vascular Diseases with Regard to Mainly Affected Vessel Types

Aorta

Mesaoritis luetica
Non-specific aortitis (include. Takayasu-Disease)

Arteries

Thrombangiitis obliterans Buerger (syn.: Endarterriitis obliterans)
Arteriitis temporalis Horton
Generalized giant cell arteriitis

Arterioles and small arteries

Polymyalgia rheumatica sine arteriitica
Polyarteriitis nodosa (syn.: Periarteriitis nodosa Kussmaul-Maier)
Wegener's disease
Granulomatosis Churg-Strauss
Hypersensitivity angiitis Zeek
Vasculitis in primary chronic polyarthritis
Panangiitis in Collagen diseases (Sclerodermia, Lupus erythematodes, Sjögren disease, Dermatomyositis)
Other forms (Cerebral Arteriitis Lindenberg-Spatz, Moya-Moya disease etc.)

Smaller vasculature

Vasculitis of capillaries and arteriolo-venules:
Thrombotic thrombocytopenic purpura Moschcowitz
Vasculitis of the superficial corium (Vasculitis allergica Ruiter, Purpura Schönlein-Henoch, Purpura rheumatica, Maladie de Gougerot etc.)
Vasculitis of the deep corium and subcutis (Erythema nodosum, Erythema induratum Bazin, Necrobiosis lipoidica, Vasculitis racemosa, Vasculitis nodularis etc.)
Concomitant vasculitis in infectious diseases (Lues, Tuberculosis, Bang, Rickettsiosis, Typhoid fever, Viral infections etc.)

of larger calibers arteritides tend to be granulomatous, and on the contrary, in the vessels of smaller calibers necrotizing arteritis is more common and the involvement of an immunological background is more obvious. It means that anatomical or structural factors are important in determining histopathological features of arterial lesions. The vasculitides of smaller vessels such as venules and/or capillaries, which are observed mostly in the skin, may be caused by a kind of Arthus' reaction.

In the following sections of this article, we are going to concentrate on the etiopathogenetic studies of the systemic arteritides. The first discussion will focus on "fibrinoid arteritides", especially those of human collagen diseases and the necrotizing arteritis in SL/Ni mice. Following this is a discussion about "granulomatous arteritides", especially that of Kawasaki Disease and the arteritis of MRL/*lpr* mice.

Fibrinoid Arteritis

Human Cases (Collagen Diseases)

The representative of this category is polyarteritis (periarteritis) nodosa. From the beginning of the 1950s researchers were already aware of the fact that in any type of collagen diseases necrotising arteritides of a similar pathologic manifestation could overlappingly develop, and these cases complicated with arteritis showed worse prognosis soon after the development of arterial lesions (Bevans *et al.*, 1954; Bywaters, 1957; Sokoloff and Bunim, 1957; Schmid *et al.*, 1961). As the histopathological features of these arteritides are quite similar to each other (Kussmaul-Maier type), it is difficult to distinguish which arterial lesions belong to which collagen diseases. For the SLE patients who received long-term glucocorticoid treatment, there is a tendency to die of arteritis instead of lupus glomerulitis. In such cases the sites of immune complex deposition move from glomeruli to arterial walls, mostly into the intermuscular spaces of vascular media, and this is followed by the conspicuous intimal thickening. In fulminant types the histopathologic features are those of necrotizing arteritides, but most of the chronic types are granulomatous (Sawai *et al.*, 1981; Kyogoku, 1985). Recently increased levels of ANCA (anti-neutrophil cytoplasmic antibody) in the sera of fulminant types are stressed as a marker of the development of necrotizing arteritis in SLE. In the cases of PSS fibroelastic intimal proliferation is a common histologic feature, but necrotizing arteritis does occur in the fulminant exsudative type. A few cases of RA with severe systemic arteritides were reported as malignant rheumatoid arthritis. According to our survey, some are granulomatous- but most belong to the necrotizing-arteritis type similar to those known as the Kussmaul-Maier type (Table 3). Patients with such complications usually die within a year of the onset of arteritis (Bevans *et al.*, 1954; Kyogoku, 1975a, 1975b, 1977a, 1983; Sawai and Kyogoku, 1982; Shiokawa, 1978).

Researchers studying collagen diseases tend to classify these cases of collagen diseases that were complicated with systemic arteritis into an overlapping syndrome, which means collagen diseases overlapped with polyarteritis nodosa (Fisher, 1957). Immunohistopathological analyses of the fibrinoid substances in affected arterial walls, however, revealed that, some of the serum components composing the fibrinoid materials are different from one disease to another, although they are quite difficult to distinguish from each other in conventionally stained histopathologic sections. For example, in arterial lesions of SLE, IgG and complements are dominant in the deposits, but in PSS, IgM and complements are dominant in the immune complex form. These results suggest that immune complexes are involved in the development of arterial lesions in both cases but the nature of the complexes is different. On the other hand, in the fibrinoid arteritis accompanied with rheumatoid arthritis, namely in malignant rheumatoid arthritis (Table 3), the deposits in the arterial

Table 3 Pathological features of clinically diagnosed malignant rheumatoid arthritis

	Type	Pathology	Clinical Sign.	Prognosis
Vasculitis (arteritis)	A. Systemic arteritis (Bevans type)	Fibrinoid polyarteritis in visceral organs	pleuritis, pericardits pneumonitis, myocarditis	poor
	B. Peripheral arteritis (Bywaters type)	Granulomatous arteritis in extremities & skin	polyneuritis, skin ulcer, spontan. gangrene, episcleritis, subcutan. nodule, suggillation	good
Non-vasculitis	C. Pneumonitis	Interstitial pneumonitis	pneumonitis, lung fibrosis	poor
	D. General infection (sepsis)	Disseminated suppurative or non-suppurative infection	sepsis?	poor
	E. Others	Amyloidosis & others		poor

(Kyogoku *et al.*, 1979)

Table 4   Different pathogenesis in apparently similar necrotizing arteritides of collagen diseases

Collagen Disease	Arteritis	Deposits
RA	RA Type (Granulomatous)	Fibrin
	PN Type (Fibrinoid necrosis)	IgM > IgG
	EA Type (Intimal thickening)	
SLE	Leucocytoclastic vascultis	IgG + C1, 4, 3, 5
	Arteritis fibrinoid	(IgM)
	intimal thickening	
PSS	Arteritis laminated	IgM + C3
	intimal thickening	Fibrin
	fibrinoid	
PN	Fibrinoid arteritis	Fibrin, IgM, C1q,
	(with intimal thickening)	(HB Type: IgG-IC)

walls are mostly composed of fibrin with some other large molecules, and the deposition of immune complexes is rarely demonstrable. The composition and ratio between these macromolecules vary from one case to another and from one stage to another. The same phenomenon is seen in the cases of genuine polyarteritis nodosa (Table 4). These findings tell us that the deposits by themselves may not be involved as the direct cause of such histopathology but must rather be a result of the augmented permeability of the endothelium (Kyogoku, 1985). If so, what causes the augmented permeability and medial necrosis?

According to our observations, the endothelial damage which induces not only the insudation of fibrinogen and/or immunoglobulins (M and G) but also extravasation of thrombocytes underneath the endothelia must be the initial phenomenon. This is accompanied by the degeneration or death of medial smooth muscle cells, and this damage lets fibrin (fibrinogen + platelet factors) and other large molecules precipitate in the sites of tissue damage and replace the media. Then, the histopathology of fibrinoid arteritis is completed. According to the Arkin's schema (Arkin 1930) the insudation of fibrin always seemed to come from the intimal side of an artery. However, in our observations fibrinoid substances sometimes deposited on the outer side of arterial walls (Sawai and Kyogoku, 1982). In such cases granulomatous changes were usually observed in the adventitia, which was explained by Arkin as a secondary reaction against fibrinoid substances. In our opinion, the granulomatous changes in the adventitia may be a cause of hyperpermeability of the small vessels in the adventitia. This interpretation can be supported by the experiment of Nishikawa (1979) and Watanabe (1984) as was mentioned in the previous section of this article.

Another characteristic of the Kussmaul-Maier type polyarteritis is the fibrocellular intimal thickening, which sometimes narrows and obliterates the lumina. This intimal thickening ends up with a fibrous sclerotic scar that looks like a kind of arteriosclerosis. Why and how do these changes occur? We will discuss this later.

Animal Models of Systemic Fibrinoid Arteritis: SL/Ni Strain of Mice

In order to analyze the process and influencing factors in the pathogenesis and histogenesis of arteritis in more detail, human specimens have limitations to manipulate. Animal models are, therefore, necessary to analyze the etiopathogenesis of fibrinoid arteritis. We had been looking for a good animal model for Kussmaul-Maier type systemic arteritis.

In 1974 very exciting news arrived at our laboratory from Dr. Yasuaki Nishizuka in the Aichi Cancer Center. He had been breeding a substrain of mice named SL, which spontaneously developed extrathymic lymphoma at a high incidence. He found that a strange pathological deviation happened among some colonies of this strain and the incidence of lymphoma became lower, and at the same time the mice started to die of glomerulonephritis and/or systemic arteritis. Histopathological features of the systemic arteritis were quite similar to those of Kussmaul-Maier type fibrinoid arteritis in humans, apart from the occasional granulomatous changes surrounding the affected arteries. This substrain of SL mice was given the name of SL/Ni (Kyogoku, 1977b, 1980).

Fully developed arterial lesions of SL/Ni mice were usually found in the mice older than 9 months. Females were affected with a higher frequency than males and almost all multiparous females had arteritis in the parametrial tissues and/or ovaries. The most surprising finding was to be the budding of a large number of C-type viral particles from plasma membranes of medial smooth muscle cells of parametrial arteries, which was observed just before or at the onset of arteritis (Kyogoku *et al.*, 1978). Shirane *et al.* (Shirane, 1979; Kizaki, 1979; Matsumoto, 1979) demonstrated the deposition of mouse immunoglobulins in the arterial wall, mostly in the intermuscular matrix spaces, and Kawashima *et al.* (Nose *et al.*, 1980; Kyogoku *et al.*, 1981; Miyazawa *et al.*, 1987) demonstrated by more precise immunoelectronmicroscopy that host IgG and C3 deposited along with the dense aggregates of virions in-between the degenerating medial muscle cells, and even on the sites of virus budding from plasma membranes. By using a XC plaque assay, Miyazawa detected infectious ecotropic viruses in the spleen from 27 of 35 SL/Ni mice tested, even as early as one month after birth. Since the ecotropic virus recovered from spleen cells of SL/Ni mice was N-tropic, NIH-3T3 cells were infected with spleen extract of an SL/Ni mouse, and then he established a highly virus-producing clone of the infected cells, A-5, which expressed on their surfaces the MuLV envelope antigen gp70. The gp70 molecule expressed on A-5 cells reacted exclusively with a monoclonal antibody specific for ecotropic viruses, and sera from SL/Ni mice specifically destroyed the cells in a complement-dependent manner (Miyazawa *et al.*, 1987). By Western blot immunoassays most of the SL/Ni sera tested showed strong immunoreactivity with the gp70 of the SL/Ni ecotropic virus.

Before we reported the SL/Ni model of arteritis, the deposition of circulating immune complexes into vascular walls had been the most frequently postulated mechanism for the production of necrotizing arteritis, and the pathogenicity of immune complexes was thought to be determined chiefly by the amount and size of the complexes (Cochrane, 1971; Cochrane and Koffler 1973). At the age when the arteritis started to appear in SL/Ni mice, however, the size and amount of circulating immune complexes were within the level of normal control mice. In the older mice, circulating immune complexes appeared in the sera and they were deposited into the vascular walls through highly permeable endothelia. Therefore, in the polyarteritis of SL/Ni mice, circulating immune complexes may act as accelerators of vascular injury rather than as initiators. These findings suggested that antibody-dependent complement-mediated membrane damage of the smooth muscle cells was the main pathogenetic mechanism producing necrotizing polyarteritis in SL/Ni mice, and that immune complex deposition into the already affected vascular walls was a secondary phenomenon (Nose *et al.*, 1980; Miyazawa *et al.*, 1987) (Figure 1).

Various experimental results have revealed that, not only the immunological mechanisms but also several other factors or mechanisms cause the pathological manifestations

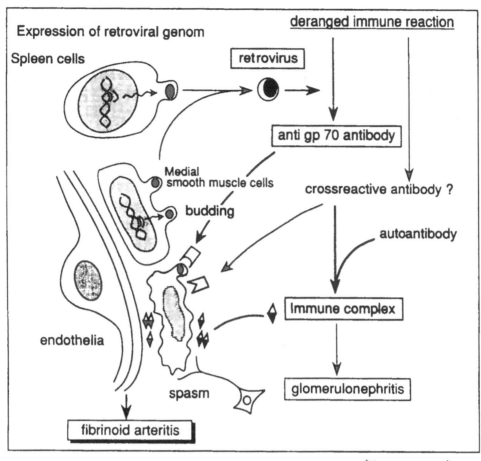

(Kyogoku 1987)

Figure 1 Possible histopathogenesis of arteritis in SL/Ni mice. In SL/Ni strain of mice, derangements in the immune system rendered the mice to make antibodies against the gp70 envelope glycoprotein of an endogenous ecotropic retrovirus. These antibodies had abilities to combine with the gp70 molecules of the retroviruses budding from the surfaces of medial smooth muscle cells. The virions and virus-producing cells were destroyed in a complement-dependent manner. This reaction facilitated the deposition of circulating immune complexes into the sites of muscle cell destruction and accelerated the process of fibrinoid necrosis in the arterial walls.

histologically similar to Kussmaul-Maier type fibrinoid arteritis. Hypertension exceeding 200 mmHg, continuous angiospasms caused by central nervous system catastrophes, or drugs such as β-stimulants could induce similar histopathological lesions. All of them can cause necrosis of medial muscle cells and let the plasma proteins insudate into and trapped within the vascular wall. In these examples no immunological mechanisms is involved to produce an arterial lesion that seems similar to necrotizing arteritis (Kyogoku, 1985).

In brief, degeneration or necrosis of medial muscle cells caused either immunologically or non-immunologically, with resultant increased permeability of the endothelium, are the primary factors that cause necrotizing (fibrinoid) arteritis.

Granulomatous Arteritis

Human Cases: Kawasaki Disease

According to the Zürich classification of vasculitides (Table 1), the arteritides in the vessels of larger calibers such as Takayasu's disease are usually granulomatous. Kawasaki disease, the pathological characteristics of which were first presented in the Zürich congress, is a common infantile febrile disease discovered in Japan. Thousands of cases of this disease have been reported since 1970. It occasionally occurs in other parts of the world. The disease affects infants and children, with 50% of the patients being younger than two years in age. The cause of the disease is still unknown. Affected children develop high fever, congestion of the conjunctiva, skin rash that looks like scarlet fever or erysipelas with edema, strawberry tongues and painless enlargement of the cervical lymph nodes. After about a week from the onset, desquamation of the skin begins on the fingers and toes. In almost all of the patients ECG is abnormal. Thirty five percent of the cases show cardiac hypertrophy, 20% pericardial effusion, and 10% show retarded cardiac output. In 60% of the patients, coronary aneurysms have been detected by angiography. Ninety-nine percent of the children recover from the disease within about two weeks, but a very small number of children, less than 1%, die of myocarditis in an early stage or die suddenly due to myocardial infarction which often attacks after the child has been regarded to be recovered. In the early stage of the disease, diffuse interstitial inflammation throughout the heart with involvement of the coronary arteries and venules was the common pathological manifestation among deceased patients at autopsy. In those cases in which children died more than 10 days after the onset of the disease, sausage-like coronary aneurysms were observed, and sometimes fresh thrombi filling the aneurysms were thought to be the cause of sudden death. Similar vasculitis and interstitial inflammation were also observed in other tissues and organs, including kidneys and pancreas (Kyogoku, 1987; Ritchie, 1990).

Histopathologically, interstitial inflammation involving capillaries and venules all over the body, including the skin, heart, and visceral organs, was the basic pathological feature of KD. Swelling of endothelial cells and adhesion of neutrophils on them were initial recognizable changes, and strangely shaped macrophages followed them (Figure 2). Most of this early inflammation disappeared within 1 or 2 weeks, but there was a tendency of inflammatory cells to accumulate around the adventitia of coronary arteries and gradually infiltrate throughout the arterial walls. The inflammation usually attacked the walls from the outside and caused the dissociation of the connections between the medial muscle cells, ultimately making lattice-like degeneration of the media (Figure 3). In severe cases neutrophils attacked the arterial walls from the intimal side, even by destroying the internal elastic laminae, allowing the thrombocytes migrate into the media (Kyogoku, 1987).

This initial change of arteritis started to heal within 2 weeks after the onset, and very active intimal thickening became remarkable. Activated medial myocytes started to migrate from the media towards the intimal side and then proliferated (Figure 4). These intimal smooth muscle cells changed their phenotypes to a synthetic form which secreted various connective tissue matrices such as hyaluronic acid, laminin, fibronectin, collagen of various types, elastin etc. Thus, fibrocellular intimal thickening developed as a sequela of arteritis. In the segment where the inflammation was quite severe the medial layer was almost completely disappeared, and under the influence of blood pressure and hemody-

Figure 2   Figure 3

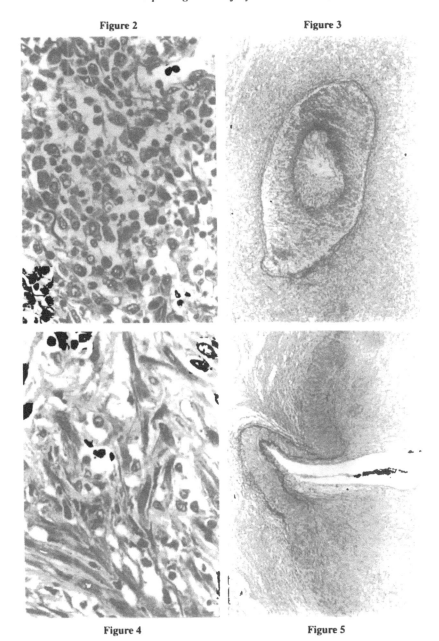

Figure 4   Figure 5

Figures 2–5   Histopathological features of the arteritis in the patients of Kawasaki Disease (KD).
Figure 2   In the early stages of KD diffuse interstitial inflammatory cell infiltration, consisting mainly of strangely-shaped macrophages, some granulocytes and lymphocytes, is the basic pathological feature.
Figure 3   Such inflammatory cells have a tendency to accumulate around the adventitia of affected arteries and gradually infiltrate throughout the arterial walls to cause the dissociation of medial smooth muscle cells.
Figure 4   Usually on the second week after the onset activated medial myocytes start to migrate from the media towards the intimal side and proliferated.
Figure 5   In this particular case, the fibrocellular intimal thickening is more remarkable in the aneurysmal lumina (right half of the picture) and it seems to compensate the widened lumen.

namics sausage-shaped aneurysms were produced. The fibrocellular intimal thickening was more remarkable in the aneurysmal lumina and it seemed to be a reasonable first-aid type repair reaction against the hemodynamics of coronary circulation (Figure 5). In angiographic examinations at this stage aneurysms apparently disappeared, but this finding was only because the luminar sizes of the affected arteries were normalized by the rapid intimal thickening. The walls were thick but had less elasticity. If such a rapid intimal thickening did not take place, the presence of aneurysms would continue for a long time, and sudden thrombosis of the aneurysms might result in acute myocardial infarction.

Experimental Models Aiming at the Mechanism of Intimal Thickening in the Arteritis of Kawasaki Disease — LPS-Induced Arteritis

Why and how does such a remarkable intimal thickening occurs in KD? Based on our precise histopathological observations made on autopsy cases, we concluded that neutrophils and macrophages attacked from the adventitial side of the arteries, and that infants had to have a tendency to over-react against the attack by making such a marked intimal thickening. Therefore, we used the bacterial LPS, a well-known granulocyte-chemotacting substance, as an inflammatory agent and performed a series of experimental studies in young kits of rabbits. Exposed femoral arteries of infantile as well as adult rabbits were wrapped with LPS-immersed oxycellulose. Histopathological examinations performed following the time course of the induced inflammation (Figure 6A) showed the sequential pictures of the development of arterial luminal narrowing. In infants the narrowing reached to the maximal level of 65% obstruction of the lumen in two weeks after application of LPS. In adults the peak of intimal thickening was observed in the fourth week, and the severity of luminal narrowing was less than 40%. After that, thickened intima started to retract, but it never came back to the initial thickness and stayed thickened for a long time. At the maximal point of luminal narrowing the thickened intima was rather cellular and myxomatous because of a large amount of hyaluronic acid. However, in later stages the matrix became acellular and compact because of polymerized collagen and elastin fibers (Figure 7A). Immunohistochemical and electron microscopical analyses revealed that medial smooth muscle cells started to migrate from the media toward the intimal side through the ruptured portions or preexisting fenestrations of the internal elastic lamina. In the intima, they proliferated with occasional mitotic figures, lost their α-smooth muscle actin filaments, and started to synthesize large amounts of extracellular matrices. Thus, smooth muscle cells changed their phenotypes from the contractile form to the synthetic fibroblastic form (Figure 6B).

Another interesting observation obtained through these experiments was that in 14% of rabbit kits, but not in adults, we could produce typical aneurysms. By a histometric study, it was revealed that about 3/4 of the media had been destroyed in such cases. In the cases where injury was not so severe the medial muscle cells reacted against the direct injury and blood pressure, and proliferated to form the reactive intimal thickening. However, if the injury was too excessive to respond by proliferation, the medial muscle cells were defeated by the blood pressure and yielded the way to form aneurysms (Fujiyama, 1986) (Figure 7B, C).

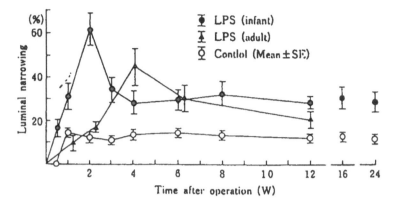

(A) Time course of intimal thickening of femoral arteriae
in the infantile & adult rabbit after stimulation of LPS.

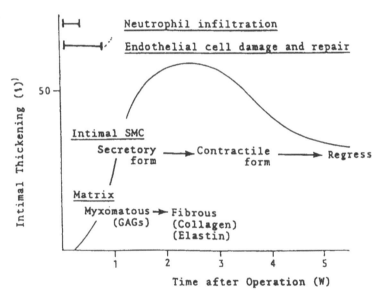

(B) Qualitative and quantitative time course of intimal thickening in
LPS arteritis

Figure 6 LPS-induced arteritis in the femoral artery of infantile and adult rabbits. In the infants the luminal narrowing reached to the maximal level of 65% obstruction in two weeks, but in the adults the peak of intimal thickening was observed in the fourth week and the narrowing was less than 40%. After the peak of obstruction the thickened intimas started to retract. However, the intimas of the LPS-treated rabbits stayed thickened for a long time, and they never came back to the initial thicknesses of the control rabbits.

In Vitro Studies Using Cultured Arterial Smooth Muscle Cells

What induces the phenotypical changes of the smooth muscle cells from the contractile to the synthetic form? By an electron microscopical examination, platelets were always observed near the migrating myocytes, and an increase in the number of platelets in the

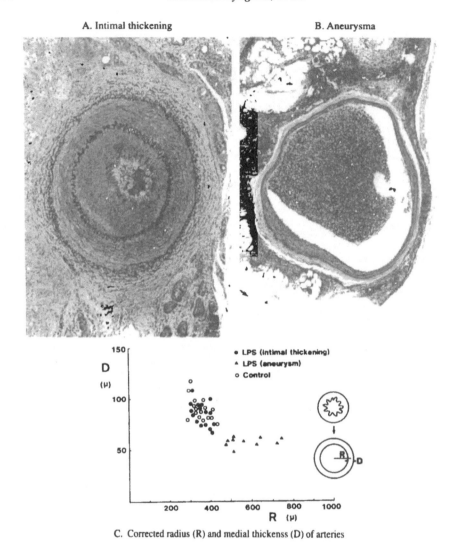

C. Corrected radius (R) and medial thickenss (D) of arteries

Figure 7 Two representative histological patterns of the LPS-induced arteritis in the femoral arteries of infantile rabbits.
(A) Severe intimal thickening of the affected artery (65% obstruction of the lumen) at the second week after application of LPS.
(B) In 14% of the LPS-treated infantile rabbits typical true aneurysms were produced.
(C) In the cases where the injury was not so severe the medial smooth muscle cells reacted by proliferation and successfully respond to bear the blood pressure. However, when the injury was excessive to respond the medial muscle cells were defeated by the blood pressure and yielded the way to form aneurysms. More than 25% of the medial smooth muscle cells should be left alive to respond to the blood pressure.

blood is a common laboratory finding of KD. Therefore, we postulated that platelets or the platelet-derived growth factor (PDGF) must have played a very important role in promoting myocyte proliferation. We, thus, started an *in vitro* experiments using freshly isolated human arterial smooth muscle cells.

The results of the experiments were as follows: 1) LPS itself had no effect on the proliferation of myocytes, 2) granulocytes had only a destructive effect, 3) platelet-rich plasma exhibited a very strong growth-inducing effect on the myocytes, and 4) lysate of smooth muscle cells also had strong proliferation-promoting effects.

In the *in vitro* studies, muscle cells immediately after isolation from the aortic media exhibited a single peak of strong reactivity with anti-α-smooth muscle actin antibody in a FACScan analysis, while no detectable specific fluorescence with anti-prolyl-4-hydroxylase antibody was observed. However, cultured muscle cells of the same origin growing exponentially in the serum-containing medium had a decreased (one tenth of the freshly isolated cells) amount of α-smooth muscle actin, and increased (about ten times more than freshly isolated cells) prolyl-4-hydroxylase (Figure 8A, B). These results

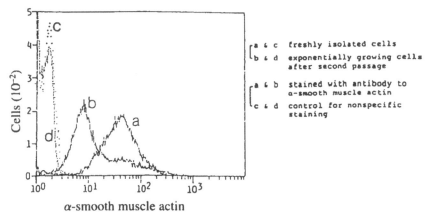

(A) α-smooth muscle actin decreaed to one tenth of the original arterial smooth muscle cells after exponential proliferation.

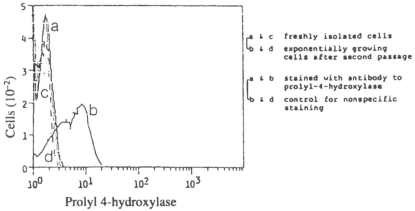

(B) On the contrary, prolyl-4-hydroxylase increase almost ten times during proliferating state.

Figure 8 Phenotypic alterations of arterial smooth muscle cells *in vitro*. Arterial smooth muscle cells show two different phenotypes with regard to their functions of contracture and matrix synthesis. Cultured arterial smooth muscle cells changed their phenotypes in association with their growth and proliferation. (cited from Kato and Kyogoku (1990) with the courtesy of New York Academy of Science)

indicated that the two different forms of the arterial smooth muscle cells had different phenotypes with regard to their functions of contraction and matrix synthesis. These cells seemed to change their phenotypes in association with their growth and proliferation. Cultured smooth muscle cells growth-arrested by serum starvation re-expressed α-smooth muscle actin with rearrangement of the filaments. Furthermore, the rearrangement of α-smooth muscle actin induced by serum starvation was completely blocked by the addition of PDGF, which is a well-known competence growth factor for smooth muscle cells. These results indicated that the expression of α-smooth muscle actin was dependent on whether the cells were growth-competent or not. However, in our experiments possible influence of other growth or transforming factors such as TGF-β or IGF, or matrix components which could be secreted by muscle cells secondary to stimulation with PDGF, could not be ruled out (Figure 9). Further confirmation is necessary to determine the role of PDGF and other growth factors. In addition to the starvation of FBS, the presence of glycosaminoglycan can also stop the proliferation of smooth muscle cells. Heparin, heparan sulfate and fibronectin are major candidates, but hyaluronic acid and chondroitin sulfate had no growth inhibitory effects on smooth muscle cells (Kato and Kyogoku, 1990).

Thus, for the induction of intimal thickening, direct contribution of immunological factors is unlikely, but we can not rule out the indirect influence through a cytokine released from immunologically competent cells.

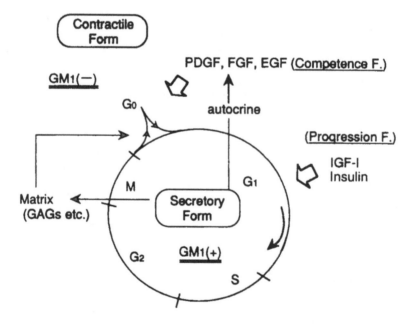

CELL CYCLE OF SMOOTH MUSCLE CELLS

Figure 9 Possible relationship between the cell cycle and the two phenotypes of arterial smooth muscle cells. (GM1, GM1 ganglioside; GAGs, glucosaminoglycane)

Spontaneously Developing Granulomatous Arteritis in MRL/Mp-lpr/lpr Mice

MRL/Mp-*lpr/lpr* mice spontaneously develop a granulomatous arteritis of medium-sized muscular arteries at an early age, in addition to severe immune complex-mediated glomerulonephritis. This disease complex is associated with massive lymphoproliferation of unusual T lymphocytes expressing cell surface antigens specified by Thy-1$^+$, Ly-1$^+$, I-A$^-$, Ly-5$^+$. MRL/Mp→+/+ mice, which have the same genetic background, except for the presence of an *lpr* gene, also develop similar arteritis in a much later stage of life with a reduced incidence and severity. Furthermore, mice of C3H/HeJ, AKR and C57BL/6 strains carrying the *lpr* gene never develop arteritis or other lupus-like lesions, although they do exhibit increased levels of rheumatoid factors, anti-gp70 and/or anti-DNA antibodies and a decrease in IL-2 production. These findings suggest that MRL/Mp→+/+ mice do have the basic disease genes, and that the *lpr* gene may simply act as an accelerator which enhances the formation of granulomatous arteritis in mice with the MRL/Mp background. We studied the effect of transferring the autosomal recessive *gld* gene into the MRL background by means of making reciprocal F$_2$ progenies between MRL→+/+ and C3H-*gld/gld* mice. The resultant MRL mice carrying the homozygous *gld/gld* genotype were almost the same in the incidence of granulomatous arteritis as the *lpr* congenic mice. Thus two distinct, non-allelic genes, *gld* and *lpr*, similarly accelerated lymphoproliferation and arteritis when transferred into the MRL/Mp background (Nose *et al.*, 1989a). Recently, the location of the *lpr* gene was identified in the chromosome 19 at 32 centi-morgan from the centriole (Watanabe *et al.*, 1991). Furthermore, its molecular nature has been identified as a mutant of the gene encoding the Fas antigen (Watanabe-Fukunaga *et al.*, 1992). Therefore, it is now postulated that autoreactive T cells are not completely eliminated in *lpr/lpr* mice, and thus can induce various autoimmune diseases. The same group (Suda and Nagata, 1994) also found that *gld* is a mutant of Fas ligand.

The most striking finding of our studies was that we were able to separate the development of arteritis from glomerulonephritis in homozygous *lpr/lpr* mice of different genetic backgrounds (Nose *et al.*, 1989a). In MRL/Mp-*lpr/lpr* mice, arteritis coincidentally developed in the nephritic mice. The incidence of the overlap of arteritis with nephritis was almost 100%. In the backcross experiments made between MRL/*lpr* and B6/*lpr* mice, however, the development of arteritis segregated from the development of glomerulonephritis. Of 29 backcross mice with arteritis, 9 had no glomerulonephritis. Thus, the predisposition to develop arteritis in these mice was not wholly identical with that to develop glomerulonephritis (Figure 10). (Nose *et al.*, 1989a, 1993)

The arteritis developed in an MRL/Mp-*lpr/lpr* strain of mice was characterized by the presence of massive macrophage infiltration in the adventitia, associated with occasional subendothelial lesions. These macrophages contained, electron-dense phagosomes (dense bodies) which were revealed to contain IgG3 immune complexes (Itoh *et al.*, 1991; Takahashi *et al.*, 1991). These macrophages were in a state of hyperingestion and at the same time in the state of hypodigestion of immune complexes, and extracellularly released large amounts of superoxide and lysosomal enzymes. They were activated and destructive against a tumor cell line *in vitro* in spite of some defects in phagocytic function. A dysfunction in phagosome-lysosome fusion may be involved in these defects, but it seemed to be normalized by adding some lymphokines and/or monokines (Nose *et al.*, 1987, 1989b; Kanno *et al.*, 1994) (Figure 11).

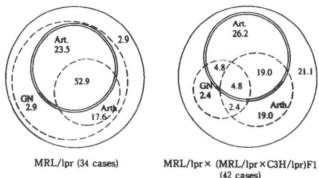

MRL/lpr (34 cases)   MRL/lpr × (MRL/lpr × C3H/lpr)F1
                                        (42 cases)

(A) Effect of rearrangement in the genetic background of MRL/Mp-*lpr/lpr* mice by
hybridization with non-autoimmune *lpr*-bearing mice. Incidence of vasculitis, glomerulonephritis and arthritis in MRL/Mp-*lpr/lpr* × reciprocal (MRL/Mp-*lpr/lpr* × C3H/HeJ-
lpr/lpr) F1 backcross mice, compared with that in MRL/Mp-*lpr/lpr* mice. Numbers in
circles indicate % of incidence of each collagen disease or overlapped collagen disease.
Art.: arteritis, GN.: glomerulonephritis, Arth.: arthritis.

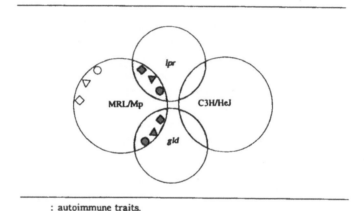

 : autoimmune traits.
○▽◇ : background genes inducing glomerulonephritis, arteritis or arthritis.
●▼◆ : development of glomerulonephritis, arteritis or arthritis.

(B) Segregating background genes inducing collagen diseases in the MRL/Mp strain
of mice.

Figure 10   Genetic segregation of arteritis and/or arthritis from glomerulonephritis in the backcross mice made
between MRL/*lpr* and B6/*lpr* strains. (cited from Nose (1993) with the courtesy of Hokkaido University Press)

These findings suggested that granulomatous arteritis of MRL/*lpr* (or *gld*) mice were
the sequela of the attacks by activated macrophages, which were unusually activated by
some cytokines probably produced from the proliferating T cell-lineage cells under the
influence of *lpr* or *gld* gene expressions and also by ingested immune complexes.

CONCLUSION

As causes of systemic arteritis, immunological mechanisms are very important, but they are
not merely the immune complexes. According to our observations, degenerative changes of

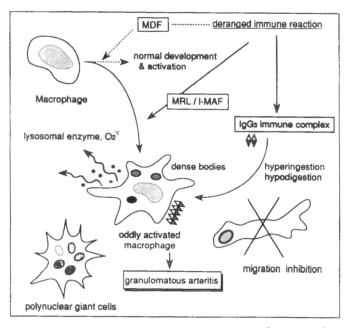

(Kyogoku 1985)

Figure 11 Possible histopathogenesis of arteritis in MRL/*lpr* mice. Oddly activated macrophages are the major component of granulomatous arteritis in MRL/*lpr* mice. They ingest a large amount of IgG3 immune complexes but cannot digest them in their cytoplasm, and thus condense them to form cytoplasmic dense bodies. These cells release various kinds of proteases, cytokines and other destructive substances extracellularly to destroy the cells nearby. (MDF, macrophage-differentiating factor(s); MAF, macrophage activating factor(s)).

medial smooth muscle cells must be more important than augmented permeability of the endothelium, although both are necessary to produce fibrinoid arteritis. In other words, anything that introduces the two above-mentioned factors can cause fibrinoid arteritis. As we have shown in this article type II allergic reaction against the medial smooth muscle cells, allowing the insudation of immune complexes into the site of medial degeneration, can induce most typical fibrinoid arteritis. However, some other factors such as continuous angiospasm or a blood pressure of over 200 mmHg can also make fibrinoid arteritis.

In the case of granulomatous arteritis, macrophage infiltration and reactive fibrocellular intimal thickening are the characteristics of the pathological features. For such macrophage infiltration immunological mechanisms are obviously most important. In most cases, macrophage are inappropriately activated to attack medial muscle cells indiscriminately. Here, the type IV allergic reaction destroying the vascular wall takes place and, immune complex seems to help in activating the macrophages.

Another characteristic of granulomatous arteritis, as well as fibrinoid arteritis, is the intimal thickening, and for that the most important factors are various growth factors including PDGF, TGF-β, IGF, FGF etc., which do not belong to the classical mediators of immune responses. However, they can be released from the cells, either parenchymatous or stromal, whichever were activated by various immunological reactions.

Thus, immunological factors are of foremost importance for the etiopathogenesis of arteritides, although they can not explain everything.

ACKNOWLEDGEMENT

The authors thank Miss K. Higuchi for her excellent secretary works, and T. Park for correcting of the manuscript.

References

Alexandersen, S., Bloom, M.E., Wolfinbergar, J. and Race, R.E. (1987). In situ molecular hybridization for detection of Aleutian mink disease parvovirus DNA by using strand-specific probes: identification of target cells for viral replication in cell cultures and in mink kits with virus-induced interstitial pneumonia. *J. Virol.,* **61**:2407–2419.

Alexandersen, S., Larsen, S., Cohn, A., Uttenthal, A., Race, R.E., Aasted, B., Hansen, M. and Bloom, M.E. (1989). Passive transfer of antiviral antibodies restricts replication of Aleutian mink disease parvovirus *in vivo. J. Virol.,* **63**:9–17.

Arkin, A. (1930). A clinical and pathological study of periarteritis nodosa. *Am. J. Pathol.,* **6**:401–426.

Bevans, M., Nadell, J., Demartini, F. and Ragan, C. (1954). The systemic lesions of malignant rheumatoid arthritis. *Am. J. Med.,* **16**:197–211.

Bywaters, E.G.L. (1957). Peripheral vascular obstruction in rheumatoid arthritis and its relationship to other vascular lesions. *Ann. Rheum. Dis.,* **16**:84.

Christiansen, P., Hansen, U., Svendsen, U.G., Strandgaard, S., Hegedus, V. and Braendstrup, O. (1983). Necrotizing vasculitis in athymic rats with infarct kidney hypertension. *J. Hypert.,* **1**:285–289.

Cochrane, C.G. and Hawkins, D. (1968). Studies on circulatory immune complexes. III. Factors govering the ability of circulating complexes to localize in blood vessels. *J. Exp. Med.,* **127**:137–154.

Cochrane, C.G. (1971). Mechanisms involved in the deposition of immune complexes in tissues. *J. Exp. Med.,* **134**:75s–89s.

Cochrane, C.G. and Koffler, D. (1973). Immune complex disease in experimental animals and man. *Adv. Immunol.,* **16**:185–264.

Dixon, F.J., Vazqnez, J.J., Weigle, W.O. and Cochrane, C.G. (1958). *Arch Pathol.,* **65**:18.

Fisher, E.R. (1957). Polyarteritis nodosa associated with rheumatoid arthritis. *Am. J. Clin. Path.,* **27**:191.

Fujiyama, J., Ogata, H., Sawai, T. and Kyogoku, M. (1986). Experimental studies on the factors to determine the prognosis of systemic arteritis -LPS arteritis-. *Jpn. Pediatric Circulation J.,* **2**:230–237.

Germuth, F.G. and Heptinstall, R.H. (1957). The development of arterial lesions following prolonged sensitization by boving gamma globulin. *Bull. Johns Hopk. Hosp.,* **100**:58.

Hansson, G.K. (1987). Pathogenetic mechanisms of arteritis in KD — a critical analysis. In *Kawasaki Disease,* S.T. Shulman (ed.), pp 383–394. New York: Alan R. Liss, Inc.

Hart, M.N., Tassell, S.K., Sadewasser, K.L., Schelper, R.L. and Moore, S.A. (1985). Autoimmune vasculitis resulting from *in vitro* immunization of lymphocyte to smooth muscle. *Am. J. Pathol.,* **119**:448–455.

Itoh, J., Nose, M. and Kyogoku, M. (1991). Pathogenic significance of serum components in the development of autoimmune polyarteritis in MRL/Mp mice bearing the lymphoproliferative gene. *Am. J. Pathol.,* **139**:511–522.

Jones, J.C., Doll, E.R. and Bryans, J.T. (1957). The lesions of equine viral arteritis. *Cornell Vet.,* **47**:52–69.

Kanno, H., Tachiwaki, O., Nose, M. and Kyogoku, M. (1994). Immune complex degradation ability of macrophages of MRL/Mp-*lpr/lpr* lupus mice and its regulation by cytokine. *Clinical and Exp. Immunol.,* **95**:115–121.

Kato, H., Fujimoto, T., Inoue, O., Kondo, M., Koga, Y., Yamamoto, S., Shingu, M., Tominaga, K. and Sasaguri, Y. (1983). Variant strain of propionibacterium acnes. — A clue to the etiology of KD. *Lancet,* **2**:1383–1388.

Kato, M., Sawai, T. and Kyogoku, M. (1989). Endoarterial proliferation and phenotype modulation of the vascular smooth muscle cell. In *Proceedings of the Third International Kawasaki Disease Symposium* (Tokyo, 1988), T. Kawasaki (ed), pp. 156–158. Tokyo: Japan Heart Foundation.

Kato, M. and Kyogoku, M. (1990). Competence growth factors evoke the phenotypic transition of arterial smooth muscle cells. *Annals of N.Y. Acad. Sci.,* **598**:232–237.

Keren, G. and Wolman, M. (1984). Can pseudomonas infection in experimental animals mimic Kawasaki's disease? *J. Infect.,* **9**:22–29.

Kizaki, T. (1979). The analysis of angitis and nephritis in SL/Ni mouse as a model of immune complex disease — Studies on SL/Ni mouse, an animal model of PN-II. *The Ryumachi,* **19**:246–259.

Kussmaul, A. and Maier, R. (1866). Ueber eine bisher nicht beschriebene eigenthumliche Arteriener Krankung (Periarteritis nodusa), die mit Morbus Brightii und rapid fortschreitender allgemeiner Muskellahmung einhergeht. *Dtsch. Arch. Klin. Med.,* **1**:484.

Kyogoku, M. (1975a). Malignant rheumatoid arthritis. *Infection Inflammation and Immunity*, 5:63–72.

Kyogoku, M. (1975b). Systemic Vascular Changes of Rheumatoid Arthritis in Japan. *Pathologia et Microbiologia*, 43:224–227.

Kyogoku, M. (1977a). Pathological Studies of Malignant Rheumatoid Arthritis (MRA) in Japan. In *Vascular Lesions of Collagen Diseases and Related Conditions*, Y. Shiokawa (ed.), pp. 99–110. Tokyo: University of Tokyo Press.

Kyogoku, M. (1977b). Studies on SL/Ni mouse: Animal model of Polyarteritis nodosa. In *Vascular Lesions of Collagen Diseases and Related Conditions*, Y. Shiokawa (ed.), pp. 356–366. Tokyo: University of Tokyo Press.

Kyogoku, M., Shimomura, R., Kizaki, T. and Shirane, H. (1978). Vasculitis and vascular permeability — as a histogenesis of fibrinoid arteritis. *Angiology*, 18:23–28.

Kyogoku, M. (1980). Pathogenesis of vasculitis in the SL/Ni mouse. In *Systemic Lupus Erythematosus*, M. Fukase (ed.), pp. 281–294. Tokyo: University of Tokyo Press.

Kyogoku, M., Kawashima, M., Nose, M. and Nagao, K. (1981). Pathological studies on the kidney of systemic arteritis. II. Animal models: Comparative studies on the pathogenesis of arteritis and glomerulonephritis of SL/Ni and MRL/l. *Jap. J. Nephrol.*, 23:913–920.

Kyogoku, M. (1983). Malignant rheumatoid arthritis. *Igaku-no-ayumi*, 126:K34–K43.

Kyogoku, M. (1985). Several Trials of Analytial Immunopathology. *Tr. Soc. Pathol. Jpn.*, 74:13–60.

Kyogoku, M. (1987). A Pathological Analysis Kawasaki Disease — With some Suggestions of its Etiopathogenesis. In *Kawasaki Disease*, S.T., Shulman (ed.), pp. 257–273. New York: Alan R. Liss, Inc. N.Y.

Kyogoku, M., Nose, M., Sawai, T. and Miyazawa, M. (1988). Animal models aiming Kawasaki Disease. In *Proceedings of the Third International Kawasaki Disease Symposium* (Tokyo, 1988), T. Kawasaki (ed.), pp. 191–196. Tokyo: Japan Heart Foundation.

Lehman, T.J., Walker, S.M., Mahnovski, V. and McCurdy, D. (1985). Coronary arteritis in mice following the systemic injection of group B lactobacillus casel cell walls in aqueous suspension. *Arthr. and Rheum.*, 28:652–659.

Leung, D.Y.M., Geha, S.R., Newburger, W.J., Burns, C.J., Fiers, W., Lapierre, A.L. and Pober, S.J. (1986). Two monokines, IL-1 and TNF, render cultured vascular endothelial cells susceptible to lysis by antibodies circulating during KD. *J. Exp. Med.*, 164:1958–1972.

Matsumoto, M. (1979). Studies on the antibody producing system of SL/Ni mouse — Studies on SL/Ni mouse, an animal model of PN-III, *The Ryumachi*, 19:297–307.

McCollum, W.H., Prickeit, M.E. and Bryans, J.T. (1971). Temporal distribution of equine arteritis virus in respiratory mucosa, tissue and body fluids of horse infected by inhalation. *Rev. Vet. Sci.*, 12:459–464.

Miyazawa, M., Nose, M., Kawashima, M. and Kyogoku, M. (1987). Pathogenesis of arteritis of SL/Ni mice. Possible lytic effect of anti-gp70 antibodies on vascular smooth muscle cells. *J. Exp. Med.*, 166:890–908.

Moyer, C.F. and Reinisch, C.L. (1984). The role of vascular smooth muscle cells in experimental autoimmune vasculitis (I). *Am. J. Path.*, 117:380–390.

Murata, H., Iijima, H., Naoe, S., Atobe, T., Uchiyama, T. and Arakawa, S. (1987). The pathogenesis of experimental arteritis induced by Candida alkali extract in mice. *Jpn. J. Exp. Med.*, 57:305–313.

Nakato, H., Shinomiya, K., Mikawa, H. (1987). Adhesion of Erysipelothrix rhusiopathiae to cultured rat aortic endothelial cells — Role of bacterial neuraminidase in the induction of arteritis. *Pathology Research and Practice*, 182:255–260.

Neild, G.H., Irony, K. and Williams, D.G. (1984). Severe systemic vascular necrosis in cyclosporin treated rabbits with acute serum sickness. *Brit. J. Exp. Path.*, 65:731–743.

Nishikawa, J. (1979). Experimental allergic angitis in hyperimmunized rabbits. The role of preexisting periarterial specific antibody in the development of vascular lesion. *Jpn. J. Allergol.*, 28:339.

Nose, M., Kawashima, M., Yamamoto, K., Sawai, T., Yaginuma, N., Nagao, K. and Kyogoku, M. (1980). Role of immune complex in the pathogenesis of arteritis in SL/Ni mice: possible effect as accelerator rather than as initiator. In *New Horizons in Rheumatoid Arthritis*, Y. Shiokawa, T. Abe and Y. Yamauchi (eds.), pp. 109–115. Amsterdam: Excerpta Medica.

Nose, M., Tachiwaki, O., Miyazawa, M., Kanno, H. and Kyogoku, M. (1987). Macrophage functions and their regulation in MRL/l lupus mice. In *New Horizons in Animal Models for autoimmune Disease*, M. Kyogoku and H. Wigzell (eds.), pp. 219–231. Orlando: Academic Press Inc.

Nose, M., Nishimura, M. and Kyogoku, M. (1989a). Analysis of granulomatous arteritis MRL/Mp autoimmune disease mice bearing lymphoproliferative genes. The use of mouse genetics to dissociate the development of arteritis and glomerulonephritis. *Amer. J. Pathol.*, 135:271–280.

Nose, M., Mori, S., Kanno, H., Taniguchi, Y., Takahashi, S., Takano, R., Kyogoku, M. and Nishimura, M. (1989b). Systemic arteritis in MRL/lpr mice giving rise to a concept of cell-mediated vasculitis not initiated by immune complexes. In *Proceedings of the Third International Kawasaki Disease Symposium* (Tokyo, 1988), T. Kawasaki (ed.), pp. 135–137. Tokyo: Japan Heart Foundation.

Nose, M. (1993). Genetic basis of vasculitis in lupus mice. In *Intractable Vascutis Syndromes*, T. Tanabe (ed.) pp. 145–153, Sapporo; Hokkaido University Press.

Ohkuni, H., Todome, Y., Yokomuro, K., Kimura, Y., Ishizaki, M., Fukuda, Y., Masugi, Y. and Hamada, S. (1987). Coronary arteritis in mice after systemic injection of bacterial cell wall peptidoglycan. *Jpn. Circ. J.*, **51**:1357–1361.

Pals, S.T., Radaszkiewicz, T., Roozendaal, L. and Gleichmann, E. (1985). Chronic progressive polyarthritis and other symptoms of collagen vascular disease induced by GvH reaction. *J. Immunol.*, **134**:1475–1482.

Porterfield, J.S., Casals, J., Chumakov, M.P., Gaidamovich, S.Y., Hannoun, C., Holmes, I.H., Horzinek, M.C., Mussgay, M., Oker-Blom, N., Russell, P.K. and Trent, D.W. (1978). Togaviridae. *Intervirology*, **9**:129–148.

Rich, A.R. and Gregory, J.E. (1943). The experimental demonstration that periarteritis nodosa is manifestation of hypersensitivity. *Bull. Johns Hopk. Hosp.*, **72**:65.

Ritchie, A.C. (1990). In Boyd's textbook of pathology, ninth edn, pp. 631–632. London: Lea & Fabiger.

Saji, T., Umezawa, T., Matsuo, N., Hashiguchi, R. and Matsuura, H. (1987). Cytotoxicity of sera from KD to rat aortic smooth muscle cells. *Prog. Clin. Biol. Res.*, **250**:559–561.

Sawai, T., Sato, N. and Kyogoku, M. (1981). Pathological studies on the kidney of systemic arteritis. *Jpn. J. Nephorol.*, **23**:905–912.

Sawai, T. and Kyogoku, M. (1982). Pathological studies on the arterial lesion of MRA — analysis of two autopsy cases — *Cinical Immunology*, **14**:389–396.

Schmid, F.R., Cooper, N.S., Ziff, M. and McEwen, C. (1961). Arteritis in rheumatoid arthritis. *Am. J. Med.*, **23**:56–83.

Shiokawa, Y. (1978). Series "Approaches to the intractable diseases through case reports" No. 6 "Malignant rheumatoid arthritis" Tokyo: Promotion of Medicine Foundation.

Shirane, H. (1979). Histopathological and immunohistological studies on the arteritis and glomerulonephritis of SL/Ni mouse — Studies on the SL/Ni mouse, an animal model of PN-I, *The Ryumachi*, **19**:228–245.

Sokoloff, L. and Bunim, J. (1957). Vascular lesions in rheumatoid arthritis. *J. Chron. Dis.*, **5**:688.

Suda, T. and Nagata, S. (1994). Purification and characterization of the Fas-ligand that induces apoptosis. *J. Exp. Med.*, **179**:873–879.

Takahashi, S., Nose, M., Sasaki, J., Yamamoto, T. and Kyogoku, M. (1991). IgG3 production in MRL/lpr mice is responsible for development of lupus nephritis. *J. Immunol.*, **147**:515–519.

Timoney, P.J., McCollum, W.H., Roberts, A.W. and Murphy, T.W. (1986). Demonstration of the carrier state in naturally acquired equine arthritis virus infection in the stallion. *Res. Vet. Sci.*, **41**:279–280.

Watanabe, Y. and Nishikawa, J. (1984). Serum sickness type arteritis. In *Experimental animal models of intractable diseases*, M. Kyogoku (ed.), pp. 527–542 Tokyo: Soft Science Inc.

Watanabe, T., Sakai, Y., Miyawaki, S., Shimizu, A., Koiwai, O. and Ohno, K. (1991). A molecular genetic linkage map of mouse chromosome-19 including the lpr, Ly-44 and T & T genes. *Biochem. Genetic.*, **29**:325–336.

Watanabe-Fukunaga, R., Brannan, I.C., Copeland, G.N., Jenkins, A.N. and Nagata, S. (1992). Lympho-proliferation disorder in mice explained by defects in Fas antigen that mediate apoptosis. *Nature*, **356**:314–317.

Werner, L.L., Gross, T.L. and Hillidge, C.J. (1984). Acute necrotizing vasculitis and thrombocytopenia in a horse. *J. Am. Vet. Med. Ass.*, **185**:87–90.

6 The Role of Autoimmunity to Myeloid Lysosomal Enzymes in the Pathogenesis of Vasculitis

Jan Willem Cohen Tervaert and Cees G.M. Kallenberg

Department of Clinical Immunology, University Hospital, Groningen, The Netherlands

INTRODUCTION

Vasculitides are an extraordinary heterogeneous group of inflammatory disorders with diverse clinical manifestations. The vasculitic process can affect blood vessels of any type, size, or location, and therefore can cause dysfunction in virtually any organ system. The disease may be infectious or noninfectious in origin; may constitute the major and primary manifestation of a number of clinical syndromes or it may represent a relatively minor component of another underlying disease; may be systemic or limited to one or only a few organs. Classification of patients suffering from primary vasculitides is based on the predominant type and caliber of the blood vessel involved (Alarcón-Segovia, 1980; Lie, 1992; Lie, 1994) (Table 1). Recently, classification criteria were published for

Table 1   Classification of systemic idiopathic vasculitides

   I.   Affecting predominantly large- and medium-sized blood vessels
       1. Takayasu's arteritis
       2. Giant cell arteritis/temporal arteritis

   II.   Affecting predominantly medium-sized blood vessels
       1. Polyarteritis nodosa
       2. Kawasaki disease

   III.   Affecting predominantly medium- and small-sized blood vessels
       1. Churg Strauss Syndrome
       2. Wegener's Granulomatosis
       3. Microscopic polyangiitis

   IV.   Affecting predominantly small-sized blood vessels
       1. Henoch-Schönlein Purpura
       2. Essential cryoglobulinemic vasculitis
       3. Cutaneous leukocytoclastic angiitis

---

major vasculitic syndromes (Hunder, 1990) and at a consensus conference names and definitions for the most common forms of vasculitis were adopted (Jennette, 1994).

In most forms of vasculitis there is some evidence that antigen-antibody complexes participate in the pathogenesis of the vascular inflammation (Savage and Ng, 1986; Haynes, 1992). Previous studies have established two pathogenetic mechanisms: deposition of circulating immune complexes with subsequent complement activation and inflammation, and local formation of immune complexes due to interactions between circulating antibodies and blood vessel wall antigens *in situ*. Unfortunately, the nature of the involved antigen is known in very few disorders only. Recently, several additional or alternative pathways have been explored (Abramson and Weissman, 1988; Kallenberg, 1991a; Cotran and Pober, 1992). Although underlying immunopathogenic mechanisms of different forms of vasculitis may be diverse, all vasculitic syndromes share a final common pathway, in which vessel wall inflammation compromises the patency of the vessel lumen and, consequently, causes ischemic tissue damage.

The demonstration of autoantibodies to myeloid lysosomal enzymes, i.e., antineutrophil cytoplasmic antibodies (ANCA), in patients with various forms of vasculitis (reviewed in Kallenberg, 1992) has facilitated the diagnostic work-up and classification of those patients (Cohen Tervaert, 1991a; Cohen Tervaert and Kallenberg, 1993a). In addition, growing evidence now indicates that autoimmune responses to myeloid lysosomal enzymes are implicated in the pathogenesis of ANCA-associated vasculitides. In this chapter, we will evaluate the current state of ANCA with respect to clinicopathologic syndromes, review current concepts concerning the pathophysiology of ANCA-associated vasculitis, and focus special attention on the role of autoimmunity to myeloid lysosomal enzymes in these disorders.

ANTI-NEUTROPHIL CYTOPLASMIC ANTIBODIES

Autoantibodies directed against cytoplasmic constituents of polymorphonuclear leukocytes and/or monocytes, i.e. antineutrophil cytoplasmic antibodies (ANCA), were first described in 1982 by Davies *et al.* in a few patients with renal vasculitis (Davies, 1982). In 1985, it became apparent that ANCA are a sensitive and specific marker for Wegener's Granulomatosis (WG), one of the granulomatous vasculitides that is characterized by chronic inflammatory lesions of the respiratory tract usually accompanied by renal and/or systemic vasculitis (Van der Woude, 1985). Since then, ANCA were also described in patients with idiopathic and/or vasculitis-associated necrotizing crescentic glomerulonephritis (NCGN) (Savage, 1987; Falk and Jennette, 1988), clinically manifesting as rapidly progressive glomerulonephritis and histologically characterized by the presence of fibrinoid necrosis of glomerular capillary loops ('renal vasculitis'), extracapillary proliferation, and absence of immunoglobulin deposits. Later on, ANCA were also described in another form of granulomatous vasculitis, i.e., the Churg Strauss syndrome (CSS), characterized by asthma, hypereosinophilia and systemic vasculitis (Cohen Tervaert, 1991b). During these studies it was recognized that ANCA in patients with vasculitis are directed against myeloid lysosomal enzymes such as proteinase 3 (PR3), myeloperoxidase (MPO), and/or elastase (Goldschmeding, 1989a; Goldschmeding, 1989b).

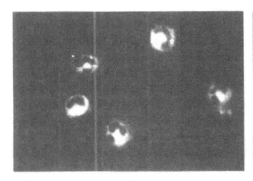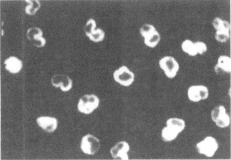

Figure 1   Staining of ethanol fixed neutrophils by indirect immunofluorescence by sera producing: (a) a characteristic cytoplasmic staining pattern with accentuation of the fluorescence intensity in the area within the nuclear lobes (c-ANCA, left), (b) a perinuclear staining pattern (p-ANCA, right).

ANCA: AUTOANTIBODIES DIRECTED AGAINST DIFFERENT ANTIGENS

ANCA are routinely detected by indirect immunofluorescence (IIF) on ethanol fixed neutrophils (Wiik, 1989). At least three different patterns of fluorescence can be distinguished: a cytoplasmic pattern with accentuation of the fluorescence intensity in the area within the nuclear lobes (cytoplasmic or c-ANCA; Figure 1A), a perinuclear pattern (p-ANCA; Figure 1B), and a more diffuse cytoplasmic staining pattern (atypical ANCA).

c-ANCA

The first pattern has been recognized as a characteristic staining pattern produced by the sera of most patients with active, untreated WG (Van der Woude, 1985; Cohen Tervaert, 1989). The antigen recognized by most sera that produce this classical ANCA pattern (c-ANCA) has been identified as PR3, a third serine protease from the azurophilic granules of neutrophils different from elastase and cathepsin G, the other two serine proteases from these granules (Goldschmeding, 1989b; Niles, 1989; Lüdemann, 1990). The full length c-DNA for PR3 has been cloned and was shown to code for a 29 kD glycoprotein of 228 aminoacids (Campanelli, 1990a) that is identical to p29b, a recently described antibiotic protein from human neutrophils (Campanelli, 1990b), and myeloblastin, a growth-promoting protein from myeloid cells (Bories, 1990). The enzyme is cationic (pI 9.0). The active sites of PR3 and elastase are very similar. PR3 degrades elastin and a variety of other matrix proteins and is physiologically inhibited by α_1-antitrypsin (Kam, 1992; Dolman, 1992). Most antibodies to PR3 recognize conformational determinants on the molecule (Bini, 1992) and interfere with the inactivation of the enzyme by α_1-antitrypsin (Van de Wiel, 1992), suggesting that the epitope(s) in question are localized at or near the catalytic domain of the molecule. PR3 is localized in the azurophilic granules from myeloid cells and is released when degranulation of neutrophils and monocytes occurs upon inflammatory stimulation by a process involving fusion of the membrane of azurophilic granules with the plasmamembrane (Calafat, 1990).

p-ANCA

P-ANCA are found in a wide variety of disorders such as vasculitis, various rheumatic diseases, inflammatory bowel diseases, autoimmune liver diseases, and infectious diseases such as HIV-infection. P-ANCA positive sera produce a cytoplasmic staining pattern when neutrophils are fixed with a cross-linking fixative such as paraformaldehyde (Charles, 1989). Several different antigens may be recognized by p-ANCA positive sera (Cohen Tervaert, 1993b). In patients with vasculitis and/or glomerulonephritis, many p-ANCA positive sera contain antibodies to myeloperoxidase (MPO) (Falk, 1988; Cohen Tervaert, 1990a; Cohen Tervaert, 1990b). MPO is a highly cationic protein (pI 11.0) with a m.w. of 146 kD, localized in the azurophilic granules from myeloid cells. The enzyme plays a critical role in the generation of reactive oxygen species (Weiss, 1989). Most anti-MPO positive sera do not seem to inactivate the enzymatic activity of the molecule (Roberts, 1991; Falk, 1992). The autoimmune response to MPO is directed against multiple epitopes as demonstrated by inhibition studies using anti-MPO positive sera and a set of different monoclonal antibodies (Cambridge, 1991). Both conformational and linear epitopes are recognized by anti-MPO positive sera (Pedrollo, 1993).

In sera that are routinely submitted for ANCA determination many p-ANCA positive sera do not contain antibodies to MPO (Cohen Tervaert, 1990b; Cohen Tervaert, 1993c). A number of these anti-MPO-negative p-ANCA sera contain antibodies to other defined granular constituents of neutrophils. In particular, autoantibodies have been demonstrated to elastase (Cohen Tervaert, 1993d) and cathepsin G (Halbwachs-Mecarelli, 1992), the two other serine proteases that are present in the azurophilic granules, to β-glucuronidase (Kaneko, 1993), another constituent of those granules, and to lactoferrin (Peen, 1993; Sinico, 1993) and lysozyme (Schmitt, 1993) which are constituents of the specific granules. In addition, autoantibodies have been detected that are directed against cytosolic components of neutrophils, in particular to α-enolase (Moodie, 1993).

Atypical Cytoplasmic ANCA

The third pattern, an atypical cytoplasmic fluorescence staining, has not been linked to particular antigens nor to specific disease entities until now. Occasionally, sera that produce this pattern contain antibodies to MPO (Cohen Tervaert, 1990b) or to elastase (Cohen Tervaert, 1993d).

ANCA: TOOLS FOR DIAGNOSIS AND FOLLOW-UP OF PATIENTS WITH VASCULITIS

Autoantibodies to myeloid lysosomal enzymes are predominantly found in the following diseases: the Churg-Strauss Syndrome, Wegener's granulomatosis, microscopic polyangiitis, and idiopathic necrotizing and/or crescentic glomerulonephritis. The most important clinical findings in these diseases will be briefly described (see also Table 2).

Churg-Strauss Syndrome

The Churg-Strauss (CSS) syndrome is a distinctive clinical syndrome characterized by asthma, allergic rhinitis, eosinophilia, and systemic vasculitis.

Table 2   Characteristics of ANCA-associated vasculitides

DISEASE	CLINICAL	BIOPSY SITE	PR 3 ANTIBODY	MPO ANTIBODY
Churg-Strauss syndrome	asthma, eosinophilia, neuropathy	skin, muscle/ nerve	+	++++
Wegener's granulomatosis	nose bleeds, nephritis, lung infiltrates	nose, kidney, lung	++++	++
microscopic polyangiitis	nephritis, purpura, haemoptysis	kidney, skin	+++	+++
idiopathic necrotizing and/or crescentic glomerulonephritis	nephritis, malaise	kidney	++	+++

++++ = > 70% of patients; +++ = 30%–70% of patients; ++ = 10–30% of patients; + = 3–10% of patients; − = < 1% of patients

Not much is known about the frequency of occurrence in different races and/or the epidemiology of CSS. Males are slightly more often affected than females. The disease has been observed at any age; its peak incidence is in the third and fourth decades.

The disease elapses in a phasic pattern (Lanham and Churg, 1991):

a. a prodromal phase characterized by allergic disease -i.e., allergic rhinitis, nasal polyposis, and asthma- and eosinophilic infiltrative disease -e.g., Löffler's syndrome and eosinophilic gastroenteritis-

b. a vasculitic phase, that follows the prodromal phase after 5–10 years (range 0–58 years).

c. a postvasculitic phase, that is dominated by allergic disease, hypertension, and incomplete recovery from major organ damage, e.g., disability due to peripheral nerve damage or recurrent cardiac failure.

Patients initially present with symptoms of rhinorrhea, nasal obstruction, and recurrent sinusitis. Nasal polyposis is frequently found; prominent mucosal ulceration -as seen in WG- is rare. Asthma appears unusually late in life (mean age of onset 35 years) and in only a minority of the patients a positive family history of atopy is recorded. Asthma may be mild initially. Attacks increase, however, in severity and frequency and many patients suffer from recurrent respiratory infections. The vasculitic phase is nearly always heralded by malaise, (often profound) weight loss, fever, (severe) disabling muscle weakness, and arthralgias. Other features of the vasculitic phase are purpura or nodular lesions, abdominal pain, pericarditis, and glomerulonephritis (Lanham and Churg, 1991). Involvement of the peripheral nervous system dominates the clinical picture in most patients. Mononeuritis multiplex or a symmetric polyneuropathy can be found in 65%–80% of the patients (Cohen Tervaert, 1993a).

Table 3   ACR criteria for Churg-Strauss syndrome

* Asthma
* Eosinophilia > 10%
* Mononeuropathy or polyneuropathy
* Pulmonary infiltrates, non-fixed
* Paranasal sinus abnormality
* Extravascular eosinophils

For classification purposes, a patient shall be said
to have Churg-Strauss syndrome if at least 4 of
these 6 criteria are positive.

CSS is a disorder affecting patients with an allergic diathesis that is atypical with
respect to the late onset of symptoms, frequent absence of family history, severity of
upper respiratory tract disease and exaggerated eosinophil response. Repeated antigenic
stimulation (e.g., hyposensitization therapy) in such patients probably triggers a self-per-
petuating vasculitic process (Lanham and Churg, 1991).

The diagnosis of CSS (Table 3) is based on the presence of asthma, peripheral eosinophilia, clinical signs of systemic vasculitis, the presence of myeloperoxidase antibodies,
histopathologic findings, and/or angiographic abnormalities. Biopsy of skin lesions, peripheral nerves, and/or muscles may reveal necrotizing vasculitis (often with many eosinophils
in the infiltrate, but only occasionally with granulomas), and kidney biopsies may show
focal necrotizing and/or crescentic glomerulonephritis (only occasionally with vasculitis).
The classic triad of necrotizing vasculitis, tissue infiltration by eosinophils, and extravascular granulomas is only seldom found in biopsy specimens (Lanham and Churg, 1991).

Wegener's Granulomatosis

Wegener's granulomatosis (WG) is a rare disease characterized by chronic necrotizing
inflammatory lesions of the respiratory tract usually accompanied by glomerulonephritis
and/or systemic vasculitis.

WG occurs more frequently in caucasians than in other races. There is an increased
incidence of the disease in Northern Europe. Males are slightly more frequently affected
than females. The disease has been observed at any age, but the peak incidence is in the
fourth and fifth decades.

Initial symptoms of the disease may vary from patient to patient. Patients may present
with rapidly progressing disease or with a more indolent progression of the disease. In
this latter group delays in diagnosis of more than 1 year are frequently observed. Most
patients initially present with upper airway illness such as serosanguinolent nasal discharge, nasal obstruction, and recurrent sinusitis. Other frequently observed symptoms
and signs are otitis media, hemoptysis, episcleritis, arthralgias, skin disease (e.g., palpable
purpura or ulcers), microscopic hematuria and asymptomatic pulmonary infiltrates. In
addition, constitutional symptoms such as low grade fever, weight loss, anorexia, muscle
weakness, and fatigue are usually present. Finally, at the time of diagnosis roughly two
out of three patients have nose, sinus, lung, kidney, and joint involvement, whereas half
of the patients have ear, eye, and skin involvement. Typical sites of involvement of
locoregional WG usually are: nasopharynx ("midline granuloma"), lungs ("limited WG"),
orbit ("pseudotumor of the orbit"), or trachea.

Table 4   ACR criteria for Wegener's granulomatosis

---

* Nasal or oral inflammation
* Abnormal chest radiograph
* Abnormal urinary sediment
* Granulomatous inflammation on biopsy

For purposes of classification, a patient shall be said
to have Wegener's granulomatosis if at least 2 of
these 4 criteria are present.

WG is a disorder affecting patients with chronic and/or recurrent upper respiratory tract infections. Most patients with WG are chronic nasal carriers of *Staphylococcus aureus*, which may trigger the vasculitic process (Stegeman, 1994).

The diagnosis of WG (Table 4) is based upon the presence of typical clinical symptoms and signs, the demonstration of antibodies to proteinase 3, and histopathologic findings. Histologic examination of nasal and/or sinus biopsies frequently shows granulomatous inflammation (often without vasculitis), kidney biopsies show pauci-immune necrotizing and/or crescentic glomerulonephritis (only occasionally with vasculitis and/or granulomas), and open lung biopsies show in more than 90% of the cases the combination of granulomatous inflammation, geographic necrosis, and vasculitis (Hoffman, 1992).

Microscopic Polyangiitis

Microscopic polyangiitis (MPA) is characterized by necrotizing and/or crescentic glomerulonephritis (NCGN) ("renal vasculitis") and a multisystem vasculitis involving small ("microscopic") and/or medium-sized vessels (Jennette, 1994).

MPA shares many features with WG (Savage, 1985). Clinically, the most important difference is the lack of respiratory tract manifestations -apart from alveolar hemorrhage- in MPA. Granulomatous inflammation of the respiratory tract is never found in MPA.

The peak incidence is in the fifth decade. Patients present with malaise, fever, arthralgias, and purpura in combination with (severely) impaired renal function, proteinuria, and microscopic hematuria. In addition, 30%–60% of the patients have hemoptysis with or without alveolar hemorrhage. The diagnosis of microscopic polyangiitis is based on clinical findings, the presence of either proteinase 3 or myeloperoxidase antibodies, and histopathologic findings. The diagnosis can only be made after exclusion of other recognized vasculitic syndromes most notably WG. Histologic examination of the kidney shows pauci-immune necrotizing glomerulonephritis with crescent formation and (in a minority of the cases) vasculitis involving arterioles and/or interlobular arteries. Skin biopsies show leukocytoclastic angiitis involving capillaries, arterioles, and venules. No immune deposits are detected by immunofluorescence.

Idiopathic Necrotizing and/or Crescentic Glomerulonephritis

This form of glomerulonephritis can be considered a form of necrotizing small vessel vasculitis limited to the kidney. The renal biopsy in these patients shows identical findings as in renal biopsies of patients with other forms of ANCA-associated vasculitides: necrotizing and/or crescentic glomerulonephritis, that is characterized by paucity of immunoglobulin and complement deposition in the glomeruli. Many patients have constitutional symptoms like fatigue, low-grade fever, and weight loss. In addition, signs suggestive of systemic involvement like arthralgias, purpura, and/or serosanguineous nasal discharge may be present during the initial phase of the disease or during a relapse. Most patients with idiopathic NCGN are positive for anti-myeloperoxidase antibodies, the remaining being positive for antibodies against proteinase 3. Both the clinical and serological findings place this disorder within one spectrum of diseases with WG and MPA (Cohen Tervaert, 1990a).

Clinical Association of Proteinase 3 Antibodies

Proteinase 3 (PR3) antibodies are highly sensitive for active WG. In cases of generalized WG PR3 antibodies are present in more than 90% of the cases (Cohen Tervaert, 1989; Nölle, 1989), whereas in patients with locoregional disease limited to one or two organs PR3 antibodies are detected in about two third of the cases (Nölle, 1989). When generalized WG and more limited forms of WG are taken together, the sensitivity of PR3 antibodies for active disease can be ascertained as 81% (Kallenberg and Cohen Tervaert, 1991b). PR3 antibodies have also been found in about 50% of patients with MPA (Gaskin, 1991; Geffriaud-Ricouard, 1993) and in a minority of patients with idiopathic NCGN (Jennette, 1989; Cohen Tervaert, 1990a). A substantial proportion of the patients that have anti-PR3 associated MPA and/or anti-PR3 associated idiopathic NCGN actually may have an incomplete form of WG since they have signs of upper airway involvement suggestive of WG either at the start of their disease or during a relapse. Some of these patients fulfill the American College of Rheumatology (ACR) 1990 criteria for the classification of WG. Several different groups have studied the specificity of PR3 antibodies both in unselected groups of patients and in selected groups of patients with a wide variety of renal, autoimmune, vasculitic, infectious, or lymphoproliferative disorders. When these data are combined, the specificity of PR3 antibodies for the WG disease spectrum can be ascertained as 98% or more (Kallenberg and Cohen Tervaert, 1991b).

Clinical Association of Myeloperoxidase Antibodies

MPO antibodies are found in about 70%–80% of patients with CSS (Cohen Tervaert, 1991a; Guillevin, 1993). MPO antibodies are found also in patients with biopsy-proven necrotizing arteritis involving small or medium-sized vessels, who have either asthma without eosinophilia or eosinophilia without asthma but do not fulfill the ACR 1990 criteria for CSS (Cohen Tervaert, 1991a). These latter patients probably suffer from an incomplete form of CSS. Finally, MPO antibodies are found in nearly all patients with pauci-immune NCGN who are negative for PR3 antibodies (Cohen Tervaert, 1990a; Niles, 1991). Only some of these latter patients have CSS; most have either idiopathic NCGN or NCGN that is associated with MPA or WG (Jennette, 1989; Cohen Tervaert, 1990a; Cohen Tervaert, 1990b).

The specificity of MPO antibodies for idiopathic renal and/or systemic vasculitis has been studied both in selected and unselected groups of patients and was found to be 98% (Cohen Tervaert, 1990a; Cohen Tervaert, 1990b; Niles, 1991; Bosch, 1992). MPO antibodies are, however, also detected in 30-50% of patients with anti-GBM disease, in patients with drug-induced systemic and/or renal vasculitis, and occasionally in patients with systemic lupus erythematosus (reviewed in Kallenberg, 1994).

Clinical Association of Other ANCA Specificities

Elastase antibodies are only infrequently found in sera from patients with (a presumptive diagnosis of) vasculitis (Cohen Tervaert, 1993d). In addition, these antibodies are also found in patients with propylthiouracil-induced vasculitis and in patients with hydralazine-induced NCGN (Nässberger, 1991; Dolman, 1993a). The low prevalence of these antibodies limits their diagnostic significance, although they appear to be rather specific for the aforementioned disorders. ANCA directed to lactoferrin, cathepsin G, lysozyme, and to as yet unknown 66/67 kd and 63/54 polypeptides occur in a wide variety of inflammatory disorders and are not specific for a particular disease (Cohen Tervaert, 1993b).

ANCA and Monitoring of Disease Activity

Titers of c-ANCA decline during treatment when remission is induced in patients with WG (Cohen Tervaert, 1989). Many patients relapse, however, either during tapering of the immunosuppressive treatment or after treatment has been stopped. Relapses occur nearly exclusively in patients that are persistently or intermittently ANCA positive (Stegeman, 1994a). Various longitudinal studies have shown that titers of ANCA rise prior to a relapse of WG (reviewed in Stegeman, 1994b). In a prospective study of 16-month duration, we found that increases in ANCA titer preceded all 17 observed relapses. The ANCA rise was detectable a mean of 49 days (range 9 to 106 days) before a relapse was clinically diagnosed (Cohen Tervaert, 1989). Based on these findings a prospective study was undertaken in 58 patients with WG in order to test whether treatment based on changes in c-ANCA-titer could prevent the occurrence of relapses (Cohen Tervaert, 1990c). In this study blood samples were tested every month for ANCA-titer. Over an observation period of 24 months titers of ANCA rose in 20 patients. None of the 9 patients who were randomized for treatment at the time of ANCA rise relapsed. In contrast, 6 of the 11 patients who were not treated at that moment, developed a relapse within 6 months of ANCA rise, and three of the remaining patients relapsed after 6 months. Patients receiving no treatment at the time of ANCA rise used more immunosuppressives and corticosteroids than the patients who were treated immediately once a significant rise of ANCA had taken place. Thus, serial quantitation of ANCA levels is useful for following patients with WG. Increasing titers of the autoantibodies should alert the clinician to the possibility of an ensuing relapse. Serial quantitation of MPO and/or elastase antibody levels may be useful as well (Cohen Tervaert, 1990b; unpublished observations). At present, however, no prospective studies have been reported in patients with MPO and/or elastase antibodies. In contrast with ANCA directed to PR3, MPO, and/or elastase, ANCA directed against other antigens do not seem to reflect disease activity and, generally, occur late during the disease process.

PATHOGENESIS OF ANCA-ASSOCIATED VASCULITIDES

The close association between anti-MPO and anti-proteinase 3 antibodies and diseaese activity in a variety of systemic vasculitides suggests a pathophysiological role for these autoantibodies. Experimental data further support the hypothesis that ANCA are intimately involved in the pathogenesis of the aforementioned diseases.

Effect of ANCA on their Target Antigens

As discussed before, binding of anti-PR3 to its target enzyme can inhibit the irreversible inactivation of the enzyme by α_1-antitrypsin, its natural inhibitor (Van de Wiel, 1992). Similarly, complex formation *in vitro* of elastase with α_1-antitrypsin is inhibited by anti-elastase antibodies (Dolman, 1993a). The inhibitory activity differs between sera and is not directly related to the amount of specific antibody (Dolman, 1993b). In a longitudinal study it has been shown that disease activity in patients with WG correlates with the amount of inhibitory activity of the serum rather than with the titer of the anti-PR3 antibodies (Dolman, 1993b). This suggests that escape of the enzyme from its inactivation may contribute to the inflammatory process. Most anti-PR3 positive sera also inhibit the enzymatic activity of PR3 (Van de Wiel, 1992). The reversible antigen-antibody binding, however, may be dissolved at sites of inflammation allowing the enzyme to display its lytic activity, locally, at these sites.

Activation of Leukocytes by ANCA

Histopathologic findings in patients with ANCA-associated vasculitides suggest that the endothelium of blood vessel walls is a major target for injury (Churg and Churg, 1989). Intravascular activation of leukocytes that are in close contact with endothelial cells are considered to play a crucial role in the development of endothelial injury (Cotran and Pober, 1992). *In vitro* studies have shown that activated neutrophils and/or monocytes can injure vascular endothelial cells in culture (Sacks, 1978; Peri, 1990). Activated PMN may play a pivotal role in ANCA-associated vasculitides. Infiltrating polymorphonuclear neutrophils (PMN) are often conspicious in histologic lesions of ANCA-associated vasculitides. Further studies have shown that these PMN are activated as demonstrated by the presence of released lysosomal enzymes and the production of hydrogen peroxide *in situ* (Brouwer, 1994a; Figure 2). These PMN may be activated by the local presence of microbial products or immune complexes localized in the vessel walls, or, alternatively, by direct activation by ANCA.

Falk *et al.* were the first to demonstrate that ANCA can activate neutrophils that are pre-treated ("primed") with low dosage TNFα to the production of reactive oxygen species and the release of lysosomal enzymes (Falk, 1990). The mechanisms underlying neutrophil activation by ANCA have only partly been elucidated. Priming of neutrophils by TNFα results in the expression of lysosomal enzymes such as MPO and proteinase 3 at the cell membrane (Charles, 1991). Those pre-activated neutrophils showing surface expression of proteinase 3 can be detected in the peripheral blood at the time of active disease in patients with WG (Csernok, 1994). Binding of ANCA to their target antigens expressed on PMN may result in internalization and subsequent activation. Alternatively, ANCA may interact with their target antigens in the microenvironment near the cell surface, followed by the engagement of a Fc-receptor known to be involved in neutrophil activation. Recent studies support this latter hypothesis and suggest that ANCA engage the FcтRII ligand binding site on the surface of the PMN (Mulder, 1993; Porges, 1993).

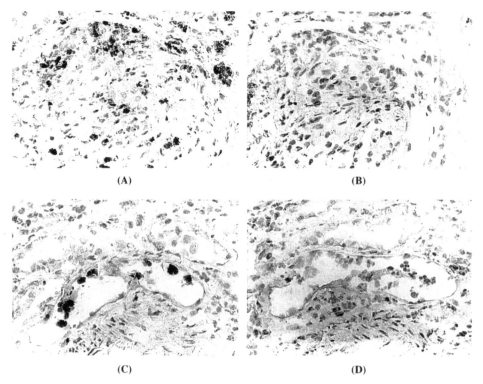

(A)   (B)

(C)   (D)

Figure 2 Precipitation of diaminobenzidine (DAB) (black staining) by endogenously produced H_2O_2 in neutrophils in cryostat sections of renal biopsies from patients with Wegener's granulomatosis. (A) Glomerulus filled up with H_2O_2 producing PMN ($\times350$). (B) Same glomerulus as in A; after the addition of 0.015% catalase all H_2O_2 is scavenged and DAB precipitates are no longer visible ($\times350$). (C) Venule within the interstitium with H_2O_2 producing PMN ($\times350$). (D) Same vessel as in C after the addition of 0.015% catalase ($\times350$). Reproduced with permission from Brouwer *et al.* Kidney Int 1994; 45:1120–1131.

Blocking of the FcγRII receptor on neutrophils inhibited ANCA-mediated activation of PMN (Mulder, 1993). The FcγRII receptor particularly interacts with IgG3-subclasses of antibodies (Van de Winkel and Capel, 1993). Interestingly, sera with relatively high levels of IgG3 subclass of ANCA preferentially activate neutrophils (Mulder, 1993), and exacerbations of WG are associated with increases of the IgG3 subclass of ANCA (Cohen Tervaert, 1994).

ANCA are also capable of stimulating PMN to damage cultured human endothelial cells *in vitro* (Ewert, 1992a; Savage, 1992). Stimulation of PMN by ANCA alone is not in itself sufficient to cause endothelial cell injury. PMN that are excessively stimulated by receiving additional priming signals with phorbol 12-myristate 13-acetate (PMA) in combination with ionomycin ór with TNF-α in combination with lipopolysaccharide (LPS), however, cause significant damage to TNF-activated cultured human endothelial cells (Ewert, 1992a; Savage, 1992). The signal transduction pathway involved in ANCA-mediated activation of neutrophils is still a matter of debate (Fujimoto and Lockwood, 1991; Lai and Lockwood, 1991; Jennette, 1993; Lai, 1994). Fujimoto and Lockwood reported that ANCA F(ab')$_2$ can initiate the translocation of protein kinase C in neutrophils (Fujimoto and Lockwood, 1991). Interestingly, Lai *et al* (Lai and Lockwood, 1991;

Lai, 1994) found that preincubation of PMN with ANCA *in vitro* blunts the subsequent activation of signal transduction by chemotactic peptide and the subsequent calcium mobilization induced by stimulation with calcium ionophore (A23187). The combination of a stimulatory effect upon the production of toxic oxygen metabolites and interference with the signal transduction pathways involved in neutrophil activation may be important in the development of chronic inflammatory lesions as observed in ANCA-associated vasculitides (Lai, 1994).

Interaction Between ANCA and Endothelial Cells

The vascular endothelium forms the biologic interface between circulating blood and all other tissues and organs. The primary event in vasculitis may be viewed as an injury to, or an activation of, the vascular endothelium (Kavanaugh and Oppenheimer-Marks, 1992). In response to these events, normal adaptive responses are generated, including the local accumulation of various blood-borne host defense factors, followed by dampening of those effector functions and activation of counterbalancing control mechanisms. In ANCA-associated vasculitides normal adaptive responses to EC activation and/or injury may be subverted and/or sustained by amplification cycles.

Endothelial Cell Activation

Recently, it has been hypothesized that activation of the vascular endothelium plays a crucial role in the pathogenesis of vasculitides (Cotran and Pober, 1992). *In vitro* studies have demonstrated that activation of cultured vascular endothelial cells renders them hyperadhesive for human PMN. Co-incubation with PMN results in EC injury, a process that is dependent upon direct neutrophil-endothelial cell contact and is mainly due to serine proteases (Westlin and Gimbrone, 1993). Furthermore, *in vitro* studies have shown that EC injury of TNF-activated endothelial cells in culture is more severe when EC cells are incubated with ANCA-stimulated primed PMN than with primed PMN that are not stimulated with ANCA (Savage, 1992). In addition, Savage *et al* (Savage, 1992) found that EC injury only occurred when EC were activated, e.g., by pretreatment with TNF-*a*, demonstrating the pivotal role of activation of EC in EC injury caused by ANCA-stimulated PMN. In *in vivo* studies it has been shown that activation of PMN in combination with endothelial activation in rabbits caused endothelial cell damage (Movat, 1987). Recently, we found evidence that EC activation occurs in vasculitis. During lesion development in an animal model of pulmonary granulomatous vasculitis, we demonstrated upregulation of vascular cell adhesion molecule-1 (VCAM-1) and intercellular cell adhesion molecule-1 (ICAM-1) on the endothelial lining of pulmonary vessels (Cohen Tervaert, 1993e; Figure 3). In addition, we found upregulation of ICAM-1 and VCAM-1 in renal biopsies of patients with ANCA-associated vasculitides (Brouwer, 1993a), and demonstrated that levels of soluble ICAM-1 and VCAM-1 are elevated in patients with active disease (Stegeman, 1994c). Moreover, levels of these soluble adhesion molecules were found to be markers of disease activity. Upregulation of endothelial-leukocyte adhesion molecules in vasculitis may reflect a complex interplay of various stimuli at the level of transcriptional regulation (Collins, 1993). Such stimuli may include cytokines (e.g., interleukin-1 and tumor necrosis factor-α), oxidant stresses, and biochemical forces

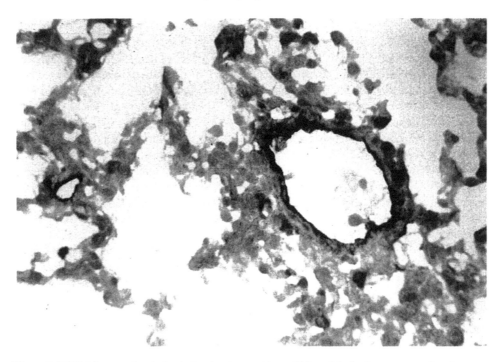

Figure 3 VCAM-1 expression during lesion development in a rabbit model of pulmonary granulomatous vasculitis. The endothelial lining of pulmonary vessels 4 hours after intravenous injection of β-glucan, shows increased staining for VCAM-1 (×100).

(Collins, 1993; Bradley, 1993; Marui, 1993; Nagel, 1994). In addition, ANCA may be such a stimulus. Mayet and Meyer zum Büschenfelde recently reported that *in vitro* ANCA stimulated the adhesion of neutrophils to cultured human endothelial cells. This effect could be partially inhibited by antibody to E-selectin. Moreover, incubation of cultured EC with affinity-purified ANCA (i.e., anti-PR3) resulted in an increased membrane expression of E-selectin (Mayet and Meyer zum Büschenfelde, 1993a). Considering these experiments one should realize that isolation of neutrophils and EC in itself may result in some degree of activation depending on the methods of isolation. This, apparently, may influence the results. Furthermore, the mechanism of ANCA-stimulated induction of E-selectin is not known.

Endothelial Cell Injury

Vascular injury in ANCA-associated vasculitides may be due to:

1. a Shwartzman-like phenomenon
2. activation by ANCA of adherent PMN that express PR3 and/or MPO
3. PMN binding to endothelial bound ANCA by Fc-interaction with subsequent PMN activation
4. local immune complex deposition and subsequent complement activation
5. cell-mediated autoimmunity to PR3 or MPO expressed on EC

1. Microvascular damage may occur in systemic lupus erythematosus in the absence of immune complex deposition particularly in vascular beds which lack fenestrations that permit trapping of immune complexes (Abramson and Weissman, 1988). Abramson and Weissman suggested that vascular damage in these conditions may occur by a mechanism involving intravascular activation and aggregation of PMN (Abramson and Weissman, 1988; Belmont, 1994). The cellular events which charaterize this mechanism of vascular injury are best modeled by the Shwartzman phenomenon. The local Shwartzman lesion requires a preparatory intradermal injection of endotoxin, which is followed (in 4–18 hours) by the intraveneous injection of endotoxin ('challenge'). It is now recognized that agents which prepare the skin for the Shwartzman response do so by promoting activation of the vascular endothelium, and that challenging agents promote activation of circulating PMN and upregulation of CD11b/CD18 expression on these PMN (Argenbright and Barton, 1992). Similar mechanisms may play a role in vascular injury in patients with ANCA-associated vasculitides. Immune cxomplexes are, generally, not detected in vascular beds in these patients. As discussed, *in vitro* studies have demonstrated that ANCA may induce both EC activation and PMN activation. Preliminary studies by Ewert *et al.* suggested that ANCA *in vitro* causes upregulation of CD11b/CD18 expression on PMN (Ewert, 1992b). Indeed, in patients with active WG both activated endothelial cells and activated circulating PMN (indicated by the up-regulation of CD11b/CD18) are present (unpublished observations).

2. Another proposed mechanism of vascular injury in ANCA-associated vasculitides is the activation of adherent PMN expressing PR3 and/or MPO by ANCA. To test this hypothesis, Khoury *et al.* incubated *in vitro* unstimulated normal donor PMN with human cultured EC that were activated with TNF-α and subsequently detected surface expression of PR3, which can be recognized and bound by ANCA (Khoury, 1993).

3. PMN binding to endothelial bound ANCA by Fc-interaction and subsequent PMN activation may also be involved in vascular injury in ANCA-associated vasculitides. In this situation ANCA target antigens released during an inflammatory response, e.g., an infection, could act as membrane ligands for interaction with ANCA. MPO and proteinase 3 are cationic proteins with an isoelectric point of 11.0 and 9.0, respectively. These cationic proteins may bind to anionic structures such as the glomerular basement membrane (GBM) and the surface of endothelial cells. It has, indeed, been shown that ANCA can bind to cultured EC incubated with MPO or proteinase 3 (Vargunam, 1992; Savage, 1993; Ballieux, 1993). Another possible mechanism by which ANCA antigens are displayed on EC was reported by Mayet *et al* (Mayet, 1993b), who identified proteinase 3 in cultured human EC. Cytokine treatment either with TNFα, IL-1, or IFN gamma resulted in increased expression of proteinase 3 with translocation of the enzyme to the cell membrane. As such the antigen is available for interaction with the autoantibody when cytokines are produced, e.g., during upper respiratory tract infections that are frequently observed in patients before the onset of vasculitis.

4. Microvascular damage as seen in vasculitides has often been considered as resulting from deposition of immune complexes in the blood vessel wall (Savage and Ng, 1986). Immune complexes, deposited from the circulation or formed *in situ* may be involved in vascular injury in ANCA-associated vasculitides. However, immunofluorescence studies

in biopsies of these patients, generally, do not reveal immune deposits in vessel walls or at other sites (Jennette, 1989; Brouwer, 1994a). These immunofluorescence findings, however, do not exclude a pathogenetic role for immune complexes. Immune complexes may be rapidly cleared as was observed in animal studies (Cream, 1971; Brouwer, 1993b). Immune complexes may be formed by ANCA and their antigens released from activated PMN, and deposited in vascular walls or formed *in situ*.

5. Finally, ANCA antigen expression on EC may trigger an autoreactive T-cell response, resulting in granulomatous vasculitis. Vascular infiltrates, lung lesions, and kidney lesions in WG show a predominance of CD4[+] T cells. The presence of activated T-cells is further suggested by the presence of elevated levels of soluble IL-2 receptors in patients with active WG (Stegeman, 1993). Recently, Brouwer *et al* have shown that lymphocytes isolated from 32% of patients with ANCA-associated vasculitis show *in vitro* reactivity with the target antigen of their ANCA (Brouwer, 1994b). In line with these findings, it is attractive to speculate that T cells directed against ANCA antigens play a pathophysiological role in ANCA-associated vasculitides. At present, the *in vivo* relevance of those *in vitro* studies still has to be established.

The *in Vivo* Role of ANCA in NCGN

The *in vivo* potential of ANCA to aggravate the inflammatory response has recently been demonstrated (Kobayashi, 1993). Rats were injected with rabbit anti-rat MPO antibodies together with rabbit anti-rat GBM antibodies. Control rats were injected with either anti-rat GBM or anti-rat MPO antibodies. In the latter group no lesions were apparent. The most severe lesions were found in rats injected with both antibodies. In these rats, MPO was found along the glomerular capillary wall and anti-MPO could be eluted from the kidneys. Thus, besides direct activation of rat neutrophils by anti-MPO, MPO released from activated neutrophils may have bound to the GBM due to charge interaction followed by in situ binding of anti-MPO. This local immune complex formation may have aggravated the passive anti-GBM nephritis. In line with these findings are the data of Brouwer *et al.* (Brouwer, 1993b). They immunized Brown Norway (BN) rats with human MPO. The rats developed anti-human MPO antibodies, which, in part, showed cross-reactivity with rat MPO, as well as delayed type hypersensitivity to human MPO. Five weeks after immunization the left kidney was perfused with products of activated neutrophils, i.e., lytic enzymes, particularly proteinase 3 and elastase, MPO, and its substrate H_2O_2. The rats developed NCGN and vasculitis. Along the GBM MPO, IgG, and C3 could be detected at 24 hrs after perfusion. Immune deposits were, however, absent at 4 and 10 days after perfusion. This finding illustrates that immune complexes are rapidly cleared in this animal model. In control immunized animals perfused with enzymes and H_2O_2 no significant lesions occurred. From these findings it is suggested that the initial step in the development of NCGN is (focal) immune complex formation. The presence of lytic enzymes, which were concomitantly perfused but may also have been released from neutrophils activated by ANCA, probably is responsible for the rapid degradation of the immune deposits that were only detected in the very early stage of the lesions.

Anti-MPO antibodies have also been demonstrated in BN rats treated with mercuric chloride (Esnault, 1992). These rats develop a polyclonal autoimmune response comprising, amongst others, antibodies to MPO. Necrotizing vasculitis, particularly involving the gut, developed in some of the animals, possibly in conjunction with a microbial infection (Mathieson, 1992). The pathophysiological role of anti-MPO in the induction of the vasculitic process is, however, not clear in this particular model. Finally, ANCA are detected in canine juvenile polyarteritis syndrome (Felsburg, 1992) and in MRL-*LPR/LPR* mice (Harper, 1993). The significance of ANCA in these animal models is at present not clear.

A schematic representation of the possible pathophysiology of ANCA-associated vasculitides which summarizes the items discussed before is shown in Figure 4.

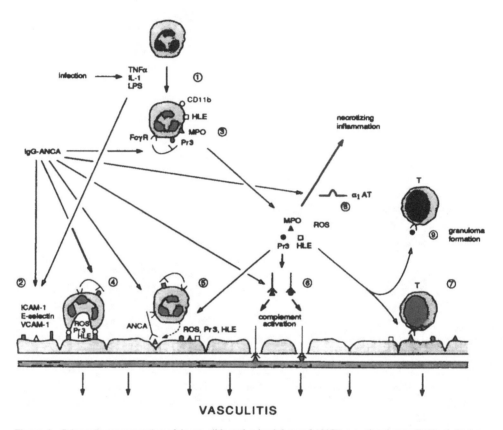

VASCULITIS

Figure 4 Schematic representation of the possible pathophysiology of ANCA-associated vasculitides. Infection induces the production of proinflammatory cytokines (e.g. TNFα and IL-1). In addition, microbially derived substances (e.g. lipopolysaccharide) may be liberated. (1) Both cytokines and microbially derived substances induce priming of neutrophils (PMN) and (local) activation of endothelial cells. (2) Activation of endothelial cells may be potentiated by ANCA. (3) Primed PMN are further activated by ANCA to the production of reactive oxygen species (ROS) and the release of lytic enzymes such as proteinase 3 (PR3) and elastase (HLE). Damage of endothelial cells may occur when PMN are in close connection with activated endothelial cells. Damage may be due to (4) a Shwartzman-like phenomenon or to (5) activated PMN that are attracted by ANCA that is bound to endothelial cells that express PR3 and/or myeloperoxidase (MPO). Damage of the endothelial cells may be further potentiated by activation of adherent PMN that express PR3 and/or MPO by ANCA. (6) Alternatively, endothelial cell damage occurs when soluble immune complexes are deposited in blood vessel walls and subsequently become trapped. PMN are attracted and activated after complement activation by these immune complexes. (7) Otherwise, ANCA antigen expression on endothelial cells may trigger an autoreactive T-cell response, resulting in granulomatous vasculitis. (8) Activated PMN are also involved in the induction of necrotizing inflammation which might be potentiated by the inhibition by ANCA of the α1-antitrypsin (α1AT) induced inactivation of PR3 and HLE. (9) Furthermore, CD4-positive T-cells, autoreactive to PR3 and/or MPO, may contribute to granuloma formation.

CONCLUSION

Our increased understanding of the interactions between circulating leukocytes and the vascular wall has provided new insights into the possible mechanisms by which vascular injury in vasculitides can occur, and it has become evident that the vascular endothelium plays a pivotal role in the development of systemic vasculitis. The discovery of ANCA in certain forms of systemic vasculitis has further increased our understanding of patho-physiological mechanisms in vasculitides. The pathophysiological role of ANCA has been studied in *in vitro* and *in vivo* models. *In vitro* anti-proteinase 3 interferes with the inactivation of proteinase 3 by α_1-antitrypsin. ANCA of diverse specificities are able to activate primed neutrophils to the production of reactive oxygen species and the release of lysosomal enzymes. In addition, ANCA are able to activate cultured endothelial cells. These effects may contribute to the inflammatory process, whereas the combination of activation of neutrophils and endothelial cells may cause vascular injury by a Shwartzman-like reaction. Furthermore, the possible expression of the ANCA antigens at the surface of (activated) endothelial cells and/or at the surface of endothelium-bound PMN might allow the respective antibodies and/or autoreactive T-cells to react with their targets. Vascular injury may be a consequence of these interactions via both direct and indirect mechanisms.

Although many questions still remain, the expanding knowledge on ANCA has greatly contributed to the diagnosis and the understanding of the pauci-immune necrotizing vasculitides.

References

Abramson, S.B. and Weissman, G. (1988). Complement split products and the pathogenesis of SLE. *Hosp Pract.*, **23**:45–55.

Alarcón-Segovia, D. (1980). Classification of the necrotizing vasculitides in man. *Clin. Rheum. Dis.*, **6**:223–231.

Argenbright, L.W. and Barton, R.W. (1992). Interactions of leukocyte integrins with intercellular adhesion molecule 1 in the production of inflammatory vascular injury *in vivo*. *J. Clin. Invest.*, **89**:259–272.

Ballieux, B.E.P.B., Zondervan, K., Hagen, E.C., van der Woude, F.J., van Es, L.A. and Daha, M.R. (1993). Differential binding of MPO and PR3 to monolayers of endothelial cells. (abstract) *Clin. Exp. Immunol.*, **93**:17.

Belmont, H.M., Buyon, J., Giorno, R. and Abramson, S. (1994). Up-regulation of endothelial cell adhesion molecules characterizes disease activity in systemic lupus erythematosus. The Shartzman phenomenon revisited. *Arthritis Rheum.*, **37**:376–383.

Bini, P., Gabay, J.E., Teitel, A., Melchior, M. Zhou, J.L. and Elkon, K.B. (1992). Antineutrophil cytoplasmic autoantibodies in Wegener's Granulomatosis recognize conformational epitope(s) on proteinase 3. *J Immunol.*, **149**:1409–1415.

Bosch, X., Mirapeix, E., Font, J., *et al.* (1992). Anti-myeloperoxidase autoantibodies in patients with necrotizing glomerular and alveolar capillaritis. *Am. J. Kidney Dis.*, **20**:231–239.

Bories, D., Raynal, M.C., Solomon, D.H., Darzynkiewicz, Z. and Cayre, Y. (1990). Down-regulation of a serine protease, myeloblastin, causes growth arrest and differentiation of promyelocytic leukemia cells. *Cell*, **59**:959-968.

Bradley, J.R., Johnson, D.R. and Pober, J.S. (1993). Endothelial activation by hydrogen peroxide. Selective increases of intercellular adhesion molecule-1 and major histocompatibility complex class I. *Am. J. Pathol.*, **142**:1598–1609.

Brouwer, E., Huitema, M.G., Heeringa, P., Cohen Tervaert, J.W., Weening, J.J. and Kallenberg, C.G.M. (1993a). Upregulation of adhesion molecules in renal biopsies from patients with Wegener's granulomatosis. (abstract) *Clin. Exp. Immunol.*, **93(suppl. 1)**:22.

Brouwer, E., Huitema, M.G., Klok, P.A., Weerd, H. de, Cohen Tervaert, J.W., Weening, J.J. and Kallenberg, C.G.M. (1993b). Anti-myeloperoxidase-associated proliferative glomerulonephritis: an animal model. *J. Exp. Med.*, **177**:905–914.

Brouwer, E., Huitema, M.G., Mulder, A.H.L., Heeringa, P., van Goor, H., Cohen Tervaert, J.W. and Weening, J.J., Kallenberg, C.G.M. (1994a). Neutrophil activation *in vitro* and *in vivo* in Wegener's granulomatosis. *Kidney Int.*, 45:1120–1131.

Brouwer, E., Stegeman, C.A., Huitema, M.G., Limburg, P.C. and Kallenberg, C.G.M. (1994b). T-cell reactivity to proteinase 3 and myeloperoxidase in patients with Wegener's granulomatosis. In *Pathogenic potential of anti neutrophil cytoplasmic antibodies*, E. Brouwer, pp. 55–71. Thesis, University of Groningen.

Calafat, J., Goldschmeding, R., Ringeling, P.L., Janssen, H. and van der Schoot, C.E. (1990). In situ localization by double-labeling immunoelectron microscopy of anti-neutrophil cytoplasmic autoantibodies in neutrophils and monocytes. *Blood*, 75:242–250.

Cambridge, G., Hall, T.J. and Leaker, B. (1991). Heterogeneity of antibodies to myeloperoxidase in sera from patients with vasculitis (abstract). *J. Am. Soc. Nephrol*, 2:590.

Campanelli, D., Melchior, M., Fu, Y., Nakata, N., Shuman, H., Nathan, C. and Gabay, J.E. (1990a). Cloning of cDNA for proteinase 3: a serine protease, antibiotic, and autoantigen from human neutrophils. *J. Exp. Med.*, 172:1709–1715.

Campanelli, D., Detmers, P.A., Nathan, C.F. and Gabay, J.E. (1990b). Azurocidin and a homologous serine protease from neutrophils. Differential antimicrobial and proteolytic properties. *J. Clin. Invest.*, 85:904–915.

Charles, L.A., Falk, R.J. and Jennette, J.C. (1989). Reactivity of anti-neutrophil cytoplasmic autoantibodies with HL-60 cells. *Clin. Immunol. Immunopathol.*, 53:243-253.

Charles, L.A., Caldas, M.L.R., Falk, R.J., Terrell, R.S. and Jennette, J.C. (1991). Antibodies against granule proteins activate neutrophils *in vitro. J. Leukocyte Biol.*, 50:539–546.

Churg, J., Churg, A. (1989). Idiopathic and secondary vasculitis: a review. *Mod. Pathol.*, 2:144–160.

Cohen Tervaert, J.W., van der Woude, F.J., Fauci, A.S., Ambrus, J.L., Velosa, J., Keane, W.F., Meijer, S., van der Giessen, M., The, T.H., van der Hem, G.K. and Kallenberg, C.G.M. (1989). Association between active Wegener's Granulomatosis and anticytoplasmic antibodies. *Arch. Int. Med.*, 149:2461–2465.

Cohen Tervaert, J.W., Goldschmeding, R., Elema, J.D., van der Giessen, M., Huitema, M.G., van der Hem, G.K., von dem Borne, A.E.G.Kr. and Kallenberg, C.G.M. (1990a). Autoantibodies against myeloid lysosomal enzymes in crescentic glomerulonephritis. *Kidney Int.*, 37:799–806.

Cohen Tervaert, J.W., Goldschmeding, R., Elema, J.D., van der Giessen, M., Huitema, M.G., Koolen, M.I., Hené, R.J., The, T.H., van der Hem, G.K., von dem Borne, A.E.G.Kr. and Kallenberg, C.G.M. (1990b). Association of autoantibodies to myeloperoxidase with different forms of vasculitis. *Arthritis Rheum*, 33:1264–1272.

Cohen Tervaert, J.W., Huitema, M.G., Hené, R.J., Sluiter, W.J., The, T.H., van der Hem, G.K. and Kallenberg, CGM. (1990c). Prevention of relapses of Wegener's Granulomatosis by treatment based on antineutrophil cytoplasmic antibody titre. *Lancet*, 336:709–711.

Cohen Tervaert, J.W., Limburg, P.C., Elema, J.D., Huitema, M.G., Horst, G., The, T.H. and Kallenberg, C.G.M. (1991a). Detection of autoantibodies against myeloid lysosomal enzymes: a useful adjunct to classification of patients with biopsy-proven necrotizing arteritis. *Am. J. Med.*, 91:59–66.

Cohen Tervaert, J.W., Goldschmeding, R., Elema, J.D., von dem Borne, A.E.G.Kr. and Kallenberg, C.G.M. (1991b). Anti-myeloperoxidase antibodies in the Churg Strauss Syndrome. *Thorax*, 46:70–71.

Cohen Tervaert, J.W. and Kallenberg, C.G.M. (1993a). Neurologic manifestations of systemic vasculitides. *Rheum. Dis. Cin. North Am.*, 19:913–940.

Cohen Tervaert, J.W. (1993b). Detection and clinical associations of autoantibodies to myeloid granular proteins. *Adv. Exp. Med. Biol.*, 336:299–302.

Cohen Tervaert, J.W., Mulder, A.H.L. and Kallenberg, C.G.M. (1993c). Perinuclear antineutrophil cytoplasmic antibodies (P-ANCA): clinical significance and relation to antibodies against myeloid lysosomal enzymes. *Adv. Exp. Med. Biol.*, 336:253–256.

Cohen Tervaert, J.W., Mulder, A.H.L., Stegeman, C.A., Huitema, M.G., The, T.H. and Kallenberg, C.G.M. (1993d). The occurrence of autoantibodies to human leukocyte elastase in Wegener's granulomatosis and other inflammatory disorders. *Ann. Rheum. Dis.*, 52:115–120.

Cohen Tervaert, J.W., Cybulsky, M.I. and Gimbrone, M.A., Jr. (1993e). Differential expression of VCAM-1 in a rabbit model of pulmonary granulomatous vasculitis. (abstract) *Faseb J.*, 7, A344.

Cohen Tervaert, J.W., Mulder, A.H.L., Kallenberg, C.G.M. and Stegeman, C.A. (1994). Measurement of IgG3 levels of anti-proteinase 3 antibodies is useful in monitoring disease activity in Wegener's granulomatosis. (abstract) *J. Am. Soc. Nephrol.*, 5:828.

Collins, T. (1993). Endothelial nuclear factor-kappa B and the initiation of the atherosclerotic lesion. *Lab. Invest.*, 68:499–508.

Cotran, R.S. and Pober, J.S. (1992). Recent insights into mechanisms of vascular injury. Implications for the pathogenesis of vasculitis. In *Endothelial cell dysfunctions*. N. Simionescu and M. Simionescu (eds.), pp. 183–189. New York: Plenum Press.

Cream, J.J., Bryceson, A.D.M. and Ryder, G. (1971). Disappearance of immunoglobulin and complement from the Arthus reaction and its relevance to studies of vasculitis in man. *Br. J. Derm.*, 84:106–109.

Csernok, E., Ernst, M., Schmitt, W.H., Bainton, D.F. and Gross, W.L. (1994). Activated neutrophils express proteinase 3 on their plasma membrane *in vitro* and *in vivo*. *Clin. Exp. Immunol.*, **95**:244–250.

Davies, D.J., Moran, J.E., Niall, J.F. and Ryan, G.B. (1982). Segmental necrotizing glomerulonephritis with antineutrophil antibody: possible arbovirus aetiology? *Br. Med. J.*, **285**:606.

Dolman, K.M., van de Wiel, B.A., Kam, C.M., Abbink, J.J., Hack, C.E., Sonnenberg, A., Powers, J.C., von dem Borne, A.E.G.Kr. and Goldschmeding, R. (1992). Determination of proteinase 3/alpha$_1$-antitrypsin complexes in inflammatory fluids. *FEBS Lett.*, **314**:117–121.

Dolman, K.M., Gans, R.O.B., Vervaart, T.H.J., Zevenbergen, G., Maingay, D., Nikkels, R.E., Donker, A.J.M., von dem Borne, A.E.G.Kr. and Goldschmeding, R. (1993a). Vasculitic disorders and anti-neutrophil cytoplasmic autoantibodies associated with propylthiouracil therapy. *Lancet*, **342**:651–652.

Dolman, K.M., Stegeman, C.A., van de Wiel, B.A., Hack, C.E., von dem Borne, A.E.G.Kr., Kallenberg, C.G.M. and Goldschmeding, R. (1993b). Relevance of classic anti-neutrophil cytoplasmic autoantibody (c-ANCA)-mediated inhibition of proteinase 3-α_1-antitrypsin complexation to disease activity in Wegener's Granulomatosis. *Clin. Exp. Immunol.*, **93**:405–410.

Esnault, V.L.M., Mathieson, P.W., Thiru, S., Oliveira, D.B.G. and Lockwood, C.M. (1992). Autoantibodies to myeloperoxidase in Brown Norway rats treated with mercuric chloride. *Lab. Invest.*, **67**:114–120.

Ewert, B.H., Jennette, J.C. and Falk, R.J. (1992a). Anti-myeloperoxidase antibodies stimulate neutrophils to damage human endothelial cells. *Kidney Int.*, **41**:375–383.

Ewert, B.H., Becker, M., Jennette, J.C. and Falk, R.J. (1992b). Anti-myeloperoxidase antibodies (αMPO) stimulate neutrophils to adhere to cultured human endothelial cells utilizing the b_2-integrin CD11/18. (abstract) *J. Am. Soc. Nephrol.*, **3**:585.

Falk, R.J. and Jennette, J.C. (1988). Anti-neutrophil cytoplasmic autoantibodies with specificity for myeloperoxidase in patients with systemic vasculitis and idiopathic necrotizing and crescentic glomerulonephritis. *N. Engl. J. Med.*, **318**:1651–1657.

Falk, R.J., Terrell, R.S., Charles, L.A. and Jennette, J.C. (1990). Anti-neutrophil cytoplasmic autoantibodies induce neutrophils to degranulate and produce oxygen radicals *in vitro*. *Proc. Natl. Acad. Sci. USA*, **87**:4115–4119.

Falk, R.J., Becker, M., Terrell, R. and Jennette, J.C. (1992). Anti-meyloperoxidase autoantibodies react with native but not denatured myeloperoxidase. *Clin. Exp. Immunol.*, **89**:274–278.

Felsburg, P.J., HogenEsch, H., Somberg, R.L., Snyder, P.W. and Glickman, L.T. (1992). Immunologic abnormalities in canine juvenile polyarteritis syndrome: a naturally occurring animal model of Kawasaki disease. *Clin. Immunol. Immunopathol*, **65**:110–118.

Fujimoto, T. and Lockwood, C.M. (1991). Antineutrophil cytoplasm antibodies (ANCA) activate protein kinase C in human neutrophils and HL-60 cells (abstract). *Am. J. Kidney Dis.*, **18**:204.

Gaskin, G., Savage, C.O.S., Ryan, J.J., *et al.* (1991). Anti-neutrophil cytoplasmic antibodies and disease activity during long-term follow-up of 70 patients with systemic vasculitis. *Nephrol. Dial Transplant*, 6:689–694.

Geffriaud-Ricouard, C., Noël, L.H., Chauveau, D., Houhou, S., Grünfeld, J.P. and Lesavre, P. (1993). Clinical spectrum associated with ANCA of defined antigen specificities in 98 selected patients. *Clin. Nephrol.*, **39**:125–136.

Goldschmeding, R., Cohen Tervaert, J.W., van der Schoot, C.E., van der Veen, C., Kallenberg, C.G.M. and von dem Borne, A.E.G.Kr. (1989a). ANCA, anti-myeloperoxydase and anti-elastase: three members of a novel class of autoantibodies against myeloid lysosomal enzymes. *APMIS*, **97(S6)**:48–49.

Goldschmeding, R., van der Schoot, C.E., ten Bokkel Huinink, D., Hack, C.E., van den Ende, M.E., Kallenberg, C.G.M. and von dem Borne, A.E.G.Kr. (1989b). Wegener's Granulomatosis autoantibodies identify a novel diisopropylfluorophosphate-binding protein in the lysosomes of normal human neutrophils. *J. Clin. Invest.*, **84**:1577–1587.

Guillevin, L., Visser, H., Noël, L.H., Pourrat, J., Vernier, I., Gayraud, M., Oksman, F. and Lesavre, P. (1993). Antineutrophil cytoplasm antibodies in systemic polyarteritis nodosa with and without Hepatitis B Virus infection and Churg-Strauss syndrome. *J. Rheumatol*, **20**:1345–1349.

Halbwachs-Mecarelli, L., Nusbaum, P., Noël, L.H., Reumaux, D., Erlinger, S., Grünfeld, J.P. and Lesavre, P. (1992). Antineutrophil cytoplasmic antibodies (ANCA) directed against Cathepsin G in ulcerative colitis, Crohn's disease and primary sclerosing cholangitis. *Clin. Exp. Immunol.*, **90**:79–84.

Harper, J.M., Lockwood, C.M. and Cooke, A. (1993). Anti-neutrophil cytoplasm antibodies in MRL-*LPR/LPR* mice. (abstract) *Clin. Exp. Immunol.*, **93(suppl. 1)**:22.

Haynes, B.F. (1992). Vasculitis: Pathogenic Mechanisms of Vessel Damage. In *Inflammation: Basic Principles and Clinical Correlates*, 2nd edn, J.I. Gallin, I.M. Goldstein and R. Snyderman (eds.), pp. 921–941. New York: Raven Press.

Hoffman, G.S., Kerr, G.S., Leavitt, R.Y., *et al.* (1992). Wegener granulomatosis: an analysis of 158 patients. *Ann. Intern. Med.*, **116**:488–498.

Hunder, G.G., Arend, W.P., Bloch, D.A., Calabrese, L.H., Fauci, A.S., Fries, J.F., Leavitt, R.Y., Lie, J.T., Lightfoot Jr., R.W., Masi, A.T., McShane, D.J., Michel, B.A., Mills, J.A., Stevens, M.B., Wallace, S.C.

and Zvaifler, N.J. (1990). The American College of Rheumatology 1990 criteria for the classification of vasculitis. *Arthritis Rheum.*, **33**:1065–1136.

Jennette, J.C., Wilkman, A.S. and Falk, R.J. (1989). Antineutrophil cytoplasmic autoantibodies-associated glomerulonephritis and vasculitis. *Am. J. Pathol.*, **135**:921–930.

Jennette, J.C., Ewert, B.H. and Falk, R.J. (1993). Do antineutrophil cytoplasmic autoantibodies cause Wegener's granulomatosis and other forms of necrotizing vasculitis? *Rheum. Dis. Clin. North America*, **19**:1–28.

Jennette, J.C., Falk, R.J., Andrassy, K., Bacon, B.A., Churg, J., Gross, W.L., Hagen, E.C., Hoffmann, G.S., Hunder, G.G., Kallenberg, C.G.M., McCluskey, R.T., Sinico, R.A., Rees, A.J., van Es, L.A., Waldherr, R. and Wiik, A. (1994). Nomenclature of systemic vasculitides: the proposal of an international consensus conference. *Arthritis Rheum.*, **37**:187–192.

Kallenberg, C.G.M., Cohen Tervaert, J.W., van der Woude, F.J., Goldschmeding, R., von dem Borne, A.E.G.Kr. and Weening, J.J. (1991a). Autoimmunity to lysosomal enzymes: new clues to vasculitis and glomerulonephritis? *Immunol. Today*, **12**:61–64.

Kallenberg, C.G.M. and Cohen Tervaert, J.W. (1991b). Anti-neutrophilic cytoplasmic antibodies: new tools in the diagnosis and follow-up of necrotizing glomerulonephritis. In *International Yearbook of Nephrology 1992*, V.E. Andreucci and L.G. Fine (eds), pp. 313–335. London: Springer-Verlag.

Kallenberg, C.G.M., Mulder, A.H.L. and Cohen Tervaert, J.W. (1992). Antineutrophil cytoplasmic antibodies: a still-growing class of autoantibodies in inflammatory disorders. *Am. J. Med.*, **93**:675–682.

Kallenberg, C.G.M., Brouwer, E., Weening, J.J. and Cohen Tervaert, J.W. (1994). Anti-neutrophil cytoplasmic antibodies: current diagnostic and pathophysiological potential. *Kidney Int.*, **46**:1–15.

Kam, C.M., Kerrigan, J.E., Dolman, K.M., Goldschmeding, R., von dem Borne, A.E.G.Kr. and Powers, J.C. (1992). Substrate and inhibitor studies on Proteinase 3. *FEBS Lett.*, **297**:119–123.

Kaneko, K., Suzuki, Y., Yamashiro, Y. and Yabuta, S. (1993). Is p-ANCA in ulcerative colitis directed against glucuronidase? *Lancet*, **341**:320.

Kavanaugh, A. and Oppenheimer-Marks, N. (1992). The role of the vascular endothelium in the pathogenesis of vasculitis. In *Systemic vasculitis. The biological basis*, E.C. LeRoy (ed.), pp. 27–48. New York: Marcel Dekker.

Khoury, N.A., Moriya, S., Csernok, E., Pratt, J.R., Cameron, J.S. and Frampton, G. (1993). Expression of proteinase 3 on neutrophils attached to cytokine stimulated HUVEC. (abstract) *Clin. Exp. Immunol.*, **93**:17.

Kobayashi, K., Shibata, T. and Sugisaki, T. (1993). Aggravation of rat Masugi nephritis by heterologous anti-rat myeloperoxidase antibody. (abstract) *Clin. Exp. Immunol.*, **93(suppl 1)**:S20.

Lai, K.N. and Lockwood, C.M. (1991). The effect of anti-neutrophil cytoplasm antibodies on the signal transduction in human neutrophils. *Clin. Exp. Immunol.*, **85**:396–401.

Lai, K.N., Leung, J.C.K., Rifkin, I. and Lockwood, C.M. (1994). Effect of anti-neutrophil cytoplasm autoantibodies on the intracellular calcium concentration of human neutrophils. *Lab. Invest.*, **70**:152–162.

Lanham, J.G. and Churg, J. (1991). Churg-Strauss syndrome. In *Systemic Vasculitides*, A. Churg and J. Churg (eds.), p. 101. New York: Igaku-Shoin.

Lie, J.T. (1992). Vasculitis, 1815 to 1991: classification and diagnostic specificity. *J. Rheumatol.*, **19**:83–89.

Lie, J.T. (1994). Nomenclature and classification of vasculitis: plus ca change, plus c'est la meme chose. *Arthritis Rheum.*, **37**:181–186.

Lüdemann, J., Utecht, B. and Gross, W.L. (1990). Anti-neutrophil cytoplasm antibodies in Wegener's Granulomatosis recognize an elastinolytic enzyme. *J. Exp. Med.*, **171**:357–362.

Marui, N., Offerman, M.K., Swerlick, R., Kunsch, C., Rosen, C.A., Ahmad, M., Alexander, R.W. and Medford, R.M. (1993). Vascular cell adhesion molecule-1 (VCAM-1) gene transcription and expression are regulated through an antioxidant sensitive mechanism in human vascular endothelial cells. *J. Clin. Invest.*, **92**:1866–1874.

Mathieson, P.W., Thiru, S. and Oliveira, D.B.G. (1992). Mercuric chloride-treated Brown Norway rats develop widespread tissue injury including necrotizing vasculitis. *Lab. Invest.*, **67**:121–129.

Mayet, W.J. and Meyer Zum Büschenfelde, K.H. (1993a). Antibodies to proteinase 3 increase adhesion of neutrophils to human endothelial cells. *Clin. Exp. Immunol.*, **94**:440–446.

Mayet, W.J., Csernok, E., Szymkowiak, C., Gross, W.L. and Meyer zum Büschenfelde, K.H. (1993b). Human endothelial cells express proteinase 3, the target antigen of anti-cytoplasmic antibodies in Wegener's Granulomatosis. *Blood*, **82**:1221–1229

Moodie, F.D.L., Leaker, B., Cambridge, G., Totty, N.F. and Segal, A.W. (1993). Alpha-enolase: a novel cytosolic autoantigen in ANCA positive vasculitis. *Kidney Int.* **43**:675–681.

Movat, H.Z., Burrowes, C.E., Cybulsky, M.I. and Dinarello, C.A.: Acute inflammation and a Schwartzman-like reaction induced by interleukin-1 and tumor necrosis factor. Synergistic action of the cytokines in the induction of inflammation and microvascular injury. *Am. J. Pathol. 1987*, **129**:463–476

Mulder, A.H.L., Horst, G., Limburg, P.C. and Kallenberg, C.G.M. (1993). Activation of neutrophils by anti-neutrophil cytoplasmic antibodies is FcR-dependent. (abstract) *Clin. Exp. Immunol.*, **93(suppl 1)**:S16.

Nagel, T., Resnick, N., Atkinson, W.J., Dewey, C.F. and Gimbrone Jr, M.A. (1994). Shear stress differentially upregulates ICAM-1 expression in cultured vascular endothelial cells. *J. Clin. Invest.*, **94**:885–891.

Nässberger, L., Johansson, A.-C., Björck, S. and Sjöholm, A.G. (1991). Antibodies to neutrophil granulocyte myeloperoxidase and elastase: autoimmune responses in glomerulonephritis due to hydralazine treatment. *J. Int. Med.*, **229**:261–265.

Niles, J.L., McCluskey, R.T., Ahmad, M.F. and Arnaout, M.A. (1989). Wegener's Granulomatosis autoantigen is a novel serine proteinase. *Blood*, **74**:1888–1893.

Niles, J.L., Pan, G., Collins, A.B., Shannon, T., Skates, S., Fienberg, R., Arnaout, M.A. and McCluskey, R.T. (1991). Antigen-specific radioimmunoassays for anti-neutrophil cytoplasmic antibodies in the diagnosis of rapidly progressive glomerulonephritis. *J. Am. Soc. Nephrol.*, **2**:27–36.

Nölle, B., Specks, V., Lüdemann, J., Rohrbach, M.S., De Remee, D.A. and Gross, W.L. (1989). Anticytoplasmic autoantibodies: their immunodiagnostic value in Wegener's Granulomatosis. *Ann. Int. Med.*, **111**:28–40.

Pedrollo, E., Bleil, L., Bautz, F.A., Kalden, J.R. and Bautz, E.K.F. (1993). Antineutrophil cytoplasmic autoantibodies (ANCA) recognizing a recombinant myeloperoxidase subunit. *Adv. Exp. Med. Biol.*, **336**:87–92.

Peen, E., Almer, S., Bodemar, G., Ryder, B.O., Sjolin, C., Tejle, K. and Skogh, T. (1993). Anti-lactoferrin antibodies and other types of ANCA in ulcerative colitis, primary sclerosing cholangitis and Crohn's disease. *Gut*, **34**:56–62.

Peri, G., Chiaffarino, F., Bernasconi, S., Padura, I.M. and Mantovani, A. (1990). Cytotoxicity of activated monocytes on endothelial cells. *J. Immunol.*, **144**:1444–1448.

Porges, A.J., Redecha, P.B., Csernok, E., Gross, W.L. and Kimberly, R.P. (1993). Monoclonal ANCA (anti-MPO and anti-Pr3) engage and activate neutrophils via Fcγ Receptor IIA. (abstract) *Clin. Exp. Immunol.*, **93(suppl 1)**:S18.

Roberts, D.E., Peebles, C., Curd, J.G., Tan, E.M. and Rubin, R.L. (1991). Autoantibodies to native myeloperoxidase in patients with pulmonary hemorrhage and acute renal failure. *J. Clin. Immunol.*, **11**:389–397.

Sacks, T., Moldow, C.F., Craddock, P.R., Bowers, T.K. and Jacob, H.S. (1978). Oxygen radicals mediate endothelial cell damage by complement-stimulated granulocytes. An *in vitro* model of immune vascular damage. *J. Clin. Invest.*, **61**:1161–1167.

Savage, C.O.S., Winearls, C.G., Evans, D.J., Rees, A.J. and Lockwood, C.M. (1985). Microscopic polyarteritis: presentation, pathology and prognosis. *Q. J. Med.*, **56**:467–483.

Savage, C.O.S. and Ng, Y.C. (1986). The aetiology and pathogenesis of major systemic vasculitides. *Postgrad. Med. J.*, **62**:627–636.

Savage, C.O.S., Winearls, C.G., Jones, S.J., Marshall, P.D. and Lockwood, C.M. (1987). Prospective study of radioimmunoassay for antibodies against neutrophil cytoplasm in diagnosis of systemic vasculitis. *Lancet*, **8**:1389–1393.

Savage, C.O.S., Pottinger, B.E., Gaskin, G., Pusey, C.D. and Pearson, J.D. (1992). Autoantibodies developing to myeloperoxidase and proteinase 3 in systemic vasculitis stimulate neutrophil cytotoxicity towards cultured endothelial cells. *Am. J. Pathol.*, **141**:335–342.

Savage, C.O.S., Gaskin, G. and Pusey, C.D. (1993). Anti-neutrophil cytoplasm antibodies (ANCA) can recognize vascular endothelial cell-bound ANCA-associated autoantigens. *J. Exp. Nephrol.*, **1**:190–195.

Schmitt, W.H., Csernok, E., Flesch, B.K., Hauschild, S. and Gross, W.L. (1993). Autoantibodies directed against lysozyme: a new target antigen for anti-neutrophil cytoplasmic antibodies. *Adv. Exp. Med. Biol.*, **336**:267–272.

Sinico, R.A., Pozzi, C., Radice, A., Tincani, A., Li Vecchi, M., Rota, S., Comotti, C., Ferrario, F. and D'Amico, G. (1993). Clinical significance of antineutrophil cytoplasmic autoantibodies with specificity for lactoferrin in renal diseases. *Am. J. Kidney Dis.*, **22**:253–260.

Stegeman, C.A., Cohen Tervaert, J.W., Huitema, M.G. and Kallenberg, C.G.M. (1993). Serum markers of T cell activation in relapses of Wegener's granulomatosis. *Clin. Exp. Immunol.*, **91**:415–420.

Stegeman, C.A., Cohen Tervaert, J.W., Sluiter, W.J., Manson, W.L., de Jong, P.E. and Kallenberg, C.G.M. (1994). Association of chronic nasal carriage of *Staphylococcus aureus* and higher relapse rates in Wegener Granulomatosis. *Ann. Int. Med.*, **120**:12–17.

Stegeman, C.A., Cohen Tervaert, J.W. and Kallenberg, C.G.M. (1994b). Anti-neutrophil cytoplasmic antibodies (ANCA): tools for diagnosis and follow-up in systemic vasculitis. *Ann. Med. Int.*, **145**:523–532.

Stegeman, C.A., Cohen Tervaert, J.W., Huitema, M.G., de Jong, P.E. and Kallenberg, C.G.M. (1994c) Serum levels of soluble adhesion molecules sICAM-1, sVCAM-1, and sE-selectin in patients with Wegener's granulomatosis. Relation with disease activity and relevance during follow-up. *Arthritis Rheum.*, **37**:1228–1235.

Vargunam, M., Adu, D., Taylor, C.M., *et al.* (1992). Endothelium myeloperoxidase interaction in vasculitis. *Nephrol. Dial. Transplant*, **7**:1077–1081.

van de Wiel, A., Dolman, K.M., van der Meer-Gerritsen, C.H., Hack, C.E., von dem Borne, A.E.G.Kr. and Goldschmeding, R. (1992). Interference of Wegener's Granulomatosis autoantibodies with neutrophil proteinase 3 activity. *Clin. Exp. Immunol.*, **90**:409–414.

van de Winkel, J.G.J. and Capel, P.J.A. (1993). Human IgG Fc receptor heterogeneity: molecular aspects and clinical implications. *Immunol. Today*, **14**:215–221.

van der Woude, F.J., Rasmussen, N., Lobatto, S., Wiik, A., Permin, H., van Es, L.A., van der Giessen, M., van der Hem, G.K. and The, T.H. (1985). Autoantibodies to neutrophils and monocytes: a new tool for diagnosis and a marker of disease activity in Wegener's Granulomatosis. *Lancet*, **ii**:425–429.

Weiss, S.J. (1989). Tissue destruction by neutrophils. *N. Engl. J. Med.*, **320**–365–376.

Westlin, W.F. and Gimbrone, M.A. (1993). Neutrophil-mediated damage to human vascular endothelium. Role of cytokine activation. *Am. J. Pathol.*, **142**:117–128.

Wiik, A. (1989). Delineation of a standard procedure for indirect immunofluorescence detection of ANCA. *APMIS*, **97**(S6):12–13.

7 Humoral Immunity and Vascular Injury in the Pathogenesis of Discordant Xenograft Rejection

Fritz H. Bach, Simon C. Robson and Wayne W. Hancock

Sandoz Center for Immunobiology and Departments of Surgery and Pathology,
New England Deaconess Hospital, Harvard Medical School, Boston, MA, 02215, USA

INTRODUCTION

Endothelial cells provide a semi-permeable barrier between the intravascular space and the parenchyma of body organs, and help maintain the normal physiologic anticoagulant condition. However, endothelial cells can be "activated" from their resting condition to undergo a series of cellular and biochemical responses which are central to inflammation. The recognition that endothelial cells can actively contribute to the inflammatory response has revolutionized our understanding of the mechanisms of many diseases. Such knowledge has important therapeutic consequences given that the acute inflammatory response appears to begin with an increase in vascular permeability, and, if more than trivial injury is produced, is typically followed shortly thereafter by leukocyte adhesion and infiltration.

Both normal endothelial cell function and activation occur within a complex milieu involving contact with adjacent parenchymal cells, circulating leukocytes and various soluble blood constituents. Endothelial cell activation is influenced by many other components of the vascular unit, including smooth muscle cells, pericytes, extracellular matrix, as well as circulating cells. Many of these interactions are the focus of other chapters in this book. This chapter arises from a perspective that there is now considerable interest in undertaking transplantation of organs or tissues from other species to humans, but that such transplantation is currently unsuccessful due to events occurring within the graft vasculature shortly after anastomosis and re-vascularization, leading to hyperacute rejection. Accordingly, we shall review knowledge of the involvement of humoral immunity in vascular injury in the context of xenotransplantation, with particular emphasis on the effects of binding of xenogeneic natural antibodies (XNA) and complement (C) to graft endothelium. While the emphasis of this chapter is on the vascular pathology of xenotransplantation, we also discuss various aspects of rejection of xenografts that are important for an understanding of comparable endothelial cell and vessel wall manifestations in other disease states.

OVERVIEW OF XENOTRANSPLANTATION

Xenotransplantation, i.e. transplantation between two phylogenetically disparate species, is frequently classified as concordant and discordant based on the immunological barriers to graft acceptance (Calne, 1970). When concordant transplants (i.e. between phylogenetically closely related species such as baboon to human) are performed, hyperacute rejection is not observed. However, transplantation between members of discordant or distantly related species, such as pig to human, results in hyperacute rejection in unmodified recipients. The tempo of hyperacute rejection can vary from 10–15 minutes post-transplantation in a discordant xenograft from guinea pig to rat, for instance, to approximately 1–2 hours if a pig heart is transplanted to a baboon or a rhesus monkey. This extremely rapid rejection process is associated with the co-deposition of XNA and C on donor endothelium (reviewed in Bach *et al.*, 1992).

There are fundamental pathophysiological differences between the transplantation of an immediately-vascularized organ, such as heart, kidney, liver or pancreas where the grafted endothelium is immediately exposed to the recipient's circulating blood containing XNA and C, and transplantation of neovascularized tissues, such as in the case of pancreatic islets, in which blood vessels from the host grow over days into the transplanted tissues. In the immediately-vascularized organ, the endothelium of the transplanted vasculature persists as donor type, and thus remains foreign to the recipient. We will consider only such primarily vascularised xenografts in this chapter, whereas the overall field is the subject of recent reviews (Bach *et al.*, in press; Dorling and Lechler, 1994).

Working Model of Hyperacute Rejection

Our working model (Bach *et al.*, 1994a) posits that following transplantation and establishment of blood flow from the recipient to the transplanted organ, recipient XNA, of both IgM and IgG classes, attach to donor endothelial cells and fix complement. The combination of the recipient's XNA plus C components lead to activation of the endothelial cells lining the vessels of the donor organ. As discussed later in this chapter, we believe that progressive endothelial cell activation is a central event in the pathogenesis of xenograft rejection. While we use hyperacute rejection associated with xenografts as our model here, a very similar reaction occurs in allografts transplanted into sensitized recipients with pre-existing anti-ABO antibodies or anti-MHC class I antibodies that react with graft endothelial cells (Sablinski *et al.*, 1990).

Concept of Delayed Xenograft Rejection (DXR)

In the few minutes that it takes for an organ to be destroyed by hyperacute rejection in some discordant species combinations, there is no time for gene up-regulation and synthesis of new proteins. We refer to these early events as type I EC activation. By contrast, in DXR, which takes place if the recipient is pre-treated in one or another way to ameliorate the initial events, the rejection process may take place over many hours or several days, permitting up-regulation of genes and its consequences (type II EC activation). We argue that hyperacute rejection involves the consequences of events occurring during type I endothelial cell activation, whereas DXR appears to involve the consequences of type II endothelial cell activation as well. From a clinical perspective, DXR is the key problem, given that we can already reliably postpone rejection of a pig heart or kidney in a primate for at least some days using therapies which interfere with the action of C.

XENOREACTIVE NATURAL ANTIBODIES (XNA)

The term "natural antibodies" refers to antibodies that are present without overt stimulation, such as the blood group (ABO) isohemagglutinins and XNA. In fact, for both of these types of antibodies, there is evidence that they are not just "naturally" present, as though there are genetically programmed B cells which produce the antibodies irrespective of the immunological exposure of the animal. Rather, it appears that the XNA are elicited in response to carbohydrates, which in the case of XNA in large measure involve terminal galactose moieties present on surface molecules of organisms in the gut and other sites (Galili, 1993; Cooper *et al.*, 1994; Neethling *et al.*, 1994).

IgM and IgG XNA

There is general agreement that IgM can function as XNA, resulting in the fixation and activation of complement at the surface of endothelial cells, and that depletion of IgM XNA can be of therapeutic significance (Soares *et al.*, 1993; Soares *et al.*, 1994), but there are less data on the role of IgG. Some studies of the immunopathology of pig hearts rejected by rhesus monkeys showed primarily, if not solely, IgM deposition on the endothelium of the donor organ (Platt *et al.*, 1991a; Bach *et al.*, 1992). IgG, when found, appeared to have the same distribution as albumin, and was thus interpreted to be present secondary to loss of vascular integrity and diffusion from the intravascular space into the sub-endothelial tissues as endothelium responded to the insult of the transplant situation.

However, there is direct evidence for a role for IgG in some discordant models. e.g. Human IgG binds to pig endothelial cells *in vitro* (Bach *et al.*, 1991b; Platt *et al.*, 1991b). Moreover, Inveradi and co-workers have shown that human IgG binds to bovine endothelial cells *in vitro*, and promotes NK cell-mediated antibody-dependent cytotoxicity towards the endothelial cells (Inverardi *et al.*, 1992) The IgG molecule presumably binds targets on the endothelial cells via its antigen-combining site (paratope); this interaction allows the Fc portion of the IgG to interact with the Fc receptor III (CD16) on NK cells. This finding may have additional importance in view of our own observations that activated NK cells and monocytes are prominent in guinea pig hearts rejected after approximately 3 days in rats in which C was depleted using cobra venom factor (Hancock *et al.*, 1993; Blakely *et al.*, 1994). It is also important to note that there can be an immune response by the recipient to the donor tissues, which results in the presence of elicited antibodies directed at targets on endothelial cells. Elicited antibodies (typically IgM but also IgG) are of central importance in the rejection of at least some concordant transplants, and will likely be an issue in discordant ones with prolonged survival as well.

Titers of XNA

The titers of XNA of IgM isotype in humans vary widely. In a study of 50 apparently healthy volunteers, the titers of serum XNA measured in an anti-porcine endothelial cells ELISA varied more than 400-fold between individuals (Vanhove and Bach, 1993). To help plan therapeutic strategies aimed at removing, or blocking, XNA, several other issues were investigated. Interestingly, XNA from individuals with relatively high titers contributed only 0.1% of total IgM, but *in vitro* about 100,000 IgM molecules bound per endothelial cell, with high affinity (Kd of 1×10^{-9} M). These results may be dependent on the methods used to obtain the XNA and the pig endothelial cells, but provide a guideline for potential therapeutic manipulations.

Targets of XNA

Targets of XNA must be considered at two levels: first, the glycoproteins and other molecules in the membranes of endothelial cells to which the XNA bind, and second, the carbohydrate epitopes on those molecules that are actually recognized by the XNA. There are a number of molecules on pig endothelial cells and platelets to which XNA bind. These include a triad of glycoproteins with molecular weights 115,000, 125,000, and 135,000 (referred to as gp115-135) (Platt *et al.*, 1990a), and a number of other prominent targets with molecular weights in the range of 45 kD to 200 kD (Thibaudeau *et al.*, 1994). These target molecules recognized by human XNA on porcine cells have mainly been defined by their relative molecular mass as analyzed by Western blotting.

Carbohydrate Binding of XNA

For the sake of potential therapeutic manipulations, it is important to define the carbohydrates recognized by XNA. Administration *in vivo* of the carbohydrate target moieties recognized by anti-AB antibodies can block access of those antibodies to the endothelium and thus prolong survival of ABO incompatible allografts (Alexandre *et al.*, 1991; Cooper *et al.*, 1993). In addition, α-galactosyl oligosaccharides block the cytotoxic effects of XNA on pig epithelial and endothelial cells *in vitro* (Neethling *et al.*, 1994), and in preliminary studies appear to prolong survival of test pig cardiac xenograft in baboon recipients to 12–18 hours (versus less than 1 hour in unmodified controls) (Cooper *et al.*, 1994). Alternatively, the sugars could be bound to a matrix on appropriate columns; passage of the plasma of the potential recipient through such columns might, as has been done for anti-AB antibodies, remove the XNA from the recipient, at least temporarily (Cooper *et al.*, 1993).

Molecules of different sizes are recognized as the predominant targets on different cells. In our own studies, the gp115-135 complexes were not detected on lymphocytes of red blood cells or lymphocytes, even though all the XNA reactive with endothelial cells could be absorbed from human serum by RBC or lymphocytes (Platt *et al.*, 1990a; Bach *et al.*, 1994a). This finding is consistent with the fact that XNA react with carbohydrate moieties, and that the same, or cross-reactive, sugars are present on different molecules on the different cells.

COMPLEMENT (C)

C can be activated by two mechanisms. The two pathways meet at the level of C3 and promote formation of the membrane attack complex (MAC), the terminal components of which (poly C9) insert into the membrane of cells. The classical pathway is initiated by antigen-bound antibody activating C1q, whereas the second, or alternative, pathway of C activation is typically activated by exposure to various carbohydrates. At various stages of activation, soluble mediators are generated that can play important roles in inflammation, including activation of endothelial cells (see below).

Classical vs. Alternate Pathway Activation *In Vivo*

The extent of activation of the alternate pathway of C following xenotransplantation appears to depend on the species combination involved. The alternative pathway is activated on transplantation of organs from guinea pig to rats, or from rabbits to pigs lacking XNA, as shown by deposition of factor B regardless of the presence or absence of IgM or IgG (Johnston *et al.*, 1992). However, on transplantation of pig organs to primates, there is no clear *in vivo* evidence of alternative pathway activation; rather, there is co-deposition of components of the classical pathway (C2 and C4) with IgM and IgG (Platt *et al.*, 1991a,; Lesnikoski *et al.*, in press).

It is still controversial whether there is alternative pathway activation *in vitro*, and whether or not workers in the field have merely failed to detect this *in vivo*. This may be a critical issue in terms of planning therapy. A major approach to control of the hyperacute rejection is to remove XNA from the potential recipient. If the alternative pathway of complement is activated, then removal of XNA will not prevent the activation of complement, although the magnitude of activation may be less. XNA appear, as discussed later in regard to endothelial cells, to have a role in xenoresponses in addition to the activation of C in certain models (Pierson *et al.*, in press).

Therapeutic Agents to Block C

The inhibition of C activation has posed a major problem for clinical medicine, since few methods are considered clinically applicable. The stimulus provided by xenograft rejection, with the special opportunity afforded by having a donor animal that might be genetically manipulated, has revitalised interest in potential methods to inhibit complement.

 • Cobra venom factor (CVF). This viperid analogue of C3 forms a physicochemically stable CVF-Bb complex and has long been used in experimental animals. Indeed, work done in xenotransplantation over three decades ago, demonstrated that administration of CVF, and the consequent inhibition of C, prolonged survival of xenografts (Reemtsma *et al.*, 1964). More recently, semi-purified CVF has been used; removal of the associated venom proteases and toxins has partly improved its biocompatibility without diminishing its efficacy. The most undesirable aspect of the use of CVF, aside from its potential toxicity, is that it works by activating C (consumptive depletion) rather than inhibiting it. It is necessary to administer CVF with great care in terms of dose and rapidity of administration, since activated products of C may precipitate major side effects such as shock and pulmonary haemorrhage. Whether recipients will make antibodies to the CVF and thus neutralize the administered material after a few days or not is unknown.

 • Soluble CR1 (sCR1). Use of soluble CR1 provides a conceptually more satisfying approach to blocking C. Work by Douglas Fearon and colleagues (Hebell *et al.*, 1991) has been shown that the administration of sCR1 effectively inhibits C and permits prolongation of xenograft survival. The attractive part of this approach is that, in contrast to CVF, it acts by inhibiting, rather than activating, C. A potential disadvantage is the residual reservoir of circulating C which could undergo activation by the described cascade should the inhibitor be less than 100% effective.

Use of Endogenous Membrane-Associated Inhibitors of C

Another approach to inhibit C involves the use of normally expressed membrane-bound inhibitors of C. Decay accelerating factor (DAF, CD55) and membrane cofactor protein (MCP, CD46) each inhibit C3, and thus interfere with both the alternative and classical pathways. Homologous restriction factor (CD59) inhibits assembly of the terminal MAC complex by preventing insertion of C8 and C9 (see reviews by Dalmasso, 1992; Rooney *et al.*, 1993; and Ryan, 1994).

Dalmasso *et al.* (1991) introduced human forms of membrane-associated inhibitors of complement into porcine endothelial cells in order to inhibit C action *in vitro*. This approach was based on two concepts. First, there is species-specificity for some of these inhibitors; thus, the pig inhibitor in the endothelial cells of the donor organ may not be particularly effective at inhibiting human C. Second, by genetically engineering the pig endothelial cells, it may be possible to express the complement-inhibitory factors at a higher density than normally found, and thus achieve greater inhibition (Dalmasso *et al.*, 1991; White *et al.*, 1992).

Based on the success of these studies *in vitro*, White and colleagues and others have recently gone on to produce pigs which are transgenic for human DAF. Such pigs express the human DAF protein and their lymphocytes are lysed to a lesser extent than are control lymphocytes by human serum (personal communication). It is the goal to derive a transgenic pig that expresses high levels of human inhibitors of complement, possibly including DAF, CD46 and CD59, at the endothelial interface. A critical issue that is not yet resolved is whether delayed xenograft rejection (DXR), mediated by factors other than T cells, would be averted or adequately treated if the action of C were blocked completely.

COAGULATION AND HEMOSTASIS

Activation of clotting is a common accompaniment of immune reactions *in vivo* (reviewed by Esmon, 1993), and fibrin deposition and platelet aggregation in vascularised xenografts are considered a consequence of activation of host immune and inflammatory responses (Hunt and Rosenberg, 1993). Various products of the coagulation pathway participate in immunologically-mediated tissue damage, and degradation products of fibrin can modify immune functions (Mosesson, 1992; Robson *et al.*, 1993). Similarly, stimulation of the immune system and C activation are crucial to key events in blood coagulation, including thrombin generation (Esmon, 1993) and platelet aggregation (Sims and Wiedmer, 1991).

Platelet Aggregation and Activation

A rapid, efficient clotting process is dependent upon platelet activation and aggregation (Figure 1). Platelet function in coagulation is modulated by leukocytes and endothelial cells, in a process which has been termed thromboregulation (Marcus and Safier, 1993).

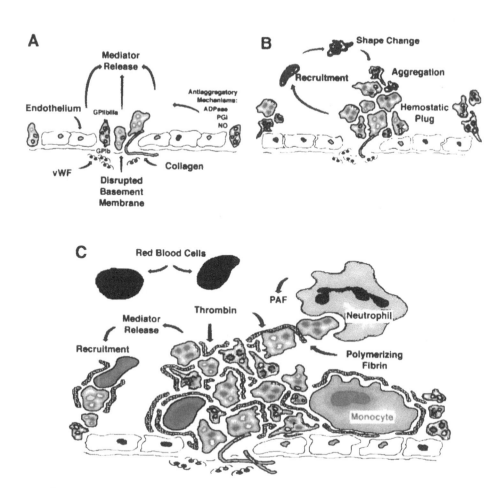

Figure 1 Diagram of platelet involvement in the pathogenesis of xenograft rejection. a) Platelets circulate in the blood in an inactive state. Following endothelial cell activation or injury, platelets adhere to and spread on the subendothelial matrix, initially by the interaction of GPIb and von Willebrand factor (vWF) which is facilitated by shear stress. Xenogeneic vWF may also have increased affinity for GPIb in the absence of stress or vascular injury. The activation of platelets with expression of P-selectin and GPIIbIIIa is accompanied by mediator release, further recruitment and promotion of the coagulation process. This process can be antagonised by the endothelial cell antiaggregatory mechanisms which include the ADPase systems, the synthesis of the prostacycline PGI2 and nitric oxide or endothelial cell derived relaxing factor (EDRF). b) Recruitment is accompanied by platelet activation, with associated shape changes and aggregation. Platelet aggregates co-localize with the initial adherent platelets to form the initial haemostatic plug. c)Thrombosis is a multicellular process, often involving neutrophils and monocytes, through their release of cytokines and platelet activating factor. Monocytes, in particular, also promote the local process of thrombogenesis by their expression of tissue factor. Red blood cells modulate platelet activation and are incorporated into the clot. The endothelial surface loses its barrier function and extravasation begins.

Platelet-derived substances are essential to the integrity of the endothelial monolayer (Kobayashi, 1992; Marcus and Safier, 1993). Platelet adhesion and activation are governed by their interaction with various components of the sub-endothelial matrix in the context of shear stresses generated by blood flow (Chow *et al.*, 1992). Shear stress is dependent upon flow and inversely related to vessel diameter, so that high shear rates are generated mainly in the microvasculature, precisely where the thrombotic insults seen in early xenograft rejection are localised (Hunt and Rosenberg, 1993; Blakely *et al.*, 1994; Lesnikoski *et al.*, 1994).

The initial binding of platelets to the endothelium is dependent on the interaction of platelet receptor GPIb with von Willebrand factor (vWF) bound to the subendothelial matrix. This process is enhanced by the binding of subendothelial collagen and fibronectin to receptors on the platelet surface (Roth, 1992; Hynes, 1992). Activation signals generated by these interactions act in concert with thrombin to enhance expression and affinity of GPIIb/IIIa and P-selectin on platelets (Kroll *et al.*, 1991; Smyth *et al.*, 1993). The platelet integrin, GPIIb/IIIa binds to both vWF (at a different site to that of GPIb) and fibrin(ogen), promoting platelet aggregation (Ruggeri and Ware, 1993). Selectin expression by platelets and leukocytes promote cell adhesion to the area of injury (Furie and Furie, 1992; Coughlan *et al.*, 1993; Coughlan *et al.*, 1994).

Platelets and Coagulation

The assembly of coagulation factors on the platelet surface is facilitated by several events. First, there is expression of specific receptors for coagulation factor V, which are upregulated as a consequence of platelet activation. Second, the platelet membrane aminophospholipids are exposed as a result of microparticle formation, which enhance the binding and assembly of the prothrombinase complex (Furie and Furie, 1992; Esmon, 1993). Third, platelets contain in their alpha granules high concentrations of fibrinogen and other coagulation proteins which, when expressed on the cell surface or secreted into the extracellular environment, promote local fibrin deposition (Harrison and Martin-Cramer, 1993). Platelet aggregation involves an initiation trigger (thrombin, exposure to collagen etc.) amplified by the release of ADP and serotonin. The generation of thrombin serves as a potent positive feed-back step. Platelet aggregation is influenced by other factors. Erythrocytes promote platelet aggregation and hemostatic plugs by co-expression of adhesion receptors, such as for thrombospondin, a large adhesion molecule, and by modulating the eicosanoid formation by platelets (Marcus and Safier, 1993).

Effects of Endothelial cells on Platelet Aggregation

Endothelial cells can potentially inhibit platelet aggregation by at least three mechanisms: (a) release of prostacyclin, (b) generation of nitric oxide, and (c) action of an ecto-ADPase. The latter binds and degrades platelet-derived ADP, thereby inhibiting amplification pathways which result in platelet plug formation (Marcus and Safier, 1993) (Figure 2).

RESTING ENDOTHELIUM

Factors associated with resting and activated endothelial cells are shown in Figure 3. Resting endothelial cells perform several functions. First, as they are tightly juxtaposed to neighbouring cells, they maintain a barrier that keeps cells and serum proteins in the intravascular space. Second, endothelial cells express several different molecules that help to maintain an anticoagulant state. Two of the most important are heparan sulfate, a

Endothelial Cell Protective Mechanisms

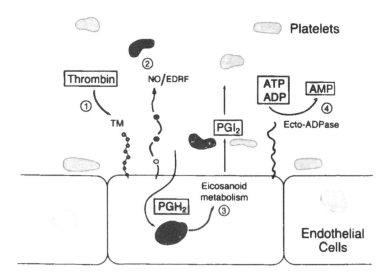

Figure 2 Endothelial cell and platelet anti-aggregatory mechanisms. Thrombomodulin (TM) expressed by the vascular endothelium is capable indirectly of abrogating platelet responses to thrombin. (1) Endothelial cells also inhibit platelet aggregation by several mechanisms which include the release of prostacyclines (2), the generation of nitric oxide (3) and the action of the ecto-ADPases (4), which efficiently degrade platelet derived ADP, thus inhibiting amplification pathways which result in platelet plug formation.

proteoglycan, and thrombomodulin, both of which are lost from the surfaces of endothelial cells during activation.

Heparan Sulphate and Antithrombin III (ATIII)

Heparan sulfate consists of a protein core with glycosaminoglycan chains attached to it. ATIII binds to appropriately substituted residues on the glycosaminoglycan chains. When ATIII attaches to the heparan sulfate, it is activated and becomes a powerful anticoagulant, interfering with the action of thrombin, a key component of the coagulation cascade, as well as other factors. Also associated with the heparan sulfate are superoxide dismutases (SOD), which break down oxygen radicals (O2-) produced, for instance, by activated neutrophils. SOD converts O2- to hydrogen peroxide plus oxygen. Although hydrogen peroxide, like oxygen radicals, is toxic to endothelial cells, endothelial cells have mechanisms to inactivate and degrade hydrogen peroxide (Esmon, 1993).

Thrombomodulin/Protein C/Protein S Pathway

Thrombomodulin present on the surface of quiescent endothelial cells, binds thrombin. As a consequence of that interaction, protein C (PC), present in blood, is converted to activated protein C (APC). APC interferes with coagulation by degrading the clotting factors Va and VIIIa (Walker and Fay, 1992; Esmon, 1993). APC has a central role in the

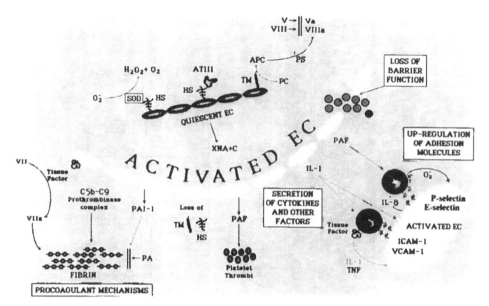

Figure 3 Model of events leading to rejection of a discordant xenograft, emphasizing the key role of endothelial cell (EC) activation, as a result of binding of XNA and/or C. Quiescent EC maintain a barrier to blood cells and proteins, and express heparan sulfate (HS) and thrombomodulin (TM) on their surfaces. HS binds the anticoagulant, antithrombin III (AT-III), and superoxide dismutase (SOD), which breaks down superoxide (O2-). TM binds thrombin, leading to generation of activated protein C (APC), which has a potent anticoagulant action, as well as anti-inflammatory effects.

Upon EC activation, there is loss of vascular integrity, resulting in hemorrhage and edema. Second, there is up-regulation of the adhesion molecules, P-selectin, E-selectin, ICAM-1 and VCAM-1, which can function as ligands for binding of PMN, monocytes, and lymphocytes, as well as MHC class I and II antigens. Third, activated EC secrete IL-1, IL-6, and IL-8 aand PAF. IL-1 is stimulatory to EC in an autocrine loop, as well as activating leukocytes. IL-8 is a chemoattractant, and has some of the functions discussed for C5a below. PAF activates neutrophils and platelets. Fourth, activated EC become procoagulant. PAF promotes formation of platelet thrombi; loss of HS and TM results in loss of the anticoagulant mechanisms of quiescent EC; secretion of plasminogen activator inhibitor (PAI-1) inhibits the naturally-occuring action of plasminogen activator (PA); vesicles shed by activated EC contain membrane attack complex (MAC, C5b-C9), which activate the prothrombinase complex, leading to clotting; and activated EC (as well as activated monocytes) produce tissue factor, perhaps the most powerful stimulus to coagulation.

Other factors also contribute to xenograft rejection. C fragments deliver signals to EC, aiding in full activation. C5a like IL-8, induces chemotaxis, chemokinesis, degranulation and respiratory bursts in PMN, as well as increasing PMN integrin affinity for EC ligands, and participating in the loss of HS from activated EC. C5a also stimulates macrophages and mast cells to release TNF and/or IL-1, which can activate (and damage) EC. Cells that bind to activated EC also participate in rejection. PMN activated by C5a and PAF secrete reactive oxygen species. The production of superoxide by activated cells bound to the EC, as well as by the EC themselves, are likely major players in the overall response, perhaps primarily by activation of NFκB; the loss of SOD aggravates these complications.

normal, physiologic inactivation of these activated procoagulant cofactors, as shown by the observation that infants born without PC usually die with massive thrombotic complications in infancy, and adults heterozygous for PC deficiency are prone to thrombotic episodes (Esmon, 1993). While thrombin alone is capable of generating APC, there is a >1000-fold increase in the activation of PC when thrombin is complexed with thrombomodulin. APC circulates in the serum with a half life of 15–30 minutes. Neutralisation of newly formed APC is controlled by at least three plasma protease inhibitors: protein C inhibitor 1 and 2, and α_1-antitrypsin, all of which act slowly, giving a long half life for

APC relative to other coagulant molecules (e.g. thrombin, whose half-life is a matter of seconds) (Walker and Fay, 1992). The inhibitory effect of α_1-antitrypsin on APC is enhanced by heparin and other glycosaminoglycans. Conversely, the anticoagulant and profibrinolytic actions of APC are enhanced by the co-factor, protein S (PS), another vitamin K-dependent serine protease (Walker and Fay, 1992).

Other Functional Molecules

Tissue factor pathway inhibitor (TFPI) is a plasma protein with potent and selective inhibitory activity for factor Xa as it is associated with the tissue factor-VIIa complex. A pool of this inhibitor is located in endothelial cells and platelets and is released by heparin infusion (Broze, 1992). In addition to specific inhibitors of coagulation, endothelial cells influence the process of fibrinolysis by the regulated secretion of plasminogen activators and their specific inhibitors, as well as thrombospondin, a large adhesion molecule which modulates plasmin generation, and hence fibrinolysis (Anonick *et al.*, 1993).

ACTIVATED ENDOTHELIUM

Changes in endothelial cells following activation can be divided into several categories (Figure 3). These will be reviewed here, whereas the following sections consider features of endothelial activation of documented relevance to xenograft responses.

First, endothelial cell retraction causes a loss of vascular integrity, exposing the sub-endothelial matrix and allowing cells and proteins to pass from the intravascular space into the tissues, resulting in hemorrhage and edema. Such retraction, stimulated by local deposition of C, histamine, PAF and possibly additional factors, may be a key initail feature of hyperacute rejection.

Second, a series of cell surface adhesion molecules are up-regulated. Some of these, such as the selectin adhesion molecules (P- and E-selectin) and tissue factor, are only expressed upon endothelial activation, whereas others are present on resting cells but are further up-regulated upon activation (e.g. ICAM-1/CD54, MHC class I). A key outcome of such activation is the increased adhesion of inflammatory cells which can themselves drive the activation process forward. e.g. Neutrophils activated by C5a and PAF, secrete reactive oxygen species. Similarly, monocytes activated by locally generated cytokines or other factors, secrete IL-1 and TNF-α which can act on adjacent endothelial cells, and these cell may also express tissue factor which can contribute to the procoagulant environment (Pober and Cotran, 1991; Murphy *et al.*, 1992).

Third, the activated endothelial cells secrete a number of cytokines and other molecules, including IL-1, IL-6, and IL-8 as well as platelet activating factor (PAF). IL-1 is likely stimulatory to the endothelial cells in an autocrine loop, as well as functioning to activate cells of blood, such as monocytes. IL-8 is a chemoattractant for leukocytes and has some of the functions discussed for C5a above. PAF serves to activate neutrophils and endothelial cell activation.

Lastly, at least six mechanisms can affect the balance between anti-coagulation (actively promoted by quiescent endothelial cells) and procoagulation (associated with activated endothelial cells): (a) PAF promotes the activation of platelets. (b) Loss of heparan sulphate results in a loss of the anticoagulant contribution of ATIII. (c) Loss of thrombomodulin results suppresses the ability to bind thrombin and rapidly generate APC. (d) Secretion of plasminogen activator inhibitor (PAI-1) inhibits the lysis of fibrin clots by plasminogen activator. (e) Endothelial membrane-derived vesicles containing components of the membrane attack complex (C5b-C9) are shed and activate the protrombinase complex, leading to clotting (Hamilton *et al.*, 1990). (f) Perhaps most important, and apparently the major pathway of induced clotting when endothelial cells are stimulated with XNA and C (Hofer *et al.*, 1993; Vanhove and Bach, 1993), is based on the production of tissue factor by the endothelial cells, leading to conversion of factor VII to factor VIIa, and then the consequent clotting cascade.

Strategies to Inhibit Endothelial Activation or Its Consequences

A number of approaches to block or attenuate endothelial cell activation are under investigation. One approach is to block expression of adhesion molecules on activated endothelial cells. Monoclonal antibodies to E-selectin, ICAM-1 and others prevent attachment of neutrophils and monocytes to the endothelial cells and thus inhibit the stimulus provided by products of these cells to the endothelial cells. Monoclonal antibodies may be aimed either at the molecule expressed on the activated endothelial cells, or the ligand on leukocytes. Antibodies to other cell surface molecules (e.g. tissue factor when expressed), or peptides that bind those same molecules, are being tested to block those molecules.

Methods that would inhibit endothelial cells activation in general, or specific aspects thereof, are still very much in developmental stages. At present the approaches fall into two categories. First, various drugs, or other inhibitory agents, interfere with one or another aspect of endothelial cell activation. Most of these drugs are selective in that they prevent expression of some aspects of endothelial cells activation but not others. Included in this list are agents that interfere with expression of adhesion molecules or with aspects of pro-coagulation. Efforts are underway to find new agents that might be useful in this regard. Second, there are efforts to manipulate pig endothelial cells genetically to avoid, or counteract, some of the undesirable consequences of endothelial cell activation. These include expression of new molecules in the endothelial cells, as well as preventing the expression of key effector molecules, such as tissue factor.

HYPERACUTE REJECTION

Hyperacute rejection of discordant xenografts, characterised by the plugging of arterioles by platelet microthrombi and widespread interstitial hemorrhages, poses a formidable barrier to clinical xenotransplantation. C depletion has the potential to dramatically modify this process but current modalities of treatment are associated with significant toxicity and morbidity, as discussed above.

Importance of C

We have studied events associated with rejection of guinea pig cardiac xenografts in untreated rats vs. recipients depleted of XNA (splenectomy, anti-μ mAb) (Hancock *et al.*, 1993; Blakely *et al.*, 1994; Soares *et al.*, 1993; Soares *et al.*, 1994). Neither splenectomy or additional depletion of IgM-XNA (<0.2% of normal rat serum) affected the tempo of HAR (rejection at 10 minutes). At the time of HAR, xenografts contained only trace levels of classical complement pathway components (C1q, C4, C2) and no IgM, indicating the functional efficacy of IgM depletion. HAR was associated with low titer, focal IgG deposition on graft venules, but dense fibrin labelling of the entire microvasculature, as well as high titer C3 deposition were noted; the latter consistent with the alternate pathway activation of C.

Type I Endothelial Activation *In Vivo*

Using rat recipients of guinea pig cardiac xenografts, we have documented type I endothelial cell activation *in vivo* during hyperacute rejection (Coughlan *et al.*, 1993; Blakely *et al.*, in press). The adhesive glycoprotein, P-selectin (GMP-140), is normally present, along with vWF, in the cytoplasmic Weibel-Palade bodies of endothelial cells and in α-granules of platelets. Stimulation of endothelial cells *in vitro* with histamine, thrombin, leukotrienes or other agents causes fusion of vesicle and plasma membranes, exposing P-selectin and vWF multimers on the endothelial surface, as well as release of PAF. We found that following transplantation, xenografts beat vigorously for several minutes and then quickly became mottled, contracted irregularly and were frankly hemorrhagic within 1–2 minutes, followed by cessation of contractions. Immunohistologic studies showed dense deposition of IgM, IgG, C3 and C5 on graft endothelial cells, in conjunction with surface labelling of endothelial cells and platelets for P-selectin.

Mechanisms of Hyperacute Rejection

Within minutes of revascularization and circulation of rat recipient blood through a guinea pig xenograft, C activation occurs via the alternative pathway (Miyagawa *et al.*, 1988; Blakely *et al.*, in press), generating the anaphylatoxins C3a and C5a. These act locally on mast cells, which are present in high concentration in rat cardiac tissues, to release histamine. The assembly of C5b-C9 on platelets, along with local histamine release, causes degranulation of platelets, releasing high levels of coagulation factors, ADP (a potent platelet agonist and vasoconstrictor) and serotonin. Within seconds, histamine and serotonin bind to receptors on endothelial cells, and stimulate surface expression of PAF as well as fusion of Weibel Palade bodies to the membrane, exposing vWF and P-selectin (Coughlan *et al.*, 1993; Blakely *et al.*, in press). Endothelial cells also retract, exposing underlying basement membranes, proteoglycans and thrombospondin to platelets and plasma components. PAF promotes the activation of platelets with a dramatic increase in vascular permeability, as evidenced by the prolongation of graft survival in this model to several hours following administration of a PAF antagonist (Coughlan *et al.*, 1993). Stasis, together with interstitial hemorrhages arising from breaches of vascular integrity, markedly and rapidly reduces vascular compliance and the heart fails within 10–15 minutes of revascularization.

DELAYED XENOGRAFT REJECTION (DXR)

Depletion of complement using CVF prolongs guinea pig cardiac xenograft survival to >70 hrs vs. 10–15 minutes in untreated rat recipients; rejection was associated with lack of C deposition, but an infiltrate of macrophages and NK cells, with associated dense expression of the cytokines TNF-α and IFN-γ (Hancock et al., 1993; Blakely et al., in press). By 48 hrs post-transplant, macrophages and graft endothelial cells expressed tissue factor, and endothelial cells showed downregulation of thrombomodulin and AT-III expression, in conjunction with widespread fibrin deposition.

Thus, it appears that once HAR is overcome, xenografts undergo a series of steps involving mononuclear and endothelial cell activation, culminating in rejection after a few days. This is a novel form of rejection in the xenograft literature, though our further data indicate that comparable events occur prior to the rejection of pig xenografts in monkeys depleted of XNA by organ perfusion (Lesnikoski et al., 1994). Mononuclear infiltrates occurring over 2–4 days post-transplant in guinea pig xenografts in CVF-treated (Leventhal et al., 1993) or C6-deficient (Brauer et al., 1993) rats have recently been noted by others, but no data on cellular activation or cytokine expression was presented. At least three scenarios may explain DXR, namely that activated mononuclear cells cause DXR; activated endothelial cells cause DXR; or that DXR occurs as a consequence of combined mononuclear and endothelial cell activation. These questions are discussed below:

(a) Mononuclear cells may be targeted to a xenograft through Fc-dependent binding to endothelial-bound XNA. Stepwise stimulation of mononuclear cells via Fc receptors could then cause cellular activation and release of products, including cytokines, which damage surrounding endothelial cells and depress myocardial contractility. Additional mechanisms for recruitment and activation of mononuclear cells may be through release of chemotactic cytokines, such as MCP-1 or IL-8, by endothelial cells and/or monocytes (Colotta et al., 1994), or, depending upon the extent of C depletion, through binding to endothelial cell-bound C3bi (Vercellotti et al., 1991). Monocytes can also be activated to produce cytokines such as TNF-α by exposure to foreign carbohydrates (Westenfelder et al., 1993).

NK cells have been implicated in xenogeneic responses in other studies. In a human to rat *ex vivo* model, Inveradi et al. (1992) showed that CD3-, CD16+ NK cells preferentially bound to vascular endothelium of rat hearts; such adherence was only partly IgG-dependent. Adhesion was inhibited by monoclonal antibodies to CD11/CD18, and adherent cells induced rapid and direct injury to xenogeneic endothelial cells, suggesting a direct role for NK cells in xenogeneic effector mechanisms. Moreover, binding of NK cells disrupts the function of guinea pig cardiac cells, and such damage is amplified by TNF-α and other cytokines (Binah et al., 1993). NK cells are important in early recognition and removal of allogeneic cells which lack self MHC class I antigens (Sheng-Tanner and Miller, 1992), and this role, alone, or in conjunction with macrophages which can be activated by IFN-γ from NK cells, may extend to xenogeneic responses during DXR. Lastly, preliminary data suggest that the absence of NK cells leads to prolongation of xenograft survival in the rodent model (Arakawa et al., 1994). Moreover, most protocols for xenotransplantation involve splenectomy, which is typically undertaken to decrease the levels of XNA, but this procedure also markedly decreases the number of circulating NK cells.

(b) Stimulation of endothelial cells following XNA deposition might cause endotheli cell activation and DXR. XNA binding by endothelial cells is known to cause upregu tion of IL-1, IL-8 and PAI-1 by cultured pig endothelial cells (Vanhove et al., 1994, However, there are no data regarding the effects of such binding in the rodent model. For this mechanism to play a key role in DXR, endothelial cells binding of XNA could stimulate a procoagulant state and local and progressive tissue ischemia and hypoxia would eventually lead to graft destruction. Indeed, hypoxia itself can induce endothelial cells to produce tissue factor, various cytokines and expression of leukocyte adhesion molecules (Shreeniwas *et al.*, 1992).

(c) The most likely scenario in our opinion is a combination of both mononuclear and endothelial cell activation. In this schema, monocyte-macrophages might be activated directly by exposure to xenogeneic carbohydrates or resulting stimuli, as envisaged for their response to certain microorganisms or tumor cells. Alternately, once again, Fc-dependent signalling might activate macrophages or NK cells and result in their mutual activation. The role of IL-12 in this step is under investigation by us. At some point, NK cells are stimulated to release IFN-γ which promotes macrophage activation and cytokine release. Such cytokines then activate endothelial cells, causing a progressive recruitment of mononuclear cells through induction of adhesion molecules, as well as stimulation of a procoagulant state through upregulation of tissue factor on macrophages and graft endothelial cells, and downregulation of anticoagulant molecules, including thrombo-modulin and AT-III. Downregulation of thrombomodulin expression, resulting in a markedly reduced capacity of endothelial cells to bind thrombin and activate protein C, may further enhance macrophage cytokine production. APC appears to have a key role in inhibition of macrophage activation *in vivo* and *in vitro* (Grey *et al.*, 1994). The cumula-tive effect of fibrin generation and local hypoxia, the toxic effects of TNF-α, IL-1 and other cytokines generated in response to activated complement components, fibrin and other coagulation products (Robson, 1994), and a potential direct effect of mononuclear cells binding to endothelial cells may be more than enough to cause DXR; see Albelda *et al.* (1994) for an excellent general review of the many complex interactions of leuco-cytes and endothelial cells during inflammation.

The issue remains open at this time whether differences between allo- and xenogeneic cell-mediated rejection with respect to the vasculature are simply quantitative, perhaps involving greater reliance on indirect sensitization of helper cells in xenogeneic responses (Bach *et al.*, in press) or whether there are truly unique mechanisms of cellular xenograft rejection that do not participate in allograft rejection. The extent to which T cell activa-tion will occur if DXR is prolonged for a further day or two and the potential conse-quences of this thus still remains to be determined.

IN VITRO MODELS OF XENOREACTIVITY

Porcine endothelial cells from the aorta, or from the microvasculature, the site at which the primary manifestations of xenograft rejection occur, can be grown in monolayer cul-tures. These cells have a characteristic morphology, express vWF and receptors for low density lipoprotein. Addition of human serum to the endothelial cell cultures, as a source of XNA and C, results in endothelial cell responses which parallel those which occur *in vivo* when blood flow to a transplanted organ is established (Vanhove *et al.*, 1994). The endothelial cells retract from one another, accompanied by changes in their actin fila-ments, resulting in increased permeability to molecules of various sizes, and presumably mimicking the leakiness that occurs *in vivo*. Heparan sulfate is lost from the surfaces of cultured endothelial cells upon stimulation with human serum (Platt *et al.*, 1990b). Loss of the heparan sulfate requires XNA plus C. However, the entire C cascade is not involved in this process; XNA and C5a are sufficient to mediate loss (Platt *et al.*, 1990b). Thrombomodulin expression is also down-regulated when the cells are stimulated with cytokines (see Pober and Cotran, 1991).

In addition, a number of the genes that are up-regulated *in vitro* following endothelial cell activation with classical stimuli such as IL-1 and TNF-α, are also up-regulated by human serum that is added to the endothelial cell monolayer (Vanhove *et al.*, 1993). Addition of human serum, presumably as a source of XNA and C, also mimics the *in vivo* situation by inducing expression of the procoagulant, tissue factor (Hofer *et al.*, 1994).

ACCOMMODATION AND XENOTRANSPLANTATION

Given the importance of XNA and C in initiating vascular rejection, many investigators have focused on methods that would inhibit one or both of these factors for the hoped-for lifetime of the graft. For instance, inhibition of recipient C by membrane-associated inhibitors of C placed in the endothelial cells of the donor organ by transgenic or other methodology might achieve this for C. There are also potential approaches that would achieve long-term depletion for XNA; two examples include: (a) B cells producing the XNA might be selectively eliminated by immunotoxins attached to antibodies recognizing the idiotypes that characterize the XNA, or (b) tolerance to the xenoantigens recognized by XNA and elicited antibodies might be achieved. However, these approaches to lower XNA and elicited antibodies for a relevant duration for clinical application need much further development.

It may not be necessary to remove XNA and compromise the C system for the life-time of the graft to prevent xenograft rejection (Bach *et al.*, 1991a; Bach *et al.*, 1994b). Based on findings in allotransplantation across the ABO barrier, it may transpire that if XNA, C and possibly other factors are depleted for some time after the transplant is in place, that it may subsequently be possible to let XNA, C and other factors return to normal without evoking endothelial cell activation and rejection. We envision that during the time that the graft is in place in the "absence" of XNA etc., the endothelial cells will have time to "heal in" and recover from the trauma of having been exposed to relative hypothermia and low oxygen tensions, with subsequent reperfusion. We have referred to the survival of a graft under such circumstances as "accommodation", and have outlined possible reasons why accommodation may be achieved (Bach *et al.*, 1993). These include possible changes in the antibodies that return after depletion, including the possibility that non-C fixing antibodies block the target sites on the endothelial cells, and/or changes in the targets themselves, e.g. addition of terminal sialic acids to the target carbohydrates might protecting them from XNA binding. However, we regard it as most likely that accommodation is based on changes in the endothelial cells, including up-regulation of inhibitors of C.

Some experimental models indicate that accommodation can be seen in xenotransplantation. We have studied one rhesus monkey recipient of a pig heart in which accommodation was achieved. More recently, White and his colleagues have attained what appears to be accommodation in some hamster to rat heart transplants (Hassan *et al.*, 1992). These findings at least encourage further studies to make accommodation a potential therapeutic goal for xenotransplantation.

Mechanisms of Endothelial Cell Accomodation

Based on the data described in the section on XNA, one can envisage that the untreated xenograft recipient, within seconds to minutes of re-vascularization, there is a sudden binding of as many as 100,000 molecules of XNA on each endothelial cell in combination with deposition of C (Vanhove and Bach, 1993; Vanhove *et al.*, 1994). The endothelial response evoked under those circumstances might be quite different compared to the situation when XNA and C are depleted prior to transplantation, and then only allowed to return slowly after the endothelial cells have had time to "heal in". We hypothesize that in the latter circumstances, the endothelial cells will accommodate, i.e. not respond, so as to lead to rejection of the graft. Recent findings, presented below, are consistent with this.

Endothelial Responses: Activation of NFκB vs. IκB and Response to Heme

An exceedingly early event following stimulation of endothelial cells is activation of the transcription factor, NFκB, which appears to play a prominent role with respect to up-regulation of many genes, including E-selectin and tissue factor, that are characteristic of endothelial cell activation. Work from our laboratories (de Martin *et al.*, 1993) has shown that following endothelial cell activation, there is not only rapid activation of NFκB, but also up-regulation of a gene coding for an IκB (inhibitor of NFκB)-like molecule. The IκB protein binds to, and inhibits, the function of NFκB. To the extent that this occurs, there would be decreased NFκB function. Thus, several of the genes that are dependent on NFκB for up-regulation, and the products of which are likely participants in hyperacute rejection, would not be up-regulated. One could imagine that under certain conditions (i.e. those leading to accommodation), IκB activity would be dominant over NFκB, and so full endothelial cell activation would be prevented, leading to accommodation rather than hyperacute rejection.

Vercellotti and colleagues have shown that a given stimulus to endothelial cells can, dependent on the conditions, induce either sensitization of the endothelial cells to a subsequent toxic challenge, or what might be considered accommodation to that same toxic challenge (Balla *et al.*, 1992). Stimulation of endothelial cells for an hour with heme leads to an increased sensitivity of the endothelial cells with regard to lysis by activated neutrophils. However, if the endothelial cells are stimulated with heme for one hour, and then left for approximately 16 hours, the cells upregulate certain metabolic pathways and synthesize ferritin. This active response of the endothelial cells apparently protects them from oxidative damage by activated neutrophils or hydrogen peroxide. In both examples, the endothelial cells respond actively by up-regulating genes that could, under the right circumstances, contribute to achieving accommodation.

Alpha-Globulins and Endothelial Activation

In addition to the active development of defence mechanisms, we suggest that normally-occurring serum inhibitory factors, such as the alpha-globulins, which inhibit up-regulation of E-selectin and other cell surface ligands, may play a role in accommodation (Stuhlmeier *et al.*, 1993). We view the potential function of the α-globulins as inhibitory factors that prevent response to low-level stimulation that, from an evolutionary point of view, would be undesirable. In this context, they might behave rather like the membrane-associated inhibitors of complement, such as DAF, discussed above. If XNA return very slowly, the stimulus to the endothelial cells may be quite weak, and these naturally-occuring inhibitors might function to protect the graft.

CONCLUDING COMMENTS

Dissection of the mechanisms of endothelial injury and endothelial cell responses which occur following xenotransplantation has begun. We anticipate that the insights arising from these studies, *in vivo* and *in vitro*, will allow development and testing of new strategies to modulate or block humoral immunity and vascular injury after engraftment. Ultimately, such strategies, combined with genetic manipulation of the endothelial cell response, are likely to provide a means for successful clinical xenotransplantation. Data derived from such studies may have relevance to understanding and modifying endothelial responses in non-xenograft settings, including vascular type rejection processes in the allograft, arteriosclerosis and other thrombotic, inflammatory vascular diseases, as well as providing a model for a role for anti-endothelial antibodies in such disorders.

References

Albelda, S.M., Smith, C.W. and Ward, P.A. (1994). Adhesion molecules and inflammatory injury. *FASEB J.*, **8**:504–512.

Alexandre, G.P.J., Latinne, D., Gianello, P. and Squifflet, J.P. (1991). Preformed cytotoxic antibodies and ABO-incompatible grafts. *Clin. Transplantation*, **5**:583–594

Anonick, P.K., Yoo, J.K., Webb, D.J. and Gonias, S.L. (1993). Characterisation of the antiplasmin activity of human thrombospondin-1 in solution. *Biochem. J.*, **289**:903–909.

Arakawa, K., Akami, T., Okamoto, M., Akioka, K., Lee, P.C., Sugano, Y., Kamei, J., Suzuki, T., Nagase, H., Tsuchihashi, Y. and Oka, T. (1994). Prolongation of heart xenograft survival in the NK-deficient rat. *Transplant. Proc.*, **26**:1266–1267

Bach, F.H., Platt, J.L. and Cooper, D. (1991a). Accommodation: the role of natural antibody and complement in discordant xenograft rejection. In: Cooper D, Kemp E, Reemtsma K, White DJG, editors. Xenotransplantation — the transplantation of organs and tissues between species. Heidelberg, Germany: Springer-Verlag, 81–100.

Bach, F.H., Turman, M.A., Vercellotti, G.M., Platt, J.L. and Dalmasso, A.P. (1991b).: Accommodation: A working paradigm for progressing toward clinical discordant xenografting. *Transplant Proc.*, **23**:205–207

Bach, F.H., Dalmasso, A.P. and Platt, J.L. (1992). Xenotransplantation: A current perspective. *Transplan. Rev.*, **6**:1–12

Bach, F.H., Blakely, M.L., Van der Werf, W.J., Vanhove, B., Stuhlmeier, K.M., Hancock, W.W., de Martin, R. and Winkler, H. (1993). Discordant xenografting: A working model of problems and issues. *Xeno*, 1:8–16.

Bach, F.H., Robson, S.C., Ferran, C., Winkler, H., Millan, M.T., Stuhlmeier, K., Vanhove, B., Blakely, M.L., van der Werf, W.J., Hofer, E., de Martin, R. and Hancock, W.W. (1994a). Endothelial cell activation and thromboregulation during xenograft rejection. *Immunol. Rev.*, **141**:5–30.

Bach, F.H., Stuhlmeier, K.M., Vanhove, B., Vanderwerf, W.J., Blakely, M.L., Demartin, R., Hancock, W.W. and Winkler, H. (1994b). Endothelial cells in xenotransplantation: do they accommodate? *Transplant. Proc.*, **26**:1167–1169

Bach, F.H., Auchincloss, H. and Robson, S.C. (1995). Xenotransplantation. *In: Transplantation Immunology*, edited by Bach, F.H. and Auchincloss, H., John Wiley and Sons, New York, NY, 305–338.

Balla, G., Jacob H.S., Balla, J., Rosenberg, M., Nath, K., Apple, F., Eaton, W.J. and Vercellotti, G.M. (1992). Ferritin: a cytoprotective antioxidant stratagem of endothelium. *J. Biol. Chem.*, **267**:18148–18153.

Binah, O., Marom, S., Rubinstein, I., Robinson, R.B., Berke, G. and Hoffman, B.F. (1992). Immunological rejection of heart transplant — How lytic granules from cytotoxic lymphocytes-T damage guinea pig ventricular myocytes. *Pflugers Arch-Eur. J. Physiol.*, **420**:172–179.

Blakely, M.L., van der Werf, W.J., Berndt, M.C., Dalmasso, A.P., Bach, F.H. and Hancock, W.W. (1994). Activation of intragraft endothelial and mononuclear cells during discordant xenograft rejection. *Transplantation*, **58**:1059–1066.

Brauer, R.B., Baldwin, W.M., Daha, M.R., Pruitt, S.K. and Sanfilippo, F. (1993). Use of C6-deficient rats to evaluate the mechanism of hyperacute rejection of discordant cardiac xenografts. *J. Immunol.*, 151:7240–7248.

Broze, G.J. (1992). The role of tissue factor pathway inhibitor in a revised coagulation cascade. *Semin. Hematol.*, 29:159–169.

Calne, R.Y. (1970). Organ transplantation between widely-disparate species. *Transplant Proc.*, 2:550–552.

Chow, T.W., Hellums, J.D., Moake, J.L. and Kroll, M.H. (1992). Shear stress induced von Willebrand factor binding to platelet glycoprotein Ib initiates calcium influx associated with aggregation. *Blood*, 80:113–120.

Colotta, F., Sciacca, F.L., Sironi, M., Luini, W., Rabiet, M.J. and Mantovani, A. (1994). Expression of monocyte chemotactic protein-1 by monocytes and endothelial cells exposed to thrombin. *Am. J. Pathol.*, 144:975–985.

Cooper, D.K.C., Ye, Y., Niekrasz, M., Kehoe, M., Martin, M., Neethling, F.A., Kosanke, S., Debault, L.E., Worsley, G., Zuhdi, N., Oriol, R. and Romano, E. (1993). Specific intravenous carbohydrate therapy — a new concept in inhibiting antibody-mediated rejection experience with ABO-incompatible cardiac allografting in the baboon. *Transplantation.*, 56:769–777.

Cooper, D.K.C., Koren, E. and Oriol, R. (1994). Natural antibodies, α-galactosyl oligosaccharides and xenotransplantation. *Xeno*, 2:22–25.

Coughlan, A.F., Berndt, M.C., Dunlop, L.C. and Hancock, W.W. (1993). *In vivo* studies of P-selectin and platelet activating factor during endotoxemia, accelerated allograft rejection and discordant xenograft rejection. *Transplant Proc.*, 25:2930–2931.

Coughlan, A.F., Hau, H., Dunlop, L.C., Berndt, M.C. and Hancock, W.W. (1994). P-Selectin and platelet–activating factor mediate initial endotoxin-induced neutropenia. *J. Exp. Med.*, 179:329–334.

Dalmasso, A.P., Vercellotti, G.M., Platt, J.L. and Bach, F.H. (1991). Inhibition of complement-mediated endothelial cell cytotoxicity by decay accelerating factor: Potential for prevention of xenograft hyperacute rejection. *Transplantation*, 52:530–535.

Dalmasso, A.P. (1992). The complement system in xenotransplantation. *Immunopharmacology*, 24:149–160

de Martin, R., Vanhove, B., Cheng, Q., Csizmadia, V., Hofer, E., Winkler, H. and Bach, F.H. (1993) Cytokine-inducible expression of IkB involves NFkB regulatory circuit for transient gene transcription. *EMBO J.*, 12:2773–2779.

Dorling, A. and R.I. Lechler. (1994). Prospects for xenografting. *Curr. Opin. Immunol.*, 6, 765–769.

Esmon C.T. (1993). Cell mediated events that control blood coagulation and vascular injury. *Annu. Rev. Cell. Biol.*, 9:1–26.

Furie, B. and Furie, B.C. (1992). Molecular and cellular biology of blood coagulation. *N. Eng. J. Med.*, 326:800–806.

Galili, U. (1993). Interaction of the natural anti-Gal antibody with alpha-galactosyl epitopes — a major obstacle for xenotransplantation in humans. *Immunol. Today.*, 14:480–482

Grey, S., Tsuchida, A., Hau, H., Orthner, C.L., Salem, H.H. and Hancock, W.W. (1994). Selective inhibitory effects of the anticoagulant activated protein C on the responses of human mononuclear phagocytes to LPS, IFN-γ or phorbol ester. *J. Immunol.*, 153:3664–3672.

Hamilton, K.K., Hattori, R., Esmon, C.T. and Sims, P.J. (1990). Complement proteins C5b-C9 induce vesiculation of the endothelial plasma membrane and expose catalytic surface for assembly of the prothrombinase enzyme complex. *J. Biol. Chem.*, 265:3809–3814.

Hancock, W.W., Blakely, M.L., Van der Werf, W.J. and Bach, F.H. (1993). Rejection of guinea pig cardiac xenografts post-cobra venom factor therapy is associated with infiltration by mononuclear cells secreting interferon-gamma and diffuse endothelial activation. *Transplant. Proc.*, 25:2932.

Harrison, P. and Martin-Cramer, E. (1993). Platelet alpha granules. *Blood Reviews*, 7, 52–62.

Hassan, R.,Van den Bogaerde, P., Forty, J., Wright, L., Wallwork, J. and White, D.J.G. (1992). Xenograft adaptation is dependent on the presence of antispecies antibody, not prolonged residence in the recipient. *Transplant. Proc.*, 24:531.

Hebell, T., Ahearn, J.M. and Fearon, D.T. (1991). Suppression of the immune response by a soluble complement receptor of B lymphocytes. *Science*, 254:102–106.

Hofer, E., Stuhlmeier, K.M., Blakely, M.L., Van der Werf, W.J., Hancock, W.W., Hunt, B.J. and Bach, F.H. (1994). Pathways of procoagulation in discordant xenografting. *Transplant. Proc.*, 26:1322–1323

Hunt, B.J. and Rosenberg, R.D. (1993). The essential role of haemostasis in hyperacute rejection. *Xeno*, 1, 16–20.

Hynes, R.O. (1992). Integrins: Versatility, modulation and signalling in cell adhesion. *Cell*, 69:11–25.

Inverardi, L., Samaja, M., Motterlini, R., Mangili, F., Bender, J.R. and Pardi, R. (1992). Early recognition of a discordant xenogeneic organ by human circulating lymphocytes. *J. Immunol.*, 149:1416–1423.

Johnston, P.S., Wang, M.W., Lim, S.M., Wright, L.J. and White, D.J. (1992). Discordant xenograft rejection in an antibody-free model. *Transplantation*, 54:573–577.

Kobayashi, M., Shimada, K. and Ozawa, T. (1992). Human platelet-derived transforming factor beta stimulates synthesis of glycosaminoglycans in cultured porcine endothelial cells. *Gerontology*, 38:36–42.

Kroll, M.H., Harris, T.S., Moake, J.L., Handin, R.I. and Schafer, A.I. (1991). von Willebrand factor binding to platelet GpIb initiates signals for platelet activation. *J. Clin. Invest.*, **88**:1568–1573.

Lesnikoski, B.A., Shaffer, D.A., Van der Werf, W.J., Hancock, W.W. and Bach, F.H. (1995). Endothelial and host mononuclear cell activation and cytokine expression during rejection of pig-to-baboon discordant xenografts. *Transplant. Proc.*, **27**:290–291.

Leventhal, J.R., Matas, A.J., Sun, L.H., Reif, S., Bolman, R.M., Dalmasso, A.P. and Platt, J.L. (1993). The immunopathology of cardiac xenograft rejection in the guinea pig-to-rat model. *Transplantation*, **56**:1–8.

Marcus, A.J. and Safier, L.B. (1993). Thromboregulation: multicellular modulation of platelet reactivity in hemostasis and thrombosis. *FASEB J.*, **7**:516–522.

Miyagawa, S., Hirose, H., Shirakura, R., Naka, Y., Nakata, S., Kawashima, Y., Seya, T., Matsumoto, M., Uenaka, A. and Kitamura, H. (1988). The mechanism of discordant xenograft rejection. *Transplantation* **46**:825–830.

Mosesson, M.W. (1992). The roles of fibrinogen and fibrin in hemostasis and thrombosis. *Semin. Hematol*, **29**:177–188.

Murphy, H.S., Shayman, J.A., Till, G.O., Mahrougui, M., Owens, C.B., Ryan, U.S and Ward, P.A. (1992). Superoxide responses of endothelial cells to C5a and TNF alpha: Divergent signal transduction pathways. *Am. J. Physiol.*, **263**:L51–L59.

Neethling, F.A., Koren, E., Ye, Y., Richards, S.V., Kujundzic, M., Oriol, R. and Cooper, D.K.C. (1994). Protection of pig kidney (PK15) cells from the cytotoxic effect of anti-pig antibodies by α-galactosyl oligosaccharides. *Transplantation*, **57**:959–963

Pierson, R.N., Kaspar-Konig, W., Tew, D.N., White, D.J.G. and Wallwork, J. (In press). Profound pulmonary vascular hypertension, characteristic of pig lung rejection by human blood, is mediated by xenoreactive antibody independent of complement. *Transplant. Proc.*

Platt, J.L., Lindman, B.J., Chen, H., Spitalnik, S.L. and Bach, F.H. (1990a). Endothelial cell antigens recognized by xenoreactive human natural antibodies. *Transplantation*, **50**:817–822

Platt, J.L., Vercellotti, G.M., Lindman, B.J., Oegama, T.R., Bach, F.H. and Dalmasso, A.P. (1990b). Release of heparan sulphate from endothelial cells: Implications for pathogenesis of hyperacute rejection. *J. Exp. Med.*, **171**:1363–1368.

Platt, J.L., Fischel, R.J., Matas, A.J., Reif, S.A., Bolman, R.M. and F.H. Bach. (1991a). Immunopathology of hyperacute xenograft rejection in a swine to primate model.*Transplantation*, **52**:214–220.

Platt, J.L., Lindman, B.J, Geller, R.L., Noreen, H.J., Swanson, J., Dalmasso, A.P. and Bach, F.H. (1991b). The role of natural antibodies in the activation of xenogeneic endothelial cells. *Transplantation*, **52**:1037–1043.

Pober, J.S. and Cotran, R.S. (1991). The role of endothelial cells in inflammation. *Transplantation*, **50**:537–544.

Reemtsma, K., McCracken, B.H. and Schlegel, J.U. (1964). Renal heterotransplantation in man. *Ann. Surg.*, **160**:384–389.

Robson, S.C., Saunders, R., de Jager, C., Purves, L. and Kirsch, R.E. (1993). Fibrin and fibrinogen degradation products with an intact D-domain C-terminal gamma chain inhibit an early step in accessory cell dependent lymphocyte mitogenesis. *Blood*, **81**:3006–3014.

Robson, S.C., Shephard, E.G. and Kirsch, R.E. (1994). Fibrin degradation product D-dimer induces the synthesis and release of biologically active IL-1β, IL-6 and plasminogen activator inhibitors from monocytes *in vitro*. *Br. J. Haem.*, **86**:322–326.

Rooney, I.A., Liszewski, M.K. and Atkinson, J.P. (1993). Using membrane-bound complement regulatory proteins to inhibit rejection. *Xeno*, **1**:29–34.

Roth, G.J. (1992). Platelets and blood vessels: the adhesion event. *Immunol. Today*, **13**:100–105.

Ruggeri, Z.M. and Ware, J. (1993). von Willebrand factor. *FASEB J.*, **7**:308–316.

Ryan, U.S. (1994) Complement inhibition: the sine qua non of xenotransplantation? *Xeno*, **2**:18–21.

Sablinski, T., Hancock, W.W., Tilney, N.L. and Kupiec-Weglinski, J.W. (1990). Biology of vascularized organ allograft rejection in sensitized recipients. *Transplant. Rev.*, **4**:108–120.

Sheng-Tanner, X. and Miller, R.G. (1992). Correlation between lymphocyte-induced donor-specific tolerance and donor cell recirculation. *J. Exp. Med.*, **176**:407–413.

Shreeniwas, R., Koga, S., Karakurum, M., Pinsky, D., Kaiser, E., Brett, J., Wolitzky, B.A., Norton, C., Plocinski, J., Benjamin, W., Burns, D.K., Goldstein, A. and Stern, D. (1992). Hypoxia-mediated induction of endothelial cell interleukin-1 alpha — an autocrine mechanism promoting expression of leukocyte adhesion molecules on the vessel surface. *J. Clin. Invest.*, **90**:2333–2339.

Sims, P.J. and Wiedmer, T. (1991). The response of human platelets to activated components of the complement system. *Immunol. Today*, **12**:338–342.

Smyth, S.S., Joneckis, C.C. and Parise, L.V. (1993). Regulation of vascular integrins. *Blood*, **81**:2827–2843.

Soares, M.P., Latinne, D., Elsen, M., Figeroa, J., Bach, F.H. and Bazin, H. (1993). *In vivo* depletion of xenoreactive natural antibodies with an anti-μ monoclonal antibody. *Transplantation*, **56**:1427–1431.

Soares, M.P., Lu, X.S., Havaux, X., Baranski, A., Reding, R., Latinne, D., Daha, M., Lambotte, L., Bach, F.H. and Bazin, H. (1994). *In vivo* IgM depeltion by anti-μ monoclonal antibody therapy — the role of IgM in hyperactive vascular rejection of discordant xenografts. *Transplantation*, **57**:1003–1007.

Stuhlmeier, K.M., Cheng, Q., Csizmadia, V., Winkler, H. and Bach, F.H. (1994). Alpha globulins selectively inhibit expression of "E-selectin" in endothelial cells. *Eur. J. Immunol.*, **24**:2186–2190.

Thibaudeau, K., Anegon, I., Lemauff, B., Soulilou, J.P. and Blanchard, D. (1994). Specificity of natural antibodies directed against cells from pigs. *Transplant. Proc.*, **26**:1003–1005.

Vanhove, B. and Bach, F.H. (1993). Human xenoreactive natural antibodies: avidity and targets on porcine endothelial cells. *Transplantation*, **56**:1251–1253.

Vanhove, B., de Martin, R., Lipp, J. and Bach, F.H. (1994). Human xenoreactive natural antibodies of the IgM isotype activate pig endothelial cells. *Xenotransplantation*, **1**:17–23.

Vercellotti, G.M., Platt, J.L., Bach, F.H. and Dalmasso, A.P. (1991). Enhanced neutrophil adhesion to xenogeneic endothelium via C3bi. *J. Immunol.*, **146**:730–736.

Walker, F.J. and Fay, P.J. (1992). Regulation of blood coagulation by the protein-C system. *FASEB J.*, **6**:2561–2567.

Westenfelder, U., Schraven, B. and Mannel, D.N. (1993). Characterization of monocyte-activating tumour cell membrane structures. *Scand. J. Immunol.*, **38**:388–394.

White, D.J., Oglesby, T. and Liszewski, M.K. (1992). Expression of human decay accelerating factor or membrane cofactor protein genes on mouse cells inhibits lysis by human complement. *Transplant. Proc.*, **24**:474–477.

8 Immune Responses in Atherosclerosis

Göran K. Hansson

Karolinska Institute, Department of Medicine and King Gustaf V Research Institute, Karolinska Hospital, S-171 76 Stockholm, Sweden

INTRODUCTION

Atherosclerosis, the leading cause of death in Western societies, is characterized by a focal, slow and progressive accumulation of cells, extracellular matrix, and lipid in the intima of medium-sized and large arteries. The resulting luminal occlusion leads to hampered blood flow to the end-organ and ischemic symptoms such as angina pectoris and intermittent claudication. In addition, thrombi often develop on the surface of the lesion and may completely obstruct the lumen. This is the most common cause of myocardial infarction (Erhardt *et al.*, 1973; Davies and Thomas, 1984). Detaching thrombi form arterial emboli that may occlude smaller arteries downstream from the lesion, leading to sudden ischemic symptoms such as transitory ischemic attacks, stroke, and acute gangrene.

Atherosclerosis is in itself a silent pathological process that precipitates dramatic clinical manifestations only late in its course (Stary, 1989). Clinical research on its pathogenesis has therefore been hampered by the lack of early indicators of the presence and progression of the disease. Furthermore, the sheer fact that atherosclerosis is one of the most common diseases that affects the human race generates substantial problems for clinical scientists attempting to identify markers of disease. Large epidemiologic studies have, however, provided important information on atherosclerosis and several risk factors have been identified which are statistically correlated to clinical manifestations of the disease. The most important among them are smoking, hypercholesterolemia, high blood pressure, and diabetes (Wilhelmsen *et al.*, 1973). It has been estimated, however, that only approximately 50% of the incidence of cardiovascular disease can be explained by these major risk factors. Consequently, there is room for substantial, as yet unknown, contributing factors. Furthermore, epidemiology has not provided an understanding of the pathophysiological mechanisms of atherosclerosis. With the exception of a small number of genetic disorders of lipid metabolism, the cause and molecular and cellular pathogenesis of atherosclerosis remain unclear.

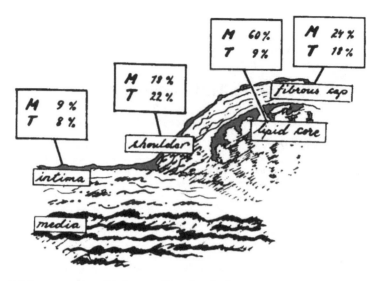

Figure 1 Cellular composition of the human atherosclerotic plaque.

The frequency of monocyte-derived macrophages (M) and T lymphocytes (T) are expressed as percentages of total cells in different regions of advanced human plaques and are based on immunohistochemical analyses of endarterectomy samples.

Reprinted with permission from Hansson, G.K., Jonasson, L., Seifert, P.S. and Stemme, S., Immune mechanisms in atherosclerosis. Arteriosclerosis 9:567–578, 1989. Copyright American Heart Association.

The discovery of activated T lymphocytes and macrophages in the atherosclerotic plaque (Jonasson *et al.*, 1985, 1986; Figure 1) together with the detection of HLA class II antigen expression (Jonasson *et al.*, 1985) and the secretion of several cytokines (Warner *et al.*, 1987; Libby and Hansson, 1991) have raised an interest in immune and inflammatory mechanisms in the pathogenesis of atherosclerosis. This has been further encouraged by the findings of autoantibody responses to plaque constituents (Salonen *et al.*, 1992; Xu *et al.*, 1993a) and there is now, as will be described here, good evidence for an involvement of the immune system in atherosclerosis.

MONOCYTE RECRUITMENT AND FOAM CELL FORMATION

The cellular events in atherogenesis have been characterized by a wide range of morphological techniques applied to human as well as experimental lesions. Early studies of atherosclerotic plaques showed the presence of macrophage-like cells filled with lipid droplets, *i.e.* the foam cells that constitute a hallmark of the disease (Anitschkoff, 1913; Leary, 1941). It was, however, unclear whether these cells were formed by transformation of vascular smooth muscle cells or derived from blood monocytes.

Poole and Florey, in the 1950s, showed in hypercholesterolemic rabbits that fatty streak-type lesions develop by infiltration of monocyte-like cells into the intima (Poole and Florey, 1958). Electron microscopic and histochemical studies (Fowler *et al.*, 1979; Schaffner *et al.*, 1980; Gerrity, 1981) later confirmed that monocytes bind to the arterial surface, enter the intima and transform into foam cells during lesion formation in hypercholesterolemic rabbits, monkeys and swine.

With the advent of the monoclonal antibody technology, it became possible to identify the cell types of the human atherosclerotic lesions with cell type-specific antibodies. Immunohistochemical studies showed that foam cells express surface antigens specific for the monocyte-macrophage lineage (Aqel *et al.*, 1984; Vedeler *et al.*, 1984; Klurfeld, 1985; Gown *et al.*, 1986; Jonasson *et al.*, 1986). The majority of foam cells therefore seem to be derived from monocytes that enter the lesion through the transendothelial route, accumulate cholesterol, and transform into lipid-laden foam cells (Faggiotto and Ross, 1984a; Rosenfeld *et al.*, 1987a). At later stages and in areas of perturbed blood flow, there is also recruitment of monocytes by Fc receptor-mediated binding to IgG in areas with endothelial injury (Hansson *et al.*, 1981).

MACROPHAGES, FOAM CELLS, AND CHOLESTEROL UPTAKE

The mechanism by which monocyte-derived macrophages accumulate cholesterol was elucidated by Brown and Goldstein, who showed that chemically modified low-density lipoprotein (LDL) — but not native LDL — is taken up by a specific macrophage receptor called the scavenger receptor (Goldstein *et al.*, 1979; Brown and Goldstein, 1983). The scavenger receptor has been cloned and its ligand-binding site characterized by blocking antibodies and the construction of truncated mutants (Kodama *et al.*, 1990; Rohrer *et al.*, 1990; Krieger *et al.*, 1993; Doi *et al.*, 1993). It is a trimeric protein with an external cysteine-rich C-terminal domain, the so-called SRCR or scavenger receptor cystein-rich domain that is shared with several cell surface molecules of the immune system, which together constitute the so called SRCR gene family (Freeman *et al.*, 1990). Surprisingly, the ligand-binding site is not located in the SRCR domain. Instead, a collagen-like coiled coil domain beneath the SRCR domain is rich in basic amino acids and binds modified LDL and several other molecules and particles with clustered negative surface charges.

The biologically most important mechanism of lipoprotein modification that makes it susceptible to uptake by the scavenger receptor, is oxidation (Steinberg *et al.*, 1989). This process occurs in the arterial intima, where macrophages and endothelial cells generate free oxygen radicals in response to activating stimuli (Steinbrecher *et al.*, 1984; Palinski *et al.*, 1989; Steinberg *et al.*, 1989). The oxidation process initially attacks double bonds in fatty acids but the fragmentation of these lipids generates small, reactive molecules such as malondialdehyde, which reacts with the ε-amino groups of lysines in the apolipoprotein (Steinbrecher *et al.*, 1987; Ylä-Herttuala *et al.*, 1991). An LDL particle that exposes such modified lysines is rapidly bound and taken up via the scavenger receptor (Parthasarathy *et al.*, 1987; Steinberg *et al.*, 1989).

In addition to the scavenger receptor, several other surface receptors have also been shown to mediate internalization of oxidized LDL. CD36 is a macrophage-specific surface protein that binds oxidized LDL as well as thrombospondin and collagen (Endemann *et al.*, 1993). It can induce foam cell transformation when transfected into a target cell that is subsequently exposed to oxidized LDL (Endemann *et al.*, 1993). Fc receptors can also induce foam cell formation, if the Fc receptor-expressing cell is exposed to antigen-antibody complexes containing LDL (Griffith *et al.*, 1988).

All these routes for LDL uptake result in a release, ester hydrolysis and re-esterification of cholesterol in the cytoplasm of the macrophage (Brown and Goldstein, 1983). In contrast to the case of the receptor for native LDL, the expression of scavenger receptors is not regulated by the intracellular cholesterol level (Brown and Goldstein, 1983). The scavenger receptor-expressing macrophage will therefore continue to internalize modified LDL, accumulate cholesterol, and develop into a foam cell (Brown and Goldstein, 1983). This process appears to continue until the cell dies.

LYMPHOCYTES IN ATHEROSCLEROTIC LESIONS

The detection of lymphocytes in the atherosclerotic plaque, in contrast to the finding of monocytes, depended entirely on the monoclonal antibody technology, as these cells are fairly inconspicuous by morphologic criteria. Using monoclonal antibodies in an immunohistochemical mapping of gene expression in human plaques, it was found (Jonasson *et al.*, 1985) that the class II histocompatibility gene, HLA-DR is expressed by many smooth muscle cells of the plaque, although these cells do not normally express the gene. Since HLA-DR is induced by the T cell cytokine, interferon-γ (IFN-γ), the obvious conclusion was that T cells present in the lesion had induced HLA-DR expression in smooth muscle cells by release of this cytokine (Jonasson *et al.*, 1985). Immunohisto-chemical analysis of the cellular composition of advanced human atherosclerotic plaques supported this interpretation (Figure 1). 10–20% of all cells in such lesions express T cell-specific antigens such as CD3, with approximately two-thirds of the T cells express-ing CD4 and one-third the CD8 antigen (Jonasson *et al.*, 1986).

The presence of T cells and monocyte-derived macrophages suggests that antigen pre-sentation and immune activation occur in atherosclerotic plaques. One might, however, argue that both cell types accumulate by nonspecific trapping and may be totally inactive. Immunophenotyping and mRNA analysis indicate to the contrary by demonstrating acti-vation of the T cells. Many T cells in atheromata bear interleukin-2 receptors and HLA-DR (Hansson *et al.*, 1989a; van der Wal *et al.*, 1989). Flow cytometric analysis of T cells isolated from plaques revealed a total dominance of the memory T cell phenotype and expression of the VLA-1 (very late activation) antigen (Stemme *et al.*, 1992a). Cytokines characteristic of activated T cells have been found in plaques by immunohistochemistry (Hansson *et al.*, 1989a) and PCR (Geng *et al.*, 1995) and the "aberrant" expression of HLA-DR in the plaque (Jonasson *et al.*, 1985) provides indirect evidence for a local IFN-γ secretion, as discussed earlier.

RECRUITMENT OF IMMUNOCOMPETENT CELLS TO THE PLAQUE

The recruitment of leukocytes to tissues is mediated by specific adhesion molecules expressed by endothelial cells. These cell surface proteins bind to "counter-receptors" on leukocytes rolling over the endothelium. Once the leukocyte is arrested on the endothe-lium, it can respond to chemotactic signals that stimulate it to migrate between interen-dothelial junctions into the underlying tissue.

T lymphocytes enter the arterial wall at a very early stage of lesion formation and are found in fatty streaks together with macrophages (Munro *et al.*, 1987; van der Wal *et al.*, 1989). The latter, however, always outnumber the T cells, with a ratio of approximately 1:10 to 1:50 between T cells and macrophages. In early lesions, CD8 cells dominate over

CD4 with a ratio of approximately 2:1 (Munro *et al.*, 1987; van der Wal *et al.*, 1989; Emeson and Robertson 1988). This contrasts with the situation in the advanced plaque (Jonasson *et al.*, 1986) and suggests that there may be a switch from a response driven by HLA class I-restricted to HLA class II-restricted antigens during the evolution of the fatty streak into a fibrofatty plaque.

Studies in cholesterol-fed rabbits shed light on the recruitment of T lymphocytes and monocytes to the arterial wall during atherogenesis. The two earliest detectable vascular events after initiation of cholesterol feeding are the expression of endothelial adhesion molecules and the deposition of complement in the intima. Focal expression of VCAM-1 (vascular cell adhesion molecule-1) occurs as early as one week after the start of the atherogenic diet (Cybulsky and Gimbrone, 1991; Li *et al.*, 1993; Richardson *et al.*, 1994), followed by the entry of monocyte-macrophages and other leukocytes during the ensuing weeks (Li *et al.*, 1993). VCAM-1 is a ligand for VLA-4, a cell surface protein expressed by lymphocytes and monocytes (Elices *et al.*, 1990). Granulocytes do not bear VLA-4, and this may explain the selective recruitment of mononuclear cells to the forming atherosclerotic lesion.

VCAM-1 is not expressed constitutively by endothelial cells but is inducible by proin-flammatory cytokines including interleukin-1 (IL-1), tumor necrosis factor (TNF), and IFN-γ (Bevilacqua *et al.*, 1987; Elices *et al.*, 1990). The production of such cytokines in the underlying atheroma likely contributes to the expression of VCAM-1 on the surface of the forming plaque. It is, however, uncertain whether nascent lesions contain sufficient local concentrations of IL-1, TNF or IFN-γ to induce VCAM-1. Surprisingly, VCAM-1 expression is also induced by lysophosphatidylcholine, which may be present in lipopro-teins and generated during lipoprotein oxidation and cell membrane injury (Kume *et al.*, 1992). In the hypercholesterolemic state, lysophosphatidylcholine might therefore induce VCAM-1 expression on the endothelium. The focal expression of VCAM-1 in lesion-prone areas of hypercholesterolemic animals may result from a combination of local flow alterations that promote influx or retention of lipoproteins and the action of a component of modified lipoprotein, either directly or by inducing a secondary cytokine. It is noteworthy in the context of T cell activation during atherogenesis (see below) that VCAM-1 not only serves as a leukocyte adhesion molecule, but by engaging VLA-4 on T cells can function as a co-stimulator or accessory molecule in the T cell activation pathway.

HUMORAL COMPONENTS OF THE IMMUNE SYSTEM

The vascular reaction in early hypercholesterolemia is characterized not only by the appearance of inflammatory cells and *de novo* gene expression in vascular cells but also by an infiltration and accumulation of plasma proteins. There is a deposition of lipopro-teins but also a prominent infiltration and deposition of immunoglobulins and comple-ment factors. IgG deposits on intracellular filaments and extracellular collagen fibers due to specific interactions between the Fc part of the immunoglobulin molecule and protein components of these filaments (Hansson *et al.*, 1984). The intracellular accumulation of IgG in injured endothelial cells is particularly striking and can be used to detect damaged endothelial cells (Hansson and Schwartz, 1983).

Several complement factors are detectable in the atherosclerotic intima, including C1 and C3b (Seifert and Kazatchkine, 1988). The accumulation of C5b-9 is particularly important since it indicates activation of the complement cascade. C5b-9 deposits are found in the rabbit aorta within two weeks after initiation of a cholesterol-rich diet and increase with the progression of the disease (Seifert *et al.*, 1989). These deposits represent membrane-anchored attack complexes with a capacity to perforate cellular membranes and they may cause cytolysis in the atherosclerotic artery. Peptide fragments such as C3a and C5a, which are released during activation of the complement cascade, exhibit chemotactic and leukocyte-activating properties and could be important for the recruitment of leukocytes to the lesion (Hansson *et al.*, 1987). The initiation of the complement cascade might occur at the IgG deposits at sites of cell injury but also in regions of cholesterol deposition. Cholesterol aggregates may, at least *in vitro*, activate the complement cascade through the alternative pathway in a reaction that is amplified by oxidative modification of the cholesterol molecule (Seifert and Kazatchkine, 1987).

To summarize, early immunologic responses of the atherosclerotic arterial wall include both expression of endothelial leukocyte-adhesion molecules and complement activation. Both of these responses could decisively influence the subsequent formation of the (macrophage-rich) fatty streak. The most comprehensive data on these processes are available in the cholesterol-fed rabbit model but there is also evidence for their involvement in the human disease (Seifert and Hansson, 1989; Poston *et al.*, 1992). It will now be important to determine whether the atherosclerotic process can be inhibited by interfering with these phenomena.

ANTIGENS

The presence of activated T cells and macrophages strongly suggests that an immunologic reaction is taking place in the atherosclerotic plaque. The antigens that elicit this response are not yet known and both microorganisms and autoantigens have been proposed to play a role.

In early lesions, the presence of T cells of the CD8 phenotype suggests that an immune response to HLA class I-restricted, endogenously synthesized antigens may be taking place. The most well-known HLA class I-restriced antigens are **viral proteins**, which are synthesized by the virus-infected cell. It is therefore possible that (at least some of) the CD8+ cells respond to viral antigens in the plaque. Antigens of Herpes simplex virus type I and cytomegalovirus are present in the arterial wall during atherosclerosis (Benditt *et al.*, 1983). These members of the herpesvirus family are, however, among the most ubiquitous viruses that infect man. The mere presence of components of such viruses therefore does not prove that they play any pathogenetic role. Non-viral microorganisms such as *Chlamydia pneumoniae*, strain TWAR, are other conceivable microbial stimuli for a local immune response during atherogenesis and they can be found in the atherosclerotic plaque (Kuo *et al.*, 1993). Recent epidemiological data are suggestive of a correlation between the systemic immune response to *Chlamydia* strain TWAR and atherosclerosis (Puolakkainen *et al.*, 1993).

The mature atherosclerotic plaque contains a large number of CD4+ T cells (Jonasson *et al.*, 1986). These cells respond to HLA class II-restricted, exogenous antigens that are taken up from the evironment by macrophages, endothelial cells and other antigen-presenting cells. The ensuing T cell responses include cytokine secretion and T cell help for antibody-producing B cells. Analysis of antibody responses to plaque components could therefore shed light on the reactivity of the CD4+ T cells.

Autoantibodies to **oxidized LDL** lipoproteins are common in man (Ylä-Herttuala *et al.*, 1989); their titer appears to correlate with the progression of atherosclerosis (Salonen *et al.*, 1992). Antibodies raised against model antigens such as malondialdehyde-(MDA)-conjugated lysine recognize oxidatively modified LDL (Palinski *et al.*, 1990) and plaques contain significant amounts of MDA-lysine crossreactive material (Ylä-Herttuala *et al.*, 1994). It is likely that the B cell response is dependent on T cell help and Frostegård *et al.* (1992) have reported that addition of oxidized LDL to peripheral blood mononuclear cells can activate some of the T cells, resulting in interleukin-2 receptor expression and DNA synthesis. We have speculated that immunospecific CD4+ T cells in the plaque might initiate an autoimmune response to oxidized LDL; this would be expected to induce both local T cell-dependent cytokine pathways, antibody production, and possibly cytotoxic responses.

To test this hypothesis, we have raised T cell clones from atherosclerotic plaques and challenged them with oxidized LDL under antigen-presenting conditions (Stemme *et al.*, 1995). Several of the clones respond by proliferation and cytokine secretion. The response shows all the characteristics of antigen-specific T cell activation since it is dependent on antigen (oxidized LDL), autologous antigen-presenting monocytes, and HLA-DR (Stemme *et al.*, 1995). Interestingly, these T cell clones respond to native LDL by a much lower degree of proliferation. Since LDL will be oxidized by the antigen-presenting monocytes present in the co-culture system, it is likely that the T cell epitope on LDL is generated by oxidation. We therefore propose that LDL when it is oxidized in the atherosclerotic lesion is converted to an autoantigen that is recognized by specific T cells present in the lesion (Figure 2) (Stemme *et al.*, 1995). It will now be important to identify the T cell epitopes on oxidized LDL and characterize their interaction with the T cell antigen receptor.

Many inflammatory and autoimmune diseases, including atherosclerosis, are associated with antibody production against **heat shock proteins**. These are intracellular chaperones that stabilize the conformation of other proteins. They are synthesized in increased amounts during cell injury and induce T cell-dependent antibody production (Kiessling *et al.*, 1991). Several heat shock proteins are found in atherosclerotic lesions (Xu *et al.*, 1993b) and the titer of autoantibodies to heat shock protein 60 appears to correlate with the extent of carotid atherosclerosis (Xu *et al.*, 1993a). In cholesterol-fed rabbits, immunization with the closely related heat shock protein 65 aggravates atherosclerosis, suggesting that this autoimmune response may be of pathogenetic significance (Xu *et al.*, 1992).

Very few B cells are found in the plaque and it is likely that B cell activation occurs in regional lymph nodes. T cells might enter the plaque, respond to antigen, and then migrate through the lymph circulation to regional lymph nodes, where B cells are activated to produce antibodies to the antigen recognized by the T cell. Such a patrolling role of the T cell is known to occur in many other situations (Mackay *et al.*, 1990) and would fit with the phenotypic characteristics of T cells isolated from plaques (Stemme *et al.*, 1992a). It probably requires that antigen is present also in the lymph node; this is likely

Göran K. Hansson

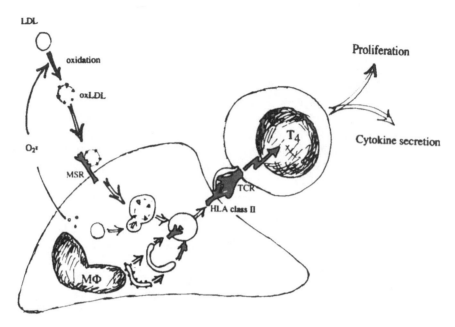

Figure 2   Hypothetic mechanism for immune recognition of oxidized LDL by specific T lymphocytes. Low density lipoprotein (LDL) is oxidized by oxygen free radicals (O_2^-) and the oxidized LDL (oxLDL) is taken up by the macrophage scavenger receptor (MSR). After intracellular processing in the macrophage (MΦ), fragments of oxLDL associate with nascent HLA class II proteins and are transported to the cell surface. Here, they are recognized by CD4+ T cells (T4) that carry T cell antigen receptors (TCR) capable of binding the (oxLDL fragment)-(HLA class II) complex. This elicits T cell activation, leading to proliferation and cytokine secretion.

to be the case for oxidized LDL. In advanced plaques, however, plasma cells are not infrequent and local IgG production has been detected (Sohma *et al.*, 1995).

Advanced cases of atherosclerosis are sometimes complicated by periadventitial inflammation. In the case of aortic atherosclerosis, this periaortitis can produce huge inflammatory infiltrates. Microscopically, the periaortitic lesion is dominated by B lymphocytes, plasma cells and macrophages together with oxidized lipid components and antibodies to oxidized LDL (Parums *et al.*, 1986; Parums *et al.*, 1990) and it is possible that the periarterial lesion represents an autoimmune response to oxidized LDL (Parums *et al.*, 1990). Therefore, although the initial B cell response probably occurs in lymph nodes, B cells may at later stages localize to and be activated in the artery and its immediate vicinity.

To conclude, the antigens of atherosclerosis remain obscure although recent data implicate oxidized LDL and heat shock proteins as likely targets for CD4+ responses and antibody production associated with atherosclerosis. In addition, it still remains to be determined whether such responses are essentially beneficial or detrimental for the artery and the patient. Recent studies of genetically immunodeficient mice of the atherosclerosis-prone C57Bl/6J strain show that an elimination of the MHC class I dependent immune response by targeted gene disruption results in severe aggravation of lesion development (Fyfe *et al.*, 1994). This contrasts with the observations in heat shock protein-immunized rabbits but goes along with the beneficial effects of T cell-derived cytokines on smooth muscle proliferation and macrophage lipid accumulation (see below).

IMMUNE EFFECTOR MECHANISMS AND THE PATHOGENESIS OF ATHEROSCLEROSIS

It is likely that a local immune reaction occurs in the atherosclerotic plaque but the patho-physiological consequences of such reactions remain largely speculative. Humoral immune mechanisms could be involved in the elimination of antigenic compounds but also initiate complement- and macrophage-dependent cytotoxic mechanisms. Cellular immune responses may initiate inflammatory reactions, cell-mediated cytotoxicity and cytokine-dependent regulatory loops in the atherosclerotic plaque.

T cell-dependent induction of antibody production to plaque antigens such as oxidized LDL could represent a mechanism for antigen elimination. Immune complexes consisting of LDL and anti-LDL antibodies are avidly taken up by Fc receptor-bearing macrophages, which may transform into cholesterol-laden foam cells (Griffith *et al.*, 1988). Antibody binding to cell surfaces may initiate cytotoxic activity since the complement cascade and Fc receptor-bearing macrophages and cytotoxic lymphocytes would attack antibody-coated target cells. The presence of membrane-bound C5b-9 complexes in experimental plaques (Seifert *et al.*, 1989) indicates that complement-mediated lysis takes place. It is, however, not clear whether this occurs as the result of antibody binding to specific antigens on the surface of cells or is due to an "innocent bystander" attack after alternative complement activation on the extracellular cholesterol deposits (Seifert and Kazatchkine, 1987).

Cellular immune reactions require T cell activation and the presence of activated CD4+ and CD8+ T cells suggests that both cytotoxic and immune-regulatory, T cell-dependent reactions could occur in the plaque. There is little direct evidence for cytotoxic immune reactions in atherosclerosis. In contrast, several reports demonstrate the presence of immune-regulatory cytokines in the atherosclerotic plaque. Proinflammatory cytokines including interleukin-1, TNF, interleukin-6, and IFN-γ are secreted in the plaque (Libby and Hansson, 1991), probably both by T lymphocytes, macrophages, endothelial cells, and smooth muscle cells. It is therefore likely that the local immune response in the plaque modulates the disease process by cytokine-mediated pathways.

IMMUNE-INDUCED CYTOKINE SECRETION IN THE ATHEROSCLEROTIC PLAQUE

Growth factors and cytokines constitute a heterogeneous group of glycoproteins and function as local hormones, controlling many aspects of cellular activity. Many of them are produced by several cell types and also act on different cell types, thus creating a network of intercellular communication pathways (Burke *et al.*, 1993). Demonstration of cytokine secretion in cultured cells is important in order to establish all potentially important signal mechanisms. However, to determine which of the different cytokine interactions are actually active *in vivo*, *in situ* detection is needed. During recent years, several cytokines and growth factors have been detected in atherosclerotic lesions by immunohistochemistry, Northern blot, *in situ* hybridization and the polymerase chain reaction (PCR).

Of T cell cytokines, IFN-γ and interleukin-2 have been detected in human plaques by immunohistochemistry and PCR (Hansson *et al.*, 1989a; Geng *et al.*, 1995). Interleukin-2 is an important mitogen during T-cell activation and may also regulate macrophage activation. Its receptor is, however, limited in expression to cells of the immune system proper.

In contrast, the receptor for IFN-γ is widespread and both endothelial and smooth muscle cells respond to this cytokine by histocompatilibity gene expression, growth inhibition and expression of adhesion molecules (Pober *et al.*, 1982; Stemme *et al.*, 1990; Hansson *et al.*, 1989b; Pober and Cotran, 1990). IFN-γ also acts to reduce the contractile capacity and tensile strength of the vessel wall, by inducing nitric oxide production (Busse and Mülsch, 1990; Wood *et al.*, 1990; Hansson *et al.*, 1994) and by inhibiting the production of α-actin (Hansson *et al.*, 1989b) and collagen (Amento *et al.*, 1991). Nitric oxide may, in fact, act as a second messenger for IFN-γ and other proinflammatory cytokines in their effects on vascular and other mesenchymal cells (Geng *et al.*, 1992a; Geng *et al.*, 1994).

In addition to its effects on vascular cells, IFN-γ is the most important macrophage-activating cytokine and stimulates cytokine production, phagocytosis, and antigen presentation in these cells (Farrar and Schreiber, 1993) In the context of the vessel wall, it is particularly interesting that IFN-γ down-regulates the expression of the scavenger receptor; this reduces cholesterol uptake and inhibits foam cell transformation of macrophages (Geng *et al.*, 1992b). This may indirectly increase the extracellular accumulation of cholesterol in the plaque, which is also enhanced by the reduced apolipoprotein E production in IFN-γ-stimulated macrophages (Brand *et al.*, 1993).

Macrophage colony stimulating factor (M-CSF) is expressed by immune and vascular cells in human plaques but not in normal vessel walls (Clinton *et al.*, 1992; Rosenfeld *et al.*, 1992). The M-CSF receptor is also expressed (Salomon *et al.*, 1992) and local M-CSF may induce macrophage proliferation and expression of the scavenger receptor, leading to foam cell formation (Clinton *et al.*, 1992).

Monocyte chemoattractant protein-1 (MCP-1) mRNA and protein were recently demonstrated in human plaques as well as in animal lesions (Nelken *et al.*, 1991; Ylä-Herttuala *et al.*, 1991). MCP-1 is produced by activated macrophages and vascular cells, functions as a chemoattractant for monocytes (Rollins *et al.*, 1990) and may promote migration of monocytes into the plaque after their initial adhesion to the endothelium.

No lymphocyte-specific, chemotactic cytokines have been detected in the plaque but it has recently been demonstrated that oxidized LDL has a prominent chemotactic effect on T lymphocytes (McMurray *et al.*, 1993). *In vitro* studies have shown that oxidized LDL also induces monocytic expression of interleukin-8, which is chemotactic for T cells and granulocytes (Terkeltaub *et al.*, 1994).

Interleukin-1α and β mRNA have been detected by *in situ* hybridization in plaques of hypercholesterolemic animals (Moyer *et al.*, 1991) and by PCR in human lesions (Wang *et al.*, 1989). It is produced by macrophages and vascular cells (Libby *et al.*, 1988) and serves as an important co-mitogen in T cell activation (Durum, Schmidt and Oppenheim). IL-1 is also a smooth muscle mitogen (Libby *et al.*, 1988) and this effect has been shown to be mediated by auto-induction of PDGF secretion (Raines *et al.*, 1989).

Tumour necrosis factor α (TNFα) mRNA can be detected in smooth muscle-like cells in the intima of human plaques by *in situ* hybridization (Barath *et al.*, 1990). It has pro-inflammatory effects on several cell types (Scheurich *et al.*, 1987; Vassalli, 1992) stimulates smooth muscle proliferation (Warner and Libby, 1989), induces adhesion molecule expression (Stemme *et al.*, 1992b; Carlos *et al.*, 1990) and may contribute to recruitment of mononuclear cells in the plaque.

CONCLUSION

Morphologic and immunologic studies of human atherosclerosis have established the T lymphocytes as important cellular components of the plaque. They have also provided evidence for a local immune activation in the arterial intima during atherosclerosis. Cell culture studies have identified potential mechanisms of interaction between lymphocytes and other cells involved in the disease process and several crucial aspects of such interactions have been evaluated in animal models of atherosclerosis.

The picture that emerges (Figure 3) is one of a cellular immune activation involving T cells and macrophages together with an antigen-independent complement activation.

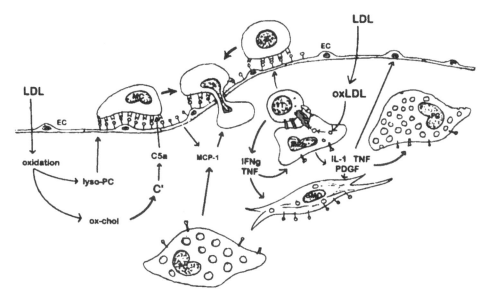

Figure 3 Hypothetic mechanism for the recruitment and activation of immunocompetent cells in atherosclerotic lesions.

Endothelial cells (EC) are stimulated to express vascular cell adhesion molecule-1 (VCAM-1?), possibly by lysophosphatidylcholine (Lyso PC) or other components of LDL oxidized in the intima (oxLDL). Monocytes (MC) and T lymphocytes (T) adhere to endothelial cells expressing VCAM-1 and other leukocyte adhesion molecules. MC are stimulated chemotactically (CTX) to enter the intima by complement-derived chemoattractants (C'), which may also be generated secondary to LDL oxidation. The cytokine, macrophage chemoattractant protein-1 (MCP-1) is another potent chemotactic agent that is produced locally in the atherosclerotic plaque. T cells may be stimulated chemotactically by oxLDL itself or components thereof. Antigen-specific T cells are activated by monocyte-derived macrophages that process and present antigens (Ag) in the lesion. Both cell types produce cytokines which act on EC, SMC, and foam cells (FC) to regulate adhesion molecule expression, chemotaxis, procoagulant activity, proliferation, contractility, and cholesterol uptake.

Activation of these two systems would in turn activate endothelial cells, inhibit smooth muscle growth, reduce the contractility of the vessel wall, and recruit more lymphocytes and monocytes to the forming lesion. Cytokines released during the cellular immune response might also reduce foam cell formation but could increase the size of the extracellular cholesterol pool. Acting in concert, the net effect of these various functions would be reduction in the size and mechanical strength of the lesion. Macrophages activated during an immune response might, however, counteract this by releasing growth factors such as PDGF. The relative importance of the various cytokine-modulated events is still unclear and may vary depending on the precise stimulus and phase of the disease process.

Finally, it should be emphasized that the antigen(s) that incite the cellular immune response are not yet identified. Recent studies suggest that heat shock proteins and oxidized lipoproteins could induce cellular immune reactions but their role as immunogens in the atherosclerotic plaque remain uncertain. If indeed important local antigens and their T cell epitopes can be identified, immunologic prevention and/or therapy could be attractive additions to the therapeutic arsenal for the treatment of atherosclerosis.

References

Amento, E.P., Ehsani, N., Palmer, H. and Libby, P. (1991). Cytokines and growth factors positively and negativley regulate interstitial collagen gene expression in human vascular smooth muscle cells. *Arterioscl. Thromb.*, **11**:1223–1230.

Anitschkoff, N.N. (1913). Über Veränderungen der Kaninchen-Aorta bei experimentelle Cholesterolinsteatose. *Beitr path Anat.*, **56**:379–391.

Aqel, N.M., Ball, R.Y., Waldmann, H. and Mitchinson, M.J. (1984). Monocytic origin of foam cells in human atherosclerotic plaques. *Atherosclerosis*, **53**:265–271.

Barath, P., Fishbein, M.C., Cao, J., Berenson, J., Helfant, R.H. and Forrester, J.S. (1990). Tumor necrosis factor expression by human vascular intimal smooth muscle cells detected by *in situ* hybridization. *Am. J. Path.*, **137**:503–509.

Benditt, E.P., Barrett, T. and McDougall, J.K. (1983). Viruses in the etiology of atherosclerosis. *Proc. Natl. Acad. Sci. USA.*, **80**:6386–6389.

Bevilacqua, M.P., Pober, J.S., Mendrick, D.L., Cotran, R.S. and Gimbrone, M.A. (1987). Identification of an inducible endothelial-leukocyte adhesion molecule *Proc. Natl. Acad. Sci. USA.*, **84**:9238–9242.

Brand, K., Mackman, N. and Curtiss, L.K. (1993). Interferon-γ inhibits macrophage apolipoprotein E production by posttranslational mechanisms. *J. Clin. Invest.*, **91**:2031–2039.

Brown, M.S. and Goldstein, J.L. (1983). Lipoprotein metabolism in the macrophage: Implications for cholesterol deposition in atherosclerosis. *Ann. Rev. Biochem.*, **52**:223–61.

Burke, F., Naylor, M.S., Davies, B. and Balkwill, F. (1993). The cytokine wall chart. *Immunol. Today*, **14**: 165–170.

Busse, R. and Mülsch, A. (1990). Induction of nitric oxide synthase by cytokines in vascular smooth muscle cells. *FEBS Letters*, **275**:87–90.

Carlos, T.M., Schwartz, R. and Kovach, N.L.K. *et al.* (1990). Vascular cell adhesion molecule-1 mediates lymphocyte adherence to cytokine-activated cultured human endothelial cells. *Blood*, **76**:695–670.

Clinton, S.K., Underwood, R., Hayes, L., Sherman, M.L. Kufe, D.W. and Libby, P. (1992). Macrophage colony-stimulating factor gene expression in vascular cells and in experimental and human atheroma. *Proc. Natl. Acad. Sci. USA.*, **89**:2814–2818.

Cybulsky, M.I. and Gimbrone, M.A. (1991). Endothelial expression of a mononuclear leukocyte adhesion molecule during atherosclerosis. *Science (Wash.)*, **251**:788–791.

Davies, M.J. and Thomas, A. (1984). Thrombosis and acute coronary-artery lesions in sudden cardiac ischemic death. *N. Engl. J. Med.*, **310**:1137–1140.

Doi, T., Higashino, K.-I., Kurihara, Y., Wada, Y., Miyazaki, T., Nakamura, H., Uesugi, S., Imanishi, T., Kawabe, Y., Itakura, H., Yazaki, Y., Matsumoto, A. and Kodama, T. (1993). Charged collagen structure mediates the recognition of negatively charged macromolecules by macrophage scavenger receptors. *J. Biol. Chem.*, **268**:2126–2133.

Durum, S.K., Schmidt, W.J. and Oppenheim, J.J. (1984). Interleukin 1: An immunological perspective. *Ann. Rev. Immunol.*, **3**:263–287.

Ehlers, S. and Smith, K.A. (1991). Differentiation of T cell lymphokine gene expression: The *in vitro* acquisition of T cell memory. *J. Exp. Med.*, 173:25–36.

Elices, M.J, Osborn, L. and Takada, Y. *et al.* (1990). VCAM-1 on activated endothelium interacts with the leukocyte integrin VLA-4 at a site distinct from the VLA-4/fibronectin binding site. *Cell*, 60:577–584.

Emeson, E.E. and Robertson, A.L. (1988). T lymphocytes in aortic and coronary intimas. Their potential role in atherogenesis. *Am. J. Pathol.*, 130:369–376.

Endemann, G., Stanton, L.W., Madden, K.S., Bryant, C.M., White, R.T. and Protter, A.A. (1993). CD36 is a receptor for oxidized low density lipoprotein. *J. Biol. Chem.*, 268:11811–11816.

Erhardt, L.R., Lundman, T. and Mellstedt, H. (1973). Incorporation of ^{125}-I-labelled fibrinogen into coronary arterial thrombi in acute myocardial infarction in man. *Lancet*, 1:387–390.

Faggiotto, A. and Ross, R. (1984a). Studies of hypercholesterolemia in the nonhuman primate. I. Changes that lead to fatty streak formation. *Arteriosclerosis*, 4:323–340.

Faggiotto, A. and Ross, R. (1984b). Studies of hypercholesterolemia in the nonhuman primate. II. Fatty streak conversion to fibrous plaque. *Arteriosclerosis*; 4:341–356.

Farrar, M.A. and Schreiber, R.D. (1993). The molecular cell biology of interferon-gamma and its receptor. *Ann. Rev. Immunol.*, 11:571–611.

Fowler, S., Shio, H. and Haley, N.J. (1979). Characterization of lipid-laden aortic cells from cholesterol-fed rabbits. IV. Investigation of macrophage-like properties of aortic cell populations. *Lab. Invest.*, 41:372–378.

Freeman, M., Ashkenas, J., Rees, J.G., Kingsley, M., Copeland, N.G., Jenkins, N.A. and Krieger, M. (1990). An ancient, highly conserved family of cysteine-rich protein domains revealed by cloning of type I and type II murine macrophage scavenger receptors. *Proc. Natl. Acad. Sci. USA*, 87:8810–8814.

Frostegård, J., Wu, R., Giscombe, R., Holm, G., Lefvert, A.K. and Nilsson, J. (1992). Induction of T-cell activation by oxidized low density lipoprotein. *Arterioscl. Thromb.*, 12:461–467.

Fyfe, A.I., Qiao, J.-H. and Lusis, A.J. (1994). Immune-deficient mice develop typical atherosclerotic fatty streaks when fed an atherogenic diet. *J. Clin. Invest.*, 94:2516–2520.

Geng, Y.J., Hansson, G.K. and Holme, E. (1992a). Interferon-γ and tumor necrosis factor synergize to induce nitric oxide production and inhibit mitochondrial respiration in vascular smooth muscle cells. *Circ. Res.*, 71:1268–1276.

Geng, Y.J. and Hansson, G.K. (1992b). Interferon-γ inhibits scavenger receptor expression and foam cell formation in human monocyte-derived macrophages. *J. Clin. Invest.*, 89:1321–1330.

Geng, Y.J., Petersson, A.-S., Wennmalm, Å. and Hansson, G.K. (1994). Cytokine-induced expression of nitric oxide synthase results in nitrosylation of heme and nonheme iron proteins in vascular smooth muscle cells. *Exp. Cell Res.*, 214:418–428.

Geng, Y.J., Holm, J., Nygren, S., Bruzelius, M., Stemme, S. and Hansson, G.K. (1995). Expression of macrophage scavenger receptor in atherosclerosis. Relationship between scavenger receptor isoforms, immunocompetent cells and T cell cytokines. *Arterioscl. Thromb. Vasc. Biol.*

Gerrity, R.G. (1981). The role of the monocyte in atherogenesis. I. Transition of blood-borne monocytes into foam cells in fatty lesions. *Am. J. Pathol.*, 103:181–190.

Goldstein, J.L., Ho, Y.K., Basu, S.K. and Brown, M.S. (1979). Binding site on macrophages that mediates uptake and degradation of acetylated low density lipoprotein producing massive cholesterol deposition *Proc. Natl. Acad. Sci. USA*, 76:168–178.

Gown, A.M., Tsukada, T. and Ross, R. (1986). Human atherosclerosis. II. Immunocytochemical analysis of the cellular composition of human atherosclerotic lesions. *Am. J. Pathol.*, 125:191–207.

Griffith, R.L., Virella, G.T., Stevenson, H.C. and Lopes-Virella, M.F. (1988). Low density lipoprotein metabolism by human macrophages activated with low density lipoprotein immune complexes. A possible mechanism of foam cell formation. *J. Exp. Med.*, 168:1041–1059.

Hansson, G.K., Björnheden, T., Bylock, A. and Bondjers, G. (1981). Fc-dependent binding of monocytes to areas with endothelial injury in the rabbit aorta. *Exp. Mol. Pathol.*, 34:264–280.

Hansson, G.K. and Schwartz, S.M. (1983). Evidence for cell death in the vascular endothelium *in vivo* and *in vitro*. *Am. J. Pathol.*, 112:278–286.

Hansson, G.K., Starkebaum, G.A., Benditt, E.P. and Schwarts, S.M. (1984). Fc-mediated binding of IgG to vimentin-type intermediate filaments in vascular endothelial cells. *Proc. Natl. Acad. Sci. USA*, 81:3103–3107.

Hansson, G.K., Lagerstedt, E., Bengtsson, A. and Heideman, M. (1987). IgG binding to cytoskeletal intermediate filaments activates the complement cascade. *Exp. Cell Res.*, 170:338–350.

Hansson, G.K., Holm, J. and Jonasson, L. (1989a). Detection of activated T lymphocytes in the human atherosclerotic plaque. *Am. J. Pathol.*, 135:169–175.

Hansson, G.K., Hellstrand, M., Rymo, L., Rubbia, L. and Gabbiani, G. (1989b). Interferon-γ inhibits both proliferation and expression of differentiation-specific α-smooth muscle actin in arterial smooth muscle cells. *J. Exp. Med.*, 170:1595–1608.

Hansson, G.K., Geng, Y.J., Holm, J., Hårdhammar, P., Wennmalm, Å. and Jennische, E. (1994). Arterial smooth muscle cells express nitric oxide synthase in response to endothelial injury. *J. Exp. Med.*, **180**:733–738.

Jonasson, L., Holm, J., Skalli, O., Gabbiani, G. and Hansson, G.K. (1985). Expression of class II transplantation antigen on vascular smooth muscle cells in human atherosclerosis. *J. Clin. Invest.*, **76**:125–131.

Jonasson, L., Holm, J., Skalli, O., Bondjers, G. and Hansson, G.K. (1986). Regional accumulations of T cells, macrophages, and smooth muscle cells in the human atherosclerotic plaque. *Arteriosclerosis*, **6**:131–138.

Kiessling, R., Grönberg, A. and Ivanyi, J., et al. (1991). Role of hsp60 during autoimmune and bacterial inflammation. *Immunol. Rev.*, **121**:91–111.

Klurfeld, D.M. (1985). Identification of foam cells in human atherosclerotic lesions as macrophages using mo noclonal antibodies. *Arch. Pathol. Lab. Med.*, **109**:445–449.

Kodama, T., Freeman, M., Rohrer, L., Zabrecky, J., Matsudaira, P. and Krieger, M. (1990). Type I macrophage scavenger receptor contains α-helical and collagen-like coiled coils. *Nature (Lond.)*, **343**:531–535.

Krieger, M., Acton, S., Ashkenas, J., Pearson, A., Penman, M. and Resnick, D. (1993). Molecular flypaper, host defense, and atherosclerosis. *J. Biol. Chem.*, **268**:4569–4572.

Kume, N., Cybulsky, M.I. and Gimbrone, M.A. (1992). Lysophosphatidylcholine, a component of atherogenic lipoproteins, induces mononuclear leukocyte adhesion molecules in cultured human and rabbit arterial endothelial cells. *J. Clin. Invest.*, **90**:1138–1144.

Kuo, C.C., Gown, A.M., Benditt, E.P. and Grayston, J.T. (1993). Detection of Chlamydia pneumoniae in aortic lesions of atherosclerosis by immunocytochemical stain. *Arteriosci. Thromb.*, **13**:1501–1504.

Leary, T. (1941). The genesis of atherosclerosis. *Arch. Pathol.*, **32**:507–518.

Libby, P., Warner, S.J.C., Salomon, R.N. and Birinyi, L.K. (1988). Production of platelet-derived growth factor-like mitogen by smooth muscle cells from human atheroma. *N. Engl. J. Med.*, **318**:1493–1498.

Libby, P. and Hansson, G.K. (1991). Involvement of the immune system in human atherogenesis: current knowledge and unanswered questions. *Lab. Invest.*, **64**:5–15.

Li, H., Cybulsky, M.I., Gimbrone, M.A. and Libby, P. (1993). An atherogenic diet rapidly induces VCAM-1, a cytokin-regulatable mononuclear leukocyte adhesion molecule, in rabbit aortic endothelium. *Arterioscl. Thromb.*, **13**:197–204.

Mackay, C.R., Marston, W.L. and Dudler, L. (1990). Naive and memory T cells show distinct pathways of lymphocyte recirculation. *J. Exp. Med.*, **171**:801–817.

McMurray, H.F., Parthasarathy, S. and Steinberg, D. (1993). Oxidatively modified low density lipoprotein is a chemoattractant for human T lymphocytes. *J. Clin. Invest.*, **92**:1004–1008.

Moyer, C.F., Sajuhti, D., Tulli, H. and Williams, J.K. (1991). Synthesis of IL-1 α and IL-1 β by arterial cells in atherosclerosis. *Am. J. Pathol.*, **138**:951–960.

Munro, J.M., van der Walt, J.D., Munro, C.S., Chalmers, J.A.C. and Cox, E.L. (1987). An immunohistochemical analysis of human aortic fatty streaks. *Hum. Pathol.*, **18**:375–380.

Nelken, N.A., Coughlin, S.R. Gordon, D. and Wilcox, J.N. (1991). Monocyte chemoattractant protein-1 in human atheromatous plaques. *J. Clin. Invest.*, **88**:1121–1127.

Palinski, W., Rosenfeld, M.E., Ylä-Herttuala, S., Gurtner, G.C., Socher, S.A., Butler, S.W., Parthasarathy, S., Carew, T.E., Steinberg, D. and Witztum, J.L. (1989). Low density lipoprotein undergoes oxidative modification *in vivo*. *Proc. Natl. Acad. Sci. USA*, **86**:1372–1376.

Palinski, W., Ylä-Herttuala, S. and Rosenfeld, M.E. (1990). Antisera and monoclonal antibodies specific for epitopes generated during oxidative modification of low density lipoprotein. *Arteriosci. Thromb.*, **10**:325–335.

Parthasarathy, S., Fong, L.G., Otero, D. and Steinberg, D. (1987). Recognition of solubilized apoproteins from delipidated, oxidized low density lipoprotein (LDL) by the acetyl-LDL receptor. *Proc. Natl. Acad. Sci. USA*, **84**:537–540.

Parums, D.V., Chadwick, D.R. and Mitchinson, M.J. (1986). The localization of immunoglobulin in chronic periaortitis. *Atherosclerosis*, **61**:117–123.

Parums, D.V., Brown, D.L. and Mitchinson, M.J. (1990). Serum antibodies to oxidized low-density lipoprotein and ceroid in chronic periaortitis. *Arch. Pathol. Lab. Med.*, **114**:383–387.

Pober, J.S., Gimbrone, M.A., Cotran, R.S., Reiss, C.S., Burakoff, S.J., Fiers, W. and Ault, K.A. (1982). Ia expression by vascular endothelium is inducible by activated T cells and by human gamma interferon. *J. Exp. Med.*, **157**:1339–1353.

Pober, J.S. and Cotran, R.S. (1990). Cytokines and endothelial cell biology. *Physiol. Rev.*, **70**:427–451.

Poole, J.C.F. and Florey, H.W. (1958). Changes in the endothelium of the aorta and the behaviour of macrohages in experimental atheroma of rabbits. *J. Pathol. Bact.*, **75**:245–252.

Poston, R.N., Haskard, D.O., Coucher, J.R., Gall, N.P. and Johnson-Tidey, R.R. (1992). Expression of intercellular adhesion molecule-1 in atherosclerotic plaques. *Am. J. Pathol.*, **140**:665–673.

Puolakkainen, M., Kuo, C.C., Shor, A., Wang, S.P., Grayston, J.T. and Campbell, L.A. (1993). Serological response to Chlamydia pneumoniae in adults with coronary arterial fatty streaks and fibrolipid plaques. *J. Clin. Microbiol.*, **31**:2212–2214.

Raines, E.W., Dower, S.K. and Ross, R. (1989). Interleukin-1 mitogenic activity for fibroblasts and smooth muscle cells is due to PDGF-AA. *Science*, **243**:393–396.

Richardson, M., Hadcock, S., DeReske, M. and Cybulsky, M. (1994). Increased expression *in vivo* of VCAM-1 and E-selectin by the aortic endothelium of normolipemic and hyperlipemic diabetic rabbits. *Arterioscl. Thromb.*, **143**:760–769.

Rohrer, L., Freeman, M., Kodama, T., Penman, M. and Krieger, M. (1990). Coiled-coil fibrous domains mediate ligand binding by macrophage scavenger receptor type II. *Nature (Lond.)*, **343**:570–572.

Rollins, B.J. Yoshimura, T., Leonard, E.J. and Pober, J.S. (1990). Cytokine-activated endothelial cells synthesize and secrete a monocyte chemoattractant MCP-1/JE. *Am. J. Pathol.*, **136**:1229–1233.

Rosenfeld, M.E., Tsukada, T., Gown, A.M. and Ross, R. (1987a). Fatty streak initiation in Watanabe heritable hyperlipemic and comparably hypercholesterolemic fat-fed rabbits. *Arteriosclerosis*, **7**:9–23.

Rosenfeld, M.E., Tsukada, T., Chait, A., Bierman, E.L., Gown, A.M. and Ross, R. (1987b). Fatty streak expansion and maturation in Watanabe heritable hyperlipemic and comparably hypercholesterolemic fat-fed rabbits. *Arteriosclerosis*, **7**:24–34.

Rosenfeld, M.E., Ylä-Herttuala, S., Lipton, B.A., Ord, V.A., Witztum, J.L. and Steinberg, D. (1992). Macrophage colony-stimulating factor mRNA and protein in atherosclerotic lesions of rabbits and humans. *Am. J. Pathol.*, **140**:291–300.

Salomon, R.N., Underwood, R., Doyle, M.V., Wang, A. and Libby, P. (1992). Increased apolipoprotein E and c-*fms* gene expression without elevated interleukin-1 or -6 mRNA levels indicates selective activation of macrophage functions in advanced human atheroma. *Proc. Natl. Acad. Sci. USA*, **89**:2814–2818.

Salonen, J.T., Ylä-Herttuala, S., Yamamoto, R., Butler, S., Korpela, H., Salonen, R., Nyyssönen, K., Palinski, W. and Witztum, J.L. (1992). Autoantibody against oxidised LDL and progression of carotid atherosclerosis. *Lancet*, **339**:883–887.

Schaffner, T., Taylor, K., Bartucci, E.J., Fischer-Dzoga, K., Beeson, J.H., Glagov, S. and Wissler, R.W. (1980). Arterial foam cells with distinctive immunomorphologic and histochemical features of macrophages. *Am. J. Pathol.*, **100**:57–80.

Scheurich, P., Thoma, B., Ücer, U. and Pfizenmaier, K. (1987). Immunoregulatory activity of recombinant hyman tumor necrosis factor (TNF)-α-mediated enhancement of T cell responses. *J. Immunol.*, **138**:1786–1790.

Seifert, P.S. and Kazatchkine, M.D. (1987). Generation of complement anaphylatoxins and C5b-9 by crystalline cholesterol oxidation derivatives depends on hydroxyl group number and position. *Mol. Immunol.*, **24**:1303–1308.

Seifert, P.S. and Kazatchkine, M.D. (1988). The complement system in atherosclerosis. *Atherosclerosis*, **73**:91–104.

Seifert, P.S., Hugo, F., Hansson, G.K. and Bhakdi, S. (1989) Prelesional complement actvation in eperimental atherosclerosis. Terminal C5b-9 complement deposition coincides with cholesterol accumulation in the aortic intima of hypercholesterolemic rabbits. *Lab. Invest.*, **60**:747–754.

Seifert, P.S. and Hansson, G.K. (1989). Complement receptors and regulatory proteins in human atherosclerotic lesions. *Arteriosclerosis*, **9**:802–811.

Sohma, Y., Sasano, H., Shiga, R., Saeki, S., Suzuki, T., Nagura, H., Nose, M. and Yamamoto, T. (1995). Accumulation of plasma cells in atherosclerotic lesions of Watanabe heritable hyperlipidemic rabbits. *Proc. Natl. Acad. Sci. USA*, **92**:4937–4941.

Stary, H.C. (1989). Evolution and progression of atherosclerotic lesions in coronary arteries of children and young adults. *Arteriosclerosis*, **9**: I, I-19-I-32.

Steinberg, D., Parthasarathy, S., Carew, T.E., Khoo, J.C. and Witztum, J.L. (1989). Beyond cholesterol: modifications of low-density lipoprotein that increase its atherogenicity. *N. Engl. J. Med.*, **320**:915–924.

Steinbrecher, U.P., Parthasarathy, S., Leake, D.S., Witztum, J.L. and Steinberg, D. (1984). Modification of low density lipoproteins by endothelial cells involves lipid peroxidation and degradation of low density lipoprotein phospholipids. *Proc. Natl. Acad. Sci. USA*, **83**:3883–3887.

Steinbrecher, U.P., Witztum, J.L., Parthasarathy, S. and Steinberg, D. (1987). Decrease in reactive amino groups during oxidation or endothelial cell modification of LDL: correlation with changes in receptor-mediated catabolism. *Arteriosclerosis*, **7**:135–143.

Stemme, S., Fager, G. and Hansson, G.K. (1990). MHC class II antigen expression in human vascular smooth muscle cells is induced by interferon-γ and modulated by tumour necrosis factor and lymphotoxin. *Immunology*, **69**:243–249.

Stemme, S., Holm, J. and Hansson, G.K. (1992a). T lymphocytes in human atherosclerotic plaques are memory cells expressing CD45RO and the integrin VLA-1. *Arterioscl. Thromb.*, **12**:206–11.

Stemme, S., Patarroyo, M. and Hansson, G.K. (1992b). Adhesion of activated T lymphocytes to vascular smooth muscle cells and dermal fibroblasts is mediated by β1- and β2-integrins. *Scand. J. Immunol.*, **36**:233–242.

Stemme, S., Faber, B., Holm, J., Wiklund, O., Witztum, J.L. and Hansson, G.K. (1995). T lymphocytes from human atherosclerotic plaques recognize oxidized LDL. *Proc. Natl. Acad. Sci. USA,* **92**:3893–3897.

Terkeltaub, R., Banka, C.L., Solan, J.M., Santoro, D., Brand, K. and Curtiss, L.K. (1994). Oxidized LDL induces monocytic cell expression of interleukin-8, a chemokine with T-lymphocyte chemotactic activity. *Arterioscl. Thromb.,* **14**:47–53.

van der Wal, A.C., Das, P.K., van de Berg, D.B., van der Loos, C.M. and Becker, A.E. (1989). Atherosclerotic lesions in humans. In situ Immunophenotypic analysis suggesting an immune mediated response. *Lab. Invest.,* **61**:166–170.

Vassalli, P. (1992). The pathophysiology of tumor necrosis factors. *Ann. Rev. Immunol.,* **10**:411–452.

Vedeler, C.A., Nyland, H. and Matre, R. (1984). In situ characterization of the foam cells in early human atherosclerotic lesions. *Acta Pathol Microbiol Immunol Scand,* **92C**:133–137.

Wang, S.A., Doyle, M.V. and Mark, D.F. (1989). Quantitation of mRNA by the polymerase chain reaction. *Proc. Natl. Acad. Sci. USA,* **86**:9717–9721.

Warner, S.J.C., Auger, K.R. and Libby, P. (1987). Interleukin-1 induces interleukin-1. II Recombinant human interleukin-1 induces interleukin-1 production by adult human vascular endothelial cells. *J. Immunol.,* **139**:1911–1917.

Warner, S.J.C. and Libby, P. (1989). Human vascular smooth muscle cells. Target for and source of tumor necrosis factor. *J. Immunol.,* **142**:100–109.

Wilhelmsen, L., Wedel, H. and Tibblin, G. (1973). Multivariate analysis of risk factors for coronary heart disease. *Circulation,* **48**:950–958.

Wood, K.S., Buga, G.M., Byrns, R.E. and Ignarro, L.J. (1990). Vascular smooth muscle-derived relaxing factor (MDRF) and its close similarity to nitric oxide. *Biochem. Biophys. Res. Commun.,* **170**:80–88.

Xu, Q., Dietrich, H. and Steiner, H.J., *et al.,* (1992). Induction of arteriosclerosis in normocholesterolemic rabbits by immunization with heat shock protein 65. *Arterioscl. Thromb.,* **12**:789–799.

Xu, Q., Willeit, J., Marosi, M., Kleindienst, R., Oberhollenzer, F., Kiechl, S., Stulnig, T., Luef, G. and Wick, G. (1993a). Association of serum antibodies to heat-shock protein 65 with carotid atherosclerosis. *Lancet,* **341**:255–259.

Xu, Q., Kleindienst, R., Waitz, W., Dietrich, H. and Wick, G. (1993b). Increased expression of heat shock protein 65 coincides with a population of infiltrating T lymphocytes in atherosclerotic lesions of rabbits specifically responding to heat shock protein 65. *J. Clin. Invest.,* **91**:2693–2702.

Ylä-Herttuala, S., Palinski, W. and Rosenfeld, M.E. *et al.* (1989). Evidence for the presence of oxidatively modified low density lipoprotein in atherosclerotic lesions of rabbit and man. *J. Clin. Invest.,* **84**:1086–1095.

Ylä-Herttuala, S., Rosenfeld, M.E., Parthasarathy, S., Sigal, E., Särkioja, T., Witztum, J.L. and Steinberg, D. (1991). Gene expression in macrophage-rich human atherosclerotic lesions: 15-lipoxygenase and acetyl low density lipoprotein receptor messenger RNA colocalize with oxidation specific lipid-protein adducts. *J. Clin. Invest.,* **87**:1146–1152.

Ylä-Herttuala, S., Palinski, W., Butler, S.W., Picard, S., Steinberg, D. and Witztum, J.L. (1994). Rabbit and human atherosclerotic lesions contain IgG that recognizes epitopes of oxidized LDL. *Arterioscl. Thromb.,* **14**:32–40.

9 Autoimmunity to Oxidized Lipoproteins

Joseph L. Witztum and Wulf Palinski

Department of Medicine, University of California, San Diego, 9500 Gilman Drive, La Jolla, CA 92093–0682

INTRODUCTION

The observation that modifications of autologous LDL rendered it immunogenic derived from serendipitous observations made many years earlier. At that time, we were studying the metabolism of LDL that had undergone non-enzymatic glycation (NEG). Glucose is known to form Amadori adducts with lysine residues of protein even in normal individuals, and this process is greatly accelerated in hyperglycemic diabetic subjects. Because lysine residues of LDL had been demonstrated to be responsible for the binding of LDL to the LDL receptor, we were interested in the possibility that increased NEG could impair the ability of LDL to bind to its receptor in diabetic subjects. We demonstrated in cell culture that heavily glycated LDL lost high affinity binding to the LDL receptor of fibroblasts and, when injected into in guinea pigs, had markedly delayed plasma clearance (Witztum, 1982). This suggested the possibility of using heavily glycated LDL as a tracer to assess the extent of the LDL receptor pathway *in vivo* in man. The rationale behind this approach was that the clearance of native LDL is due to both receptor-dependent and receptor-independent pathways, while the clearance of a heavily glycated LDL would be mediated only via receptor-independent pathways. At the time we initiated these studies, there were no accurate measurements of the extent of the LDL receptor pathway in man. Studies performed with cyclohexanedione-modified LDL greatly underestimated the extent of the pathway as this modification was reversible *in vivo*. Therefore, we isolated LDL from subjects, glycated half of it and injected both the native LDL and the glycated LDL radiolabeled with different isotopes. In most normal subjects, the clearance of the native LDL was rapid and biphasic whereas that of the glycated LDL was much slower and usually monoexponential. These studies revealed that up to 75% of LDL clearance was mediated by the LDL receptor pathway (Kesaniemi, 1983). We then sought to determine the percent of the LDL receptor pathway that occurred in diabetic subjects, since with a deficiency of insulin one might predict a decrease in the extent of this pathway. However, in a number of diabetic and normal subjects, while the clearance of the native LDL tracer was as expected, the clearance of the glycated LDL tracer was extraordinarily rapid and the shape of the disappearance curve suggested an immune mediated clearance (Kesaniemi, 1983; Witztum, 1984). Because of this result, we tested the hypothesis that glycation of autologous LDL rendered it immunogenic, even though traditional immunological theory suggested that simply covalently linking a monosaccharide to an autologous protein would not induce immunogenicity. To accomplish this, LDL was isolated from guinea pigs, subjected to NEG, and then used to immunize guinea pigs. As a control, native LDL was subject to the same manipulations in the absence of glucose and also used to immunize guinea pigs. These studies demonstrated unequivocally that very high titered antisera that recognized glycated LDL were generated, and that in these immunized guinea pigs there was a rapid, immune-mediated clearance of an injected glycated tracer, but no increased turnover of native LDL. Furthermore, the antisera were capable of recognizing the glycated lysine residue on any similarly modified protein (Witztum, 1984). Similarly, if *murine* LDL was isolated, glycated, and used to immunize mice, murine monoclonal antibodies could be produced that specifically recognized glucitollysine when present on a variety of similar modified proteins (Curtiss and Witztum, 1983). We subsequently showed that autoantibodies to glycated LDL were present in the serum of diabetic subjects. In further studies, we showed that many other such minimal modifications of autologous LDL also were immunogenic (Steinbrecher, 1984). Methylation, ethylation, acetylation, or carbamylation of autologous guinea pig LDL rendered that LDL immunogenic and the monospecific antisera produced with each antigen recognized not only the respective immunogen, but also other similarly modified proteins. An example of the fine specificity of such antisera is shown in Figure 1, which depicts a competition radioimmunoassay (RIA) of an antiserum to methylated LDL with

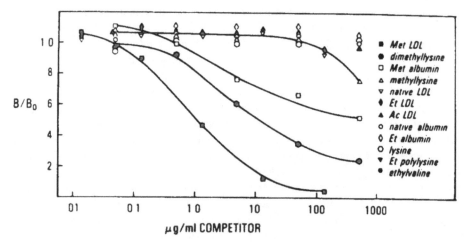

Figure 1 Competition RIA for binding of antiserum to methylated LDL. Methylated LDL was plated as solid phase antigen on microtiter wells and a fixed and limited dilution of antiserum to methylated LDL was added in the absence (B_0) or presence (B) of indicated concentrations of competitors. See text for explanations. Met LDL (albumin) = methylated LDL (albumin); Et LDL (albumin) = ethylated LDL (albumin); Et polylysine = ethylated polylysine. Reproduced with permission from Steinbrecher, 1984.

a variety of competitors. Note that when methyllysine was added as a competitor, it was relatively weak competitor. However, when we examined the literature, we discovered that the technique used for methylation yields predominantly dimethyllysine as the product. When dimethyllysine was added to the RIA as a competitor, it was quite effective. This figure demonstrates the exquisite ability of LDL to present even the most minute adduct as a highly immunogenic epitope. It should be noted that in these same studies we also demonstrated that modifications of other autologous proteins were immunogenic as well, though the titers developed were lower and the specificities of antibodies produced were more restricted. For example, an antiserum to carbamylated guinea pig albumin recognized carbamylated albumin, but had little ability to recognize carbamylated LDL.

HUMORAL IMMUNE RESPONSE TO OXIDIZED LDL

Years later, we sought to develop antibodies that would recognize epitopes of oxidized LDL and allow us to determine if oxidized LDL exists *in vivo*. We utilized the same principles as outlined above, reasoning that any modifications of autologous LDL that would occur as a result of the oxidation should also render the LDL immunogenic. We therefore took autologous LDL from guinea pigs and mice, oxidized them by exposure to copper, and immunized the appropriate host animal to generate antisera specific for epitopes of oxidized LDL (Palinski, 1989, 1990). In addition, we generated model epitopes that we predicted should be present on oxidized LDL. This was done by taking advantage of the fact that breakdown products of oxidized polyunsaturated fatty acids, such as malondialdehyde (MDA) and 4-hydroxynonenal (4-HNE) are highly reactive compounds that could derivatize lysine residues in apolipoprotein B, similar to modifications which occurred with NEG of lysine residues in hyperglycemia. To this end, we prepared autologous MDA-LDL and 4-HNE-LDL, and generated antisera and monoclonal antibodies in guinea pigs and mice, respectively (Palinski, 1989, 1990). These reagents were then used to demonstrate that these epitopes, which we termed "oxidation-specific" epitopes, could be found in atherosclerotic lesions of rabbits, humans and, most recently, mice. In every case, there was colocalization of the immunostaining obtained with the different antisera developed against the different oxidation-specific epitopes. These results have been described in detail (Palinski, 1989, 1994, 1995; Rosenfeld, 1990). Haberland and colleagues (1988) were actually the first to demonstrate that an antibody to MDA-LDL stained atherosclerotic lesions, and Boyd *et al.* (1989) also obtained similar results with an antibody to oxidized LDL. Because all of these antibodies were not absolutely specific for oxidized LDL, i.e., the antibodies recognized the same epitopes on other similarly modified proteins, it was necessary to demonstrate that oxidized *LDL* actually existed *in vivo*. This was accomplished by eluting LDL from atherosclerotic tissues and demonstrating that it possessed the physical and biological properties of *in vitro* oxidized LDL, and in particular that it contained the oxidation-specific epitopes our antibodies recognized (Palinski, 1989; Ylä-Herttuala, 1989).

The demonstration that many different epitopes of oxidized LDL were present in lesions, and the knowledge that modifications of autologous LDL (as well as other autologous proteins) rendered them immunogenic suggested that autoantibodies ought to be present in human sera. Indeed, we demonstrated that this was the case (Palinski, 1989). IgG isolated from the plasma of a human subject could be used to stain the atherosclerotic lesion of a rabbit in a manner quite identical to that achieved by the use of the monoclonal antibody MDA-2, which had been generated against the MDA-LDL antigen. In our initial studies, we found the presence of such antibodies in the sera of both normal and atherosclerotic rabbit models, as well as in the sera of all human subjects tested (Palinski, 1989). To determine if there might be a difference in titer in individuals who developed atherosclerosis versus those who didn't, we collaborated with Dr. Salonen and colleagues in Finland who had collected sera from 300 normal individuals during a baseline study at which carotid artery ultrasound measurements were also made (Salonen, 1992). These subjects were then studied two years later and carotid artery ultrasound measurements repeated. In a matched case-control study, individuals who exhibited the most progression of the carotid intima/medial thickness over the two-year interval were studied versus those who exhibited the least progression. We found that the titer of autoantibodies binding to MDA-LDL (as a representative epitope of oxidized LDL) was highly predictive of the rate of progression of disease. In fact, in a multivariant logistic regression analysis of multiple risk factors, the antibody titer and the presence of smoking were found to be the only independent risk factors predictive of progression. Since that study, an increasing number of reports have appeared in the literature demonstrating a relationship between various manifestations of atherosclerosis and increased titers of autoantibodies to epitopes of oxidized LDL (Table 1).

To determine if we could observe a change in autoantibody titer in an animal model developing atherosclerotic lesions, LDL receptor-negative mice were placed on a high fat diet and prospectively followed over a period of six months. Autoantibody titers to epitopes of oxidized LDL progressively rose, and at the end of the experiment the titer of such autoantibodies correlated with the extent of lesion formation as determined by morphometric analysis (Palinski, 1995c) (Figure 2).

Table 1   Increased Titers of Autoantibodies to Epitopes of Oxidized LDL in Human Subjects with:

Condition:	Reference:
Chronic periaortitis	Parums 1990
Carotid atherosclerosis (predictive)	Salonen 1992
Coronary artery disease	Maggi 1993
Pre-eclampsia	Branch 1994
Uremia	Maggi 1994a
Severe carotid atherosclerosis	Maggi 1994b
Coronary artery disease and other pathology	Armstrong 1994
Essential hypertension	Maggi 1995
Early onset peripheral vascular disease	Bergmark 1995
Myocardial infarction (predictive)	Vaarala 1995
NIDDM patients	Bellomo 1995

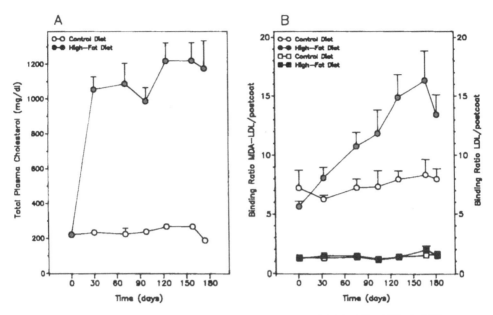

Figure 2 Development of autoantibodies to an epitope of oxidized LDL, MDA-LDL, in LDL receptor-negative mice fed a high fat diet. Sex- and litter-matched LDL receptor-negative mice were fed either a control chow diet or a high fat diet for a period of six months. Plasma cholesterol levels are shown in Panel A. In animals on the high fat diet approximately 18% of the aortic surface showed atherosclerotic lesions, compared to less than 0.5% in animals on the control diet. Panel B demonstrates a progressive rise in antibody titer to MDA-LDL in the mice on the high fat diet, while the titer did not change in the control mice (circles, left scale). Neither group showed any change in antibody titer to "native" LDL (squares, right scale). At the end of the experiment the antibody titer correlated with the plasma cholesterol level (r = 0.93, p < 0.0001), as well as with the extent of atherosclerosis (r = 0.62, p < 0.01). Reproduced with permission from Palinski, 1995c.

PRESENCE OF IgG SPECIFIC FOR OXIDIZED LDL IN ATHEROSCLEROTIC LESIONS

It has been well known for many years that immunoglobulins specifically accumulate in atherosclerotic lesions. We have also documented this in lesions of rabbits, mice and humans (Ylä-Herttuala, 1994; Palinski, 1995). Given the existence of circulating autoantibodies to oxidized LDL and the presence of oxidized LDL in lesions, we next addressed the issue of whether or not there were populations of antibodies specific for the epitopes of oxidized LDL among the immunoglobulins present in atherosclerotic lesions. To examine this question, IgG was eluted from atherosclerotic lesions of WHHL rabbits by sequential salt extraction, purified by protein-G chromatography and then tested for specificity by solid phase RIA and Western Blot analysis. These studies demonstrated a relatively high titer of IgG antibodies binding to MDA-LDL, as well as to copper-oxidized LDL itself, while the same purified IgG fraction exhibited no binding to native LDL. Similarly, by Western Blot analysis, it could be shown that this IgG specifically recognized epitopes of MDA-LDL and copper-oxidized LDL, but not native LDL. The isolated IgG could also be used to immunostain human atherosclerotic lesions in a manner identical to that of MDA-2 and other induced antibodies against oxidation-specific epitopes. In further studies, we demonstrated that immune complexes were present in human atherosclerotic lesions and that these immune complexes contained OxLDL. Similarly, when IgG extracted from human lesions was used to stain rabbit atheroslcerotic lesions, it gave a pattern identical to that of MDA-2, and could be shown to be specific by preabsorption studies (Ylä-Herttuala, 1994).

POTENTIAL ROLE OF HUMORAL RESPONSE IN ATHEROGENESIS

The data presented so far indicate that autologous modifications of LDL are immunogenic, that oxidation of LDL does occur *in vivo*, and that subsequently there is a humoral immune response. As noted above, preliminary epidemiological data indicate that there is an increased titer of antibodies to epitopes of oxidized LDL in subjects with varying manifestations of atherosclerotic disease or increased risk factors for disease. An obvious question is whether or not this humoral immunity might play any role in the modulation of the atherogenic process. In an initial approach to this question, we hyperimmunized spontaneously hypercholesterolemic WHHL rabbits to achieve very high titers of autoantibodies to a specific epitope of oxidized LDL (Palinski, 1995b). We chose MDA-LDL as such a model, because the MDA-LDL antigen can be generated quite reproducibly, whereas the oxidation of LDL with copper yields highly variable preparations, and less extensively modified preparations may continuously oxidize over time. In addition, the MDA-lysine epitope is abundantly present in lesions and circulating autoantibodies to MDA-LDL are prevalent. Thus, LDL was isolated from WHHL rabbits, modified with MDA such that greater than 75% of lysine residues were derivatized, and used to immunize WHHL rabbits using complete Freund's adjuvant for the initial injection, and incomplete Freund's adjuvant for subsequent boosts. As a control, saline with adjuvant was used to immunize litter-matched controls, and as a second control, an additional group was immunized with keyhole limpet hemocyanin (KLH). The choice of the latter antigen was dictated by the desire to use a known stimulant of the immune response, but because this protein does not have a homologue in mammalian physiology, any antibodies produced would not react with any tissue antigens. The protocol for the study is shown in Figure 3.

In normal WHHL rabbits, autoantibody titers of several thousand against MDA-LDL are found at four to six months of age (Palinski, 1989). In contrast, in the hyperimmunized rabbits, titers greater than 100,000 were achieved after the primary immunization and two boosts. These high titers were maintained at that level over a six-month period of time by monthly boosts, and the specificity of the induced antibodies was very similar to that of naturally occurring antibodies. After six months of intervention, the animals were sacrificed, and to our surprise, we noted that there was a consistent decrease in the extent of atherosclerosis in all portions of the aorta in the animals immunized with MDA-LDL, compared to control groups (Figure 4). There was no difference in atherosclerosis between control animals immunized with KLH or PBS. Immunohistochemical analysis of lesions of comparable stages from control and treated rabbits did not reveal obvious differences with respect to morphology, the presence of immune-competent cells or oxidized LDL epitopes. There were significant numbers of MHC-II positive macrophages

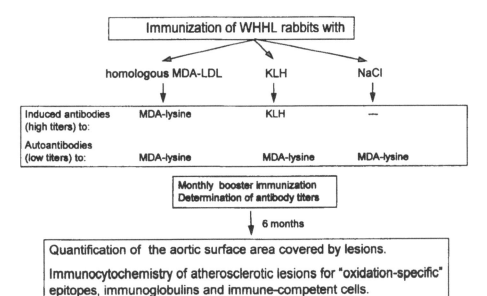

Figure 3 Protocol of the initial experiment conducted to study the potential modulation of atherogenesis by the humoral immune system.

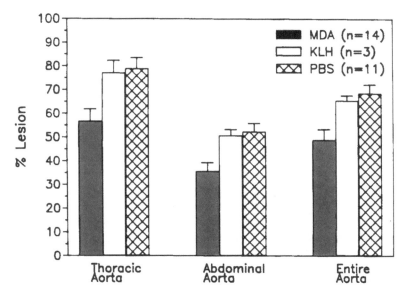

Figure 4 Comparison of extent of atherosclerosis in rabbits immunized with malondialdehyde-modified LDL (MDA-LDL), phosphate buffered saline (PBS), or keyhole limpet hemocyanin (KLH), as explained in text. Data represent percent of the entire aortic surface examined that was covered by atherosclerotic lesions. Values for MDA-LDL-immunized rabbits were significantly different from controls. Reproduced with permission from Palinski, 1995b.

multiple modifications of LDL. Similarly, it is likely that there is also an analogous response to similar modifications of other lipoproteins as well as structural proteins. This involves both humoral and cell-mediated components. Although the data presented above suggest that the humoral immune response might be protective, it must of course be understood that these experiments were conducted under a highly artificial setting in which extreme elevations of autoantibodies occurred at a relatively early stage in the atherosclerotic process. In other settings, an immune response might actually be adverse. For example, Wick and colleagues have reported that heat shock protein 60 is expressed in antherosclerotic lesions and that a humoral (and cell-mediated) response to this antigen may lead to adverse consequences (Xu, 1994). Indeed, they reported that immunization of non-hypercholesterolemic rabbits with heat shock protein 65 leads to an inflammatory type lesion in rabbit aortic tissue (Xu, 1992). Conversely, there are multiple reports that suppression of cell-mediated immunity can lead to enhancement of atherosclerotic lesions, suggesting a beneficial role for the cellular responses (Hansson, 1991; Emeson, 1993, Fyfe, 1994; Roselaar, 1995). In order to sort out the many and potentially conflicting roles that the immune response can play, it would be useful to have an animal model that has a more defined immune system than that of the rabbit and which could be more readily subject to genetic manipulation. The recent demonstration that several different murine models display atherosclerotic quite typical of those found in other animal models and in man suggests that this species is such a candidate. The immune system of the mouse has been under intensive scrutiny for many years, and not only are there many reagents available to characterize their immune system, but there are now many genetic models of specific and generalized immune deficiency available as well. It would therefore be valuable to be able to use murine models to study the role of immunity in atherosclerosis.

As noted above, we have documented previously that atherosclerotic lesions of apo E-deficient mice contain oxidation-specific epitopes in a manner quite similar to that seen in other animal models and humans. To determine if there is an autoantibody response, as in man and rabbits, sera from apo E-deficient mice were tested for autoantibody titers to MDA-LDL. In fact, it was found that they had a remarkably high titer of autoantibodies to this particular epitope and that they show similar high titers against oxidized LDL as well as to a variety of other model epitopes that are present in oxidized LDL (Palinski, 1994). The high titers of autoantibodies found in these mice (for example, >50,000 toward MDA-LDL) may make it possible to clone natural (noninduced) monoclonal antibodies from these mice directed against epitopes of oxidized LDL. These could be invaluable in identifying epitopes that actually occur *in vivo*. A better definition of these epitopes could lead to more specific reagents that might exclusively recognize oxidized *LDL* for example, and antigens which in turn could lead to more specifically targeted intervention (e.g., by immunization as described above). As noted earlier, we have also observed that autoantibody titers to epitopes of oxidized LDL progressively rise in plasma of LDL receptor-negative mice developing atherosclerosis in response to an atherogenic diet. Thus, this murine model may also be an excellent candidate for study.

Studies are already underway in a number of laboratories to determine the impact on atherosclerosis of altered immune function using murine models. When apo E-deficient mice are crossed with various murine models of cell-mediated immune deficiency, in several such models, notably that of the MHC Class 1-deficient mice, there was greatly exaggerated atherosclerotic lesions (Fyfe, 1994). Thus it seems likely that studies of the role of the immune system can be accomplished in murine models and should be rewarding in defining the potential role that the immune system can play in modulating the development of the atherosclerotic lesion. It is conceivable that the lessons gained could lead to new insights that could be exploited in ways that might have important therapeutic implications.

References

Armstrong, V.W., Wieland, E., Diedrich, F., Renner, A., Rath, W., Kreuzer, H., Kuhn, W. and Oellerich, M. (1994). Serum antibodies to oxidised low-density lipoprotein in pre-eclampsia and coronary heart disease [letter]. *Lancet*, 343:1570.

Bellomo, G., Maggi, E., Poli, M., Agosta, F.G., Bollati, P. and Finardi, G. (1995). Autoantibodies against oxidatively modified low-density lipoproteins in NIDDM. *Diabetes*, 44:60–66.

Bergmark, C., Wu, R., de Faire, U., Lefvert, A.K. and Swedenborg, J. (1995). Patients with early-onset peripheral vascular disease have increased levels of autoantibodies against oxidized LDL. *Arterioscler. Thromb. Vasc. Biol.*, 15:441–445.

Berliner, J.A., Territo, M., Almada, L., Carter, A., Shafonsky, E. and Fogelman, A.M. (1986). Monocyte chemotactic factor produced by large vessel endothelial cells *in vitro*. *Arteriosclerosis*, 6:254–258.

Berliner, J.A., Territo, M.C., Sevanian, A., Ramin, S., Kim, J.A., Bamshad, B., Esterson, M. and Fogelman, A.M. (1990). Minimally modified low density lipoprotein stimulates monocyte endothelial interactions. *J. Clin. Invest.*, 85:1260–1266.

Boyd, H.C., Gown, A.M., Wolfbauer, G. and Chait, A. (1989). Direct evidence for a protein recognized by a monoclonal antibody against oxidatively modified LDL in atherosclerotic lesions from a Watanabe Heritable Hyperlipidemic rabbit. *Am. J. Pathol.*, 135:815–826.

Branch, D.W., and Mitchell, M.D., Miller, E., Palinski, W. and Witztum, J.L. (1994). Pre-eclampsia and serum antibodies to oxidized low density lipoprotein. *Lancet*, 343:645–646.

Curtiss, L.K. and Witztum, J.L. (1983). A novel method for generating region specific monoclonal antibodies to modified proteins: Application to the identification of human glucosylated low density lipoproteins. *J. Clin. Invest.*, 72:1427–1438.

Emeson, E.E. and Shen, M.-L. (1993). Accelerated atherosclerosis in hyperlipidemic C57BL/6 mice treated with cyclosporine A. *Am. J. Pathol.*, 142:1906–1915.

Fyfe, A., Qiao, J.H. and Lusis, A.J. (1994). Immune deficient mice develop typical atherosclerotic fatty streaks when fed an atherogenic diet. *J. Clin. Invest.*, 94:2516–2520.

Haberland, M.E., Fong, D. and Cheng, L. (1988). Malondialdehyde-altered protein occurs in atheroma of Watanabe heritable hyperlipidemic rabbits. *Science*, 241:215–218.

Hansson, G.K., Holm, J., Holm, S., Fotev, Z., Hedric, H.J. and Fingerle, J. (1991). T lymphocytes inhibit the vascular response to injury. *Proc. Natl. Acad. Sci. USA*, 88:10530–10534.

Hodis, H.N., Kramsch, D.M., Avogaro, P., Bittolo-Bon, G., Cazzolato, G., Hwang, J., Peterson, H. and Sevanian, A. (1994). Biochemical and cytotoxic characteristics of an *in vivo* circulating oxidized low density lipoportein (LDL). *J. Lipid. Res.*, 35:669–677.

Holvoet, P., Perez, G., Zhao, Z., Brouwers, E., Bernar, H. and Collen, D. (1995). Malondialdehyde-modified low density lipoproteins in patients with atherosclerotic disease. *J. Clin. Invest.*, 95:2611–2619.

Houglum, K., Filip, M., Witztum, J.L. and Chojkie, M. (1990). Malondialdehyde and 4-hydroxynonenal protein adducts in plasma and liver of rats with iron overload. *J. Clin. Invest.*, 86:1991–1998.

Kesaniemi, Y.A., Witztum, J.L. and Steinbrecher, U.P. (1983). Receptor-mediated clearance of LDL in man — new estimates using glucosylated LDL. *J. Clin. Invest.*, 71:950–959.

Khoo, J.C., Miller, E., McLoughlin, P. and Steinberg, D. (1988). Enhanced macrophage uptake of low density lipoprotein after self-aggregation. *Arteriosclerosis*, 8:348–358.

Maggi, E., Marchesi, R., Ravetta, V., Martignoni, A., Finardi, G. and Bellomo, G. (1995). Presence of autoantibodies against oxidatively modified low density lipoprotein in essential hypertension — A biochemical signature of an enhanced *in vivo* low density lipoprotein oxidation. *J. Hyperten.*, 13:129–138.

Maggi, E., Bellazzi, R., Gazo, A., Seccia, M. and Bellomo, G. (1994a). Autoantibodies against oxidatively modified LDL in uremic patients undergoing dialysis. *Kidney International*, 46:869–76.

Maggi, E., Chiesa, R., Melissano, G., Castellano, R., Astore, D., Grossi, A., Finardi, G. and Bellomo, G. (1994b). LDL oxidation in patients with severe carotid atherosclerosis. A study of *in vitro* and *in vivo* oxidation markers. *Arterioscler. Thromb.*, 14:1892–1899.

Maggi, E., Finardi, G., Poli, M., Bollati, P., Filipponi, M., Stefano, P.L., Paolini, G., Grossi, A., Clot, P., Albano, E. and Bellomo, G. (1993). Specificity of autoantibodies against oxidized LDL as an additional marker for atherosclerotic risk. *Coron. Artery Dis.*, 4:1119–1122.

Neale, T.J., Ojha, P.P., Exner, M., Poczewski, H., Rüger, B., Witztum, J.L., Davis, P. and Kerjaschki, D. (1994). Proteinuria in passive Heymann nephritis is associated with lipid peroxidation and formation of adducts on Type IV collagen. *J. Clin. Invest.*, **94**:1577–1584.

Newcombe, J., Li, H. and Cuzner, M.L. (1994). Low density lipoprotein uptake by macrophages in multiple sclerosis plaques: implications for pathogenesis. *Neuropath. App. Neurobiol.*, **20**:52–162.

Palinski, W. and Witztum, J.L. (1995a). Oxidative stress and diabetes mellitus. In: *New Horizons In Diabetes Mellitus And Coronary Heart Disease*. Born, G.V.R. and Schwartz, C.D. (eds), pp. 111-123. London: Current Science.

Palinski, W., Miller, E. and Witztum, J.L. (1995b). Immunization of LDL receptor-deficient rabbits with homologous malondialdehyde-modified LDL reduces atherogenesis. *Proc. Natl. Acad. Sci. USA*, **92**:821–825.

Palinski, W., Tangirala, R., Miller, E., Young, S.G. and Witztum, J.L. (1995c). Increased autoantibody titers against epitopes of oxidized low density lipoprotein in LDL receptor-deficient mice with increased atherosclerosis. *Arterioscler. Thromb. Vasc. Biol.*, **15**:1569–1576.

Palinski, W., Ord, V., Plump, A.S., Breslow, J.L., Steinberg, D. and Witztum, J.L. (1994). ApoE deficient mice are a model of lipoprotein oxidation in atherogenesis: Demonstration of oxidation-specific epitopes in lesions and high titers of autoantibodies to malondialdehyde-lysine in serum. *Arterioscler. Thromb.*, **14**:605–616.

Palinski, W., Ylä-Herttuala, S., Rosenfeld, M.E, Butler, S., Socher, S.A., Parthasarathy, S., Curtiss, L.K. and Witztum, J.L. (1990). Antisera and monoclonal antibodies specific for epitopes generated during the oxidative modification of low density lipoprotein. *Arteriosclerosis*, **10**:325–335.

Palinski, W., Rosenfeld, M.E., Ylä-Herttuala, S., Gurtner, G.C., Socher, S.A., Butler, S., Parthasarathy, S., Carew, T.E., Steinberg, D. and Witztum, J.L. (1989). Low density lipoprotein undergoes oxidative modification *in vivo*. *Proc. Natl. Acad. Sci. USA*, **86**:1372–1376.

Parums, D.V., Brown, D.L. and Mitchinson, M.J. (1990). Serum antibodies to oxidized low density lipoprotein and ceroid in chronic periaortits. *Arch. Pathol. Lab. Med.*, **114**:383–387.

Roselaar, S.E., Schonfeld, G. and Daugherty, A. (1995). Enhanced development of atherosclerosis in cholesterol-fed rabbits by suppression of cell-mediated immunity. *J. Clin. Invest.*, **96**:1389–1394.

Rosenfeld, M.E., Palinski, W., Ylä-Herttuala, S., Butler, S. and Witztum, J.L. (1990). Distribution of oxidation specific lipid-protein adducts and apolipoprotein B in atherosclerotic lesions of varying severity from WHHL rabbits. *Arterioscleosis*, **10**:336–349.

Salonen, J.T., Ylä-Herttuala, S., Yamamoto, R., Butler, S., Korpela, H., Salonen, R., Nyyssönen, K., Palinski, W. and Witztum, J.L. (1992). Autoantibody against oxidised LDL and progression of carotid atherosclerosis. *Lancet*, **339**:883–887.

Sambrano, G. and Steinberg, D. (1995). Recognition of oxidatively damaged and apoptotic cells by an oxidized low density lipoprotein receptor on mouse peritoneal macrophages: Role of membrane phosphatidylserine. *Proc. Natl. Acad. Sci. USA*, **92**:1396–1400.

Steinbrecher, U.P., Fisher, M., Witztum, J.L. and Curtiss, L.K. (1984). Immunogenicity of homologous low density lipoprotein after methylation, ethylation, acetylation or carbamylation: Generation of antibodies specific for derivatyzed lysine. *J. Lipid Res.*, **25**:1109–1116.

Stemme, S., Rymo, L. and Hansson, G.K. (1991). Polyclonal origin of T-lymphocytes in human atherosclerotic plaques. *Lab. Invest.*, **65**:654–660.

Stemme, S., Faber, B., Holm, J., Bondjers, G., Witztum, J. and Hansson, G.K. (1995). T-lymphocytes from human athercletoric plaques recognize oxidized low density lipoprotein. *Proc. Natl. Acad. Sci. USA*, **92**:3893–3897.

Vaarala, O., Mänttäri, M., Manninen, V., Tenkanen, L., Puurunen, M., Aho, K. and Palosuo, T. (1995). Anti-cardiolipin antibodies and risk of myocardial infarction in a prospective cohort of middle-aged men. *Circulation*, **91**:23–27.

Watson, A.D., Navab, M., Hama, S.Y., Sevanian, A., Prescott, S.M., Stafforini, D.M., McIntyre, T.M., La Du, B.N., Fogelman, A.M. and Berliner, J.A. (1995). Effect of platelet activating factor-acetylhydrolase on the formation and action of minimally oxidized low density lipoprotein. *J. Clin. Invest.*, **95**:774–782.

Wiklund, O., Witztum, J.L., Carew, T.E., Pittman, R.C., Elam, R.L. and Steinberg, D. (1987). Turnover and tissue sites of degradation of glucosylated low density lipoproteins in normal and immunized rabbits. *J. Lipid Res.*, **28**:1098–1109.

Witztum, J.L., Mahoney, E.M., Branks, M.J., Fisher, M., Elam, R. and Steinberg, D. (1982). Nonenzymatic glucosylation of low-density lipoprotein alters its biological activity. *Diabetes*, **31**:283–291.

Witztum, J.L., Steinbrecher, U.P., Kesaniemi, Y.A. and Fisher, M. (1984). Autoantibodies to glucosylated proteins in the plasma of patients with diabetes mellitus. *Proc. Natl. Acad. Sci. USA*, **81**:3204–3208.

Witztum, J.L. (1994). The oxidation hypothesis of atherosclerosis. *Lancet*, **344**:793–795.

Xu, Q., Dietrich, H., Steiner, H.J., Gown, A.M., Mikuz, G., Kaufmann, S.H.E. and Wick, G. (1992). Induction of atherosclerosis in normocholesterolemic rabbits by immunization with heat shock protein 65. *Arterioscler. Thromb.*, **12**:789–799.

Xu, Q., Schett, G., Seitz, C.S., Hu, Y., Gupta, R.S. and Wick, G. (1994). Surface staining and cytotoxic activity of heat shock protein 60 antibody on stressed aortic endothelial cells. *Circ. Res.*, **75**:1079–1085.

Yan, S.-D., Chen, X., Schmidt, A.-M., Brett, J., Godman, G., Zou, Y.-S., Scott, C.W., Caputo, C., Frappier, T., Smith, M.A., Perry, G., Yen, S.-H. and Stern, D. (1994a). Glycated tau protein in Alzheimer disease: A mechanism for induction of oxidant stress. *Proc. Natl. Acad. Sci. USA*, **91**:7787-7791.

Yan, S.-D., Schmidt, A.-M., Anderson, G.M., Zhang, J., Brett, J., Zou, Y.S., Pinsky, D. and Stern, D. (1994b). Enhanced cellular oxidant stress by the interaction of advanced glycosylation endproducts with their receptors/binding proteins. *J. Biol. Chem.*, **269**:9889–9897.

Ylä-Herttuala, S., Palinski, W., Rosenfeld, M.E., Parthasarathy, S., Carew, T.E., Butler, S., Witztum, J.L. and Steinberg, D. (1989). Evidence for the presence of oxidatively modified low density lipoprotein in atherosclerotic lesions of rabbit and man. *J. Clin. Invest.*, **84**:1086–1095.

Ylä-Herttuala, S., Palinski, W., Butler, S., Picard, S., Steinberg, D. and Witztum, J.L. (1994). Rabbit and human atherosclerotic lesions contain IgG that recognizes epitopes of oxidized low density lipoprotein. *Arterioscler. Thromb.*, **14**:32–40.

10 The Role of Heat Shock Protein 65/60 in the Initial Immune-Mediated Stages of Atherosclerosis

Georg Wick*°, Roman Kleindienst°, Albert Amberger°, Georg Schett°, Cornelia Seitz°, Hermann Dietrich* and Qingbo Xu°

°*Institute for Biomedical Aging Research, Austrian Academy of Sciences and*
**Institute for General and Experimental Pathology, University of Innsbruck,*
Medical School, 6020 Innsbruck, Austria

INTRODUCTION

The multifactorial pathogenesis of atherosclerosis is well-established. However, the exact nature and relative weight of different essential and modulatory factors contributing to the final outcome of the disease are not yet unequivocally determined. It is, of course, also conceivable that different major causes of vascular alterations lead to the same final result. Due to the slowly progressive nature of the disease, its possible initiation in childhood (Stary, 1989) and manifestation in adult age, clarification of the initiating processes is difficult, if not impossible, in humans. On the other hand, only very few animal models are available to determine the etiology of atherosclerosis, and there is a special need for small rodent models in in- and outbred strains. The transgenic mouse technology has partially overcome this limitation by recreating certain aspects of the disease in mice. These models have demonstrated the interrelationship of genetic and epigenetic factors contributing to atherogenesis (Breslow, 1994). However, as in the past, these transgenic studies were so far focused primarily on genes of cholesterol metabolism, i.e. conventional avenues of thinking, and have not been the basis for new, unconventional approaches to solve this multifaceted problem. In several of these transgenic models, the animals develop fatty streaks that are considered to be early stages that later will result in severe atherosclerosis.

In this chapter we would like to present a completely new concept for atherogenesis that postulates an autoimmune reaction against stress protein 65/60 to be the initiating event leading to an inflammatory reaction in the arterial intima that may subsequently develop into classical severe atherosclerotic lesions, provided that appropriate additional risk factors come into play. Furthermore, we will attempt to show that the "immunologic hypothesis" of atherogenesis can accommodate the main classical hypotheses, such as the "response-to-injury" and the "altered lipoprotein" theories. The former is based on the concept that the initial trigger for the development of atherosclerosis is an injury to the arterial endothelium that can be induced by many different factors, such as shear stress, oxygen radicals, oxidized low density lipoproteins (oxLDL), homocysteine, infections, toxins, etc (Ross, 1993). The latter concept postulates that LDL that is chemically altered, e.g. oxidized, is taken up via the scavenger-receptor by endothelial cells, macrophages and smooth muscle cells in the subendothelial arterial space and initiates the disease (Steinberg *et al.*, 1990).

During the past few years increasing, often anecdotal evidence has been provided that humoral and/or cellular immune reactions do occur during atherogenesis, but it was not possible to determine if these were of primary or secondary nature (Emeson *et al.*, 1988; Hansson *et al.*, 1989; Libby *et al.*, 1991). Our interest in autoimmune reactions possibly contributing to the pathogenesis of atherosclerosis emerged from our previous work on the role of an altered lipid metabolism of lymphocytes for the declining immune response in the elderly on one hand, and on spontaneous and experimentally-induced animal models for organ-specific and systemic autoimmune disease on the other hand (Wick *et al.*, 1989; 1991).

EARLIER DATA SUPPORTING THE PARTICIPATION OF IMMUNE REACTIONS IN THE FORMATION OF ATHEROSCLEROTIC LESIONS

The clear-cut evidence for humoral and cellular immune reactions that occur during all stages of the development of atherosclerotic lesions has, surprisingly, been neglected for many years by laboratories involved in classical atherosclerosis research and if recognized at all, these immunologic phenomena were considered to be secondary in nature. Thus, atherosclerotic lesions contain deposits of immunoglobulins, while non-atherosclerotic arteries are devoid of such changes. Complement factors are co-localized with immunoglobulins in these lesions (Hollander *et al.*, 1979). They include the lytic C5b-9 complex, suggesting a possible involvement of complement-mediated immunopathological mechanisms in atherogenesis. Furthermore, the expression of the C3b receptor (CR1) and C3bi receptor (CR3) was observed on macrophages within atherosclerotic lesions, but not in non-atherosclerotic vascular areas (Seifert *et al.*, 1989). We have shown previously that very few B-cells occur within all stages of atherosclerotic lesions and it is, thus, rather improbable that these locally deposited immunoglobulins are produced *in situ*. So far, it is still not clear against which antigens such antibodies are directed, but several candidates, such as chemically altered, e.g. oxidized LDL, viral components, stress proteins and other antigens will be discussed later in this chapter.

As detailed elsewhere in this volume several reports showed that large numbers of T cells are present within atherosclerotic lesions of experimental animals and man. The majority of these express major histocompatibility complex (MHC) class II antigens as well as the interleukin-2 (IL-2) receptor, thus proving that they are activated (Hansson *et al.*, 1988; van der Wal, 1989). In addition, recent studies have shown that an overwhelming majority of T cells in human atherosclerotic plaques is expressing the low molecular weight form of the leukocyte common antigen (CD45RO) (partly indicative for memory cells) and the integrin very late activation antigen-1 (VLA-1) (Stemme *et al.*,

1992). Based on phenotypic and molecular biological analyses of their T cell receptors α/β (TCR α/β) and TCR γ/δ, it was shown that these T cells are polyclonal in origin (Stemme *et al.*, 1991). However, since these studies were performed on material derived from atherosclerotic plaques they do not yet give clear-cut information about the conditions during the very early stages of the disease that are of high interest for an experimental immunopathologist. These T cells in early lesions may either function as effector cells, or produce factors that attract and activate other cells, such as monocytes, macrophages and smooth muscle cells, that are known to participate in the development of atherosclerotic lesions.

We have undertaken an elaborate immunohistological study aimed at identifying the first cells immigrating into the intima at those sites of the arterial tree that are known to be prone for the emergence of atherosclerotic changes. An unexpected by-product of these studies was the observation of considerable numbers of T cells in the intima of arteriae at sites of major haemodynamic stress even without concomitant macroscopically determinable atherosclerotic changes (Xu *et al.*, 1990). Arteries known to be relatively resistant against atherosclerosis, such as the *arteria mammaria interna*, were devoid of such pre-existent intimal accumulations of lymphocytes (Kleindienst *et al.*, 1993). Based on these data we have put forward the concept of the existence of a vascular-associated lymphoid tissue (VALT) in analogy to the mucosa-associated lymphoid tissue (MALT) (Wick *et al.*, 1992). While the latter is known to serve as a first line of defense against antigenic material that comes into contact with internal bodily surfaces being part of the local immune system, the former may serve a similar function with respect to monitoring blood for possible dangerous foreign or pathologically altered autologous components. The above mentioned immunohistological study of arterial specimens from young (under 30 years) and old (over 60 years) persons gave the following results: those areas that most probably present the earliest stages of the disease, i.e. the transition zone between normal intima and fatty streaks in young people that were not afflicted by clinically manifest vascular disease, contained a majority of T cells among the mononuclear cell infiltrate in the intima, followed by macrophages and a small number of smooth muscle cells. Only later, i.e. in fatty streaks, and even more pronounced in fully developed atherosclerotic plaques, macrophages became the most prominent sub-population within the infiltrate (Xu *et al.*, 1990). Most of these T cells carried the TCR α/β but TCR γ/δ^+ cells were also found in a considerably higher proportion (about 10 %) as compared to peripheral blood (1 to 3 %) (Kleindienst *et al.*, 1993). TCR γ/δ^+ cells within atherosclerotic lesions were identified by anti-TCRδ1 framework antibody. The sub-population that is characteristic for circulating TCR γ/δ^+ cells, i.e. the TCR Vγ9δ2 variety, was not increased. TCR γ/δ^+ T cells preferentially react with certain stress inducible cell proteins (heat shock proteins — HSP) (Jindal *et al.*, 1989; Kaufmann, 1990), a fact the relevance of which in the present context became clearer in subsequent animal experiments that are discussed in the next section. Furthermore, the occurrence of TCR γ/δ^+ cells within the arterial intima again parallels the feature in the MALT and lends additional support to our analogous concept of the existence of a VALT.

Endothelial cells as well as the cells that constitute the intimal infiltrates produce a variety of immune and inflammatory mediators, such as interleukin-1 (IL-1; endothelial cells, smooth muscle cells, macrophages), tumor necrosis factor-α (TNFα: smooth muscle cells, macrophages, T cells), lymphotoxin (LT: T cells), IL-2 (T cells), IL-6 (endothelial cells, smooth muscle cells, macrophages), IL-8 (endothelial cells, macrophages), interferon-γ (IFN-γ: T cells), platelet-derived growth factor (PDGF: endothelial cells, smooth muscle cells, macrophages), etc (Libby and Hansson, 1991; Ross, 1993). These factors have a modulatory effect on the local cellular immune response and growth factors, such as PDGF, have a mitogenic effect on mesenchymal cells, such as smooth muscle cells, and stimulate leukocyte migration, thus playing a major role in the perpetuation of the inflammatory/immune process.

Several groups, including our own, have also addressed the question which cells could possibly function as antigen processing and antigen presenting cells for the activated T cells that are found within atherosclerotic lesions. As mentioned, TCR γ/δ^+ cells can exert the effects without MHC restriction, but CD4$^+$ and CD8$^+$, TCR α/β^+ cells can only react in an MHC-restricted fashion. MHC class I molecules (i.e. HLA-A, -B and -C) are expressed on all nucleated cells, including endothelial cells. We did, however, not find any evidence for a primary, aberrant expression of MHC class II molecules, such as HLA-DR, -DQ and -DP on arterial endothelial cells. Endothelial MHC class II expression was, however, found in the neighbourhood of infiltrates containing activated T cells, that were able to produce IFN-γ (Xu *et al.*, 1990). *In vitro* treatment of cultured endothelial and smooth muscle cells with IFN-γ also entails the expected expression of MHC class II molecules. Furthermore, the demonstration of the invariant HLA-DR γ-chain within these MHC class II positive endothelial cells *in vivo* and *in vitro* provide proof that HLA-DR is actually produced by these cells themselves. Taken together, these results suggest that the activation of intima-infiltrating T cells, by whatever antigen, is not achieved via presentation of these antigens by endothelial cells but rather at more distant sites, e.g. the regional para-aortic lymph nodes. The secondary expression of MHC class II molecules by endothelial cells does, however, point to the possibility that they may play an important role as antigenic presenting cells for perpetuation of the disease. All these data supported the notion that humoral and/or cellular immune reactions may be involved during the pathogenesis of atherosclerosis.

The most important open questions at that stage of the game were the following:

- Are the observed cellular and humoral immune phenomena the cause or sequel of the development of atherosclerotic lesions?
- Irrespective of which of these possibilities turns out to be true, which is/are the antigen/s that leads to the emergence of intralesional T cells or the formation of immune complexes deposited at these sites.
- How can activated T cells that recognize a putative antigen on endothelial cells adhere to the vessel wall under the conditions of rapid pulsatile blood flow?
- Why do we get atherosclerosis but no venosclerosis?
- How can immunological processes be accommodated among the well-known risk factors for atherosclerosis, such as high blood cholesterol levels, high blood pressure, smoking, overweight, etc.?
- Will it be possible to establish one or several animal models that could serve to prove or disprove the involvement of immune reactions in atherogenesis?

DEVELOPMENT OF AN ANIMAL MODEL FOR IMMUNOLOGICALLY MEDIATED ATHEROSCLEROSIS

In an attempt to identify one or several candidate antigens that may be responsible for the sensitisation of T cells that then infiltrate the intima we decided to follow the classical approach for the induction of autoimmune diseases by immunization of normal animals with appropriate antigenic material together with complete Freund's adjuvant (CFA). For this purpose, we isolated total human atherosclerotic plaque proteins and proteins derived from atherosclerotic lesions of Watanabe rabbits with hereditary, spontaneous atherosclerosis due to a deficiency of the LDL-receptor, as well as appropriate control antigens, such as ovalbumin. The rabbits were immunized three times in five week intervals and sacrificed 16 weeks after the first immunization. We reasoned that if atherosclerotic lesions would develop with this approach it should be possible to then identify the culprit protein(s) or peptide(s) within the plaque protein mixture (Xu *et al.*, 1992). As a matter of fact, macroscopically visible atherosclerotic lesions did develop at predilection sites for the disease in the aorta, i.e. the aortic arch and the branching points of larger vessels. Surprisingly, however, these lesions occurred irrespective of the antigen used as long as CFA was present in the immunization mixture. Since HSP 65 is quantitatively one of the major protein constituents of *M. tuberculosis* contained in CFA as well as its major antigenic component, we then immunized rabbits in a similar way with recombinant mycobacterial HSP 65 (rHSP 65) and obtained the same results as with CFA. Injection of incomplete Freund's adjuvant (IFA) and adjuvants that do not contain HSPs, such as Ribi and lipopeptide, were without effect. Control rabbits that were fed a cholesterol-rich diet for 16 weeks also developed severe lesions at the same locations. However, the most frequent and severe forms of the disease developed in animals that were both immunized with HSP65 containing material and fed a cholesterol-rich diet. Pathohistologically, the lesions of animals immunized only consisted of mononuclear cell infiltrates with a large proportion of T cells and monocytes and a lower number of smooth muscle cells as well as the deposition of extracellular matrix proteins. The immunized only group remained normocholesterolemic throughout the experiment and foam cells were lacking. In contrast, the cholesterol-rich diet fed group showed lesions that consisted predominantly of foam cells but also included a smaller number of T cells. Animals that were immunized and received the cholesterol-rich diet developed lesions that exactly paralleled those in man, i.e. contained foam cells, mononuclear cell infiltration by lymphocytes and monocytes, considerable numbers of smooth muscle cells and deposition of extracellular matrix proteins in the cap region.

Recent data from our laboratory provide evidence that the initial inflammatory stage of atherosclerosis is still reversible, while the more severe lesions that develop in rabbits additionally receiving a cholesterol-rich diet seem to be irreversible.

T cells prepared from atherosclerotic lesions of immunized only or immunized plus cholesterol-fed animals showed a significantly increased frequency of HSP 65 reactivity as compared to peripheral blood T cells from the same animals. Furthermore, T cells isolated from lesions of rabbits that had received the cholesterol-rich diet only also showed a significant increase of HSP 65 reactivity as compared to their peripheral blood (Xu *et al.*, 1993b).

At this point it must be emphasized that certain strains of rats develop arthritis (so called adjuvant arthritis) after immunization with HSP 65 containing material and the relevant arthritogenic epitope of HSP 65 in this instance has been shown to be localized in the aminoacid 180–188 residue of the 573 amino acid long HSP 65 (van Eden *et al.*, 1988). A similar epitope seems to be also involved in the pathogenesis of human rheumatoid arthritis. Interestingly, rats with adjuvant arthritis do not develop atherosclerosis and, *vice versa*, rabbits with HSP 65-induced atherosclerosis do not develop arthritis, presumably because the immune system of these two species recognizes different epitopes on the whole HSP molecule. In any case, rats and mice are notoriously resistant against the development of atherosclerosis after feeding a cholesterol-rich diet. One of the reasons for this behaviour seems to be the lack of the cholesterol ester transfer protein (CETP) that mediates the exchange of cholesterol esters between high density lipoproteins (HDL) and LDL in humans. We are now attempting to induce atherosclerosis by immunization with HSP 65 plus feeding of high fat diet in mice that are transgenic for simian CETP (Marotti *et al.*, 1993).

In a separate series of experiments we are attempting to reproduce our rabbit model in rats using a variety of different immunization and dietary schedules. As a first step in this direction we wanted to determine the distribution pattern and phenotypes of leukocytes adhering to the aortic endothelium of rats that were stressed by an intravenous injection of *E. coli* lipopolysaccharide (LPS). In essence, this treatment led to the adherence of leukocytes to exactly those sites that are known to be prone to the development of atherosclerotic lesions in other species (Figure 1). The major population of adhering cells in this instance were monocytes and a lower proportion of lymphocytes. When arterial endothelial cells were cultured *in vitro*, stressed with LPS and overlaid with syngeneic rat spleen cells, the majority of adhering cells were T cells, monocytes being significantly less frequent. It is, however, doubtful if LPS can be considered an atherogenic form of stress and we are, therefore, now combining this treatment with an immunization with rHSP 65 in ongoing experiments. An important observation during the above mentioned studies was the demonstration of a simultaneous and coordinated expression of HSP 60 and adhesion molecules (intracellular adhesion molecule-1 — ICAM-1 and vascular cell adhesion molecule — VCAM-1) by endothelium of LPS treated rats. These findings have been corroborated in the human system, both, on the protein and mRNA level using venous and arterial endothelial cells that were heat-stressed or treated with IL-1α (Figure 2) *in vitro*, thus providing the prerequisites that would be necessary for the prolonged binding of activated, HSP 65/60 specific T cells to the arterial wall. It remains to be determined if the expression of chemoattractants that are responsible for the immigration of mononuclear cells from the vascular lumen and smooth muscle cells from the media into the intima is also induced by these same stress factors.

The adhesion of leukocytes to the arterial endothelial cells of rats stressed *in vivo* or *in vitro* could be partially inhibited by monoclonal antibodies against either ICAM-1 or its ligands LFA-1α and LFA-1β. The partial inhibition indicates that other adhesion molecules besides ICAM-1 and its ligand are involved in this process.

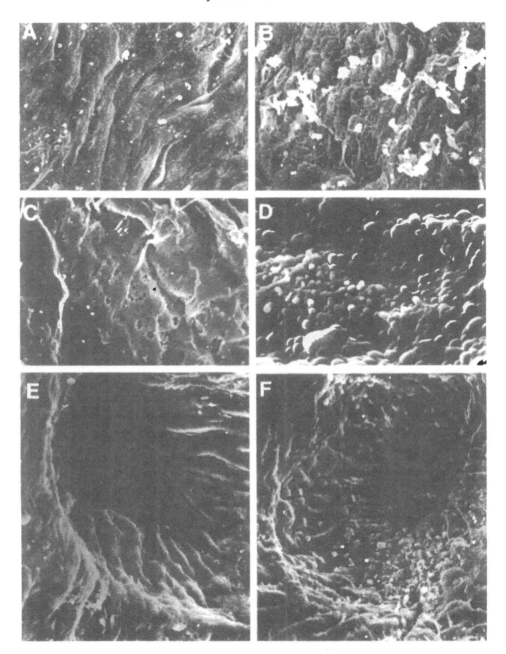

Figure 1   Scanning electron photomicrographs from lipopolysaccharide-stressed and unstressed rat aorta.
Aorta from untreated control rats (A, C, E); intravenously lipopolysaccharide (LPS) -stressed animals (B, D, F)
show increased adhesion of leucocytes (B, F) and changes of endothelial cell surface after LPS application (D).
At branching sites of intercostal arteries with increased hemodynamic stress (E, F), adhesion is a common phenomenon after LPS injury of the arterial wall. Preferential accumulation of leukocytes at predilection-sites of
atherosclerosis may be responsible for the initiation of this disease.
Original magnification 500× (A, B), 5000× (C, D), and 350× (E, F), respectively .

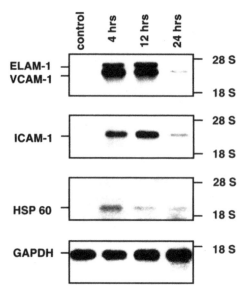

Figure 2   Northern-blot analysis of adhesion-molecules (ELAM-1, VCAM-1, ICAM-1) and heat shock protein 60 expresion on human venous endothelial cells (HVEC) after addition of IL-1α (10 ng/ml). HVEC were isolated from male saphenous veins and cultivated in endothelial cell medium. Monolayers of HVEC between passages 3–5 were washed and medium supplemented with IL-1α was added. After indicated timepoints cells were harvested, RNA was isolated and Northern-blots were performed, hybridized with ^{32}P-labelled cDNA-probes for ICAM-1, VCAM-1, ELAM-1, HSP 60 and GAPDH, washed and exposed to X-ray films. Concomitant expression of HSP 60 and adhesion molecules appear after 4 hours Il-1α incubation and decreases after 24 hours.

INVESTIGATIONS IN HUMAN ATHEROSCLEROSIS

Preliminary data with human T cell lines prepared either from peripheral blood or from atherosclerotic lesions from the same patient provided similar observations as those made in rabbits, i.e. a preponderance of HSP 65 reactive cells in the latter. The majority of these T cells were CD4+CD8−, but a considerable portion also showed the CD4−CD8+ phenotype. So far, HSP 65 reactive human T cells were only stimulated by autologous peripheral blood mononuclear antigen presenting cells and the stimulatory potential of endothelial cells has not yet been assessed in this system.

With respect to humoral antibodies we have shown in a large number of clinically healthy volunteers that had undergone Doppler sonography for determination of atherosclerotic lesions in their carotid arteries, that probands carrying such lesions had significantly higher titers of HSP 65 antibodies as compared to persons without lesions (Xu *et al.*, 1993a). The determination of HSP 65 antibodies may be a new prognostic and diagnostic parameter for atherosclerosis, independent of classical risk factors, such as the male sex, high blood pressure, smoking and total cholesterol and LDL serum levels. The presence and titer of HSP 65 antibodies did not correlate with that of antinuclear antibodies, rheumatoid factors, autoantibodies against thyroid antigens that were determined simultaneously for control purposes. The HSP 65 antibodies cross-react with recombinant human HSP 60 (Xu *et al.*, 1993c). Furthermore, we have recently shown that these antibodies are not only of diagnostic significance but may also play a pathogenetic role:

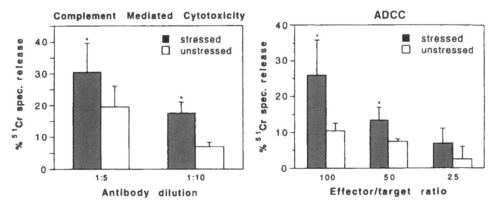

Figure 3 Endothelial cytotoxicity. Confluent human umbilical vein endothelial cells (HUVEC) in 96 well plates were incubated at 37°C or heat stressed at 42°C for 30 min, followed by 90 min incubation at 37°C. After three washes with medium 199, 5 mCi ^{51}Cr in 100 ml of medium 199 containing 10% FCS were added to each well, and incubated at 37°C for 1.5 h. After two further washes, high titer anti-hsp65 antiserum in 100 μl of medium 199 was added, and incubated at 37°C for 6 hours either in the presence of guinea pig serum as a source of complement (complement mediated cytotoxicity) or peripheral blood mononuclear cells from healthy donors as effector cells (antibody mediated cellular cytotoxicity-ADCC). Specific release of radioactivity of the supernatants was measured in a gamma-counter. The values are means of three experiments, each performed in triplicates.
* Significant difference from untreated cells, p < 0.01.

human anti-HSP 65/60 antibodies are able to lyse heat-stressed but not unstressed human endothelial cells by complement-mediated and antibody-dependent cellular cytotoxicity (ADCC) due to surface-expression of HSP 60 by stressed endothelial cells (Figure 3 Schett *et al.*, 1995).

We are now in the process of trying to identify the epitopes of HSP 65/60 that are recognized by lesion-derived human T cell lines and humoral antibodies, respectively. Furthermore, we are using internal labeling procedures to answer the question if the reactivity of polyclonal anti-HSP 65/60 rabbit and human antisera as well as certain monoclonal antibodies with the surface of stressed human macrophages and endothelial cells due to the recognition of a HSP 60 epitope is autoimmune proper or based on antigenic mimicry (Xu *et al.*, 1994).

CONCLUSION

Based on data obtained in experimental animals and in man we are proposing a new "primary immunologic" hypothesis for the development of atherosclerosis (Wick *et al.*, 1992; 1995). According to this concept the first stages of the disease consist in an inflammatory reaction in the aortic intima at sites of major haemodynamic stress based on an autoimmune reactivity against (a) certain, still unidentified epitope(s) expressed on the surface of stressed endothelial cells. Stress factors entailing this expression may include high blood pressure, toxic factors (e.g. smoking), virus infections, cytokines and — importantly — chemically altered LDL. This hypothesis does not contradict but rather encompasses previous conventional theories, such as the "response-to-injury" and "altered LDL" hypotheses. In this early inflammatory stage foam cells are not yet necessarily present and it is still reversible. At this point we do not yet know if humoral antibodies or T cells are the initiating factors at the very earliest stages of the disease. We have proposed that the intimal accumulations of mononuclear cells that, albeit to a lesser extent, have also been found in veins, may constitute a vascular associated lymphoid tissue (VALT), that — in analogy to the MALT — may have the task to monitor the blood for potentially harmful foreign or autologous components. The observation that athero-sclerosis rather then venosclerosis develops may be due to the fact that expression of adhesion molecules and HSP 60 in unaffected vessels has, so far, only been shown at sites of major haemodynamic stress, i.e. in arteries but not in veins. As a matter of fact, the *A. mammaria interna*,, known to be notoriously resistant to atherosclerosis and there-fore used for bypass operations, does not express HSP 60 constitutively. At present it is also not yet clear if anti-HSP 65/60 antibodies and T cells, respectively, are induced by exogenous bacterial HSP 65 and thus lead to a cross-reaction with human HSP 60 via antigenic mimicry or if we deal with a *bona fidae* autoimmune reaction.

Progression of the early inflammatory stage into more severe, classical atherosclerotic changes only occur if risk factors are present for prolonged period of times, high serum cholesterol levels perhaps being the most important one. It should be reemphasized, however, that oxLDL not only leads to the production of foam cells but also is a potent inducer of both HSP 60 and adhesion molecules, thus possibly playing a role not only in later stages but already in the initiation stages of endothelial injury. Finally, this new concept may open new avenues not only for the treatment but also for the prevention of atherosclerosis.

ACKNOWLEDGMENTS

The own work of the authors summarized in this review was supported by grants from the Austrian Research Council (project no. 10677), the Sandoz Foundation for Gerontological Research and the State of Tyrol. We acknowledge the technical support by Mrs. A. Mair and Mr. E. Rainer and are grateful to Drs. B. Grubeck-Loebenstein and R. Sgonc for critically reading of the manuscript.

References

Breslow, J.L. (1994). Insights into lipoprotein metabolism from studies in transgenic mice. *Annu. Rev. Physiol.*, **56**:797–810.

Emeson, E.E. and Robertson, A.L. (1988). T lymphocytes in aortic and coronary intimas. Their potential role in atherogenesis. *Am. J. Pathol.*, **130**:369–376.

Hansson, G.K., Holm, J. and Jonasson, L. (1989). Detection of activated T lymphocytes in the human athero-sclerotic plaque. *Am. J. Pathol.*, **135**:169–175.

Hansson, G.K., Jonasson, L., Holm, J., Clowes, M.K. and Clowes, A. (1988). Gamma interferon regulates vas-cular smooth muscle proliferation and Ia expression *in vivo* and *in vitro*. *Circ. Res.*, **63**:712–719.

Hollander, W., Colombo, M.A., Kirkpatrick, B. and Paddock, J. (1979). Soluble proteins in the human athero-sclerotic plaque. *Atherosclerosis*, **34**:391–405.

Jindal, S., Dudani, A.K., Singh, B., Harley, C.B. and Gupta, R.S. (1989). Primary structure of a human mito-chondrial protein homologous to the bacterial and plant chaperonins and to the 65-kilodalton mycobacter-ial antigen. *Mol. Cell Biol.*, **9**:2279–2283.

Kaufmann, S.H.E. (1990). Heat shock proteins and the immune response. *Immunol Today*, **11**:129–136.

Kleindienst, R., Xu, Q., Willeit, J., Waldenberger, F.R., Weimann, S. and Wick, G. (1993). Immunology of atherosclerosis: demonstration of heat shock protein 60 expression and T lymphocytes bearing alpha/beta or gamma/delta receptor in human atherosclerotic lesions. *Am. J. Pathol.*, **142**:1927–1937.

Libby, P. and Hansson, G.K. (1991). Involvement of the immune system in human atherogenesis: current knowledge and unanswered questions. *Lab. Invest.*, **64**:5–15.

Marotti, K.R., Castle, C.K., Boyle, T.P., Lin, A.H., Murray, R.W. and Melchior, G.W. (1993). Severe atherosclerosis in transgenic mice expressing simian cholesteryl ester transfer protein. *Nature*, **364**:73–75.

Ross, R. (1993). The pathogenesis of atherosclerosis: a perspective for the 1990s. *Nature*, **362**:801–809.

Schett, G., Xu, Q., Amberger, A., van der Zee, R., Recheis, H. and Wick, G. (1995). Autoantibodies against heat shock protein 60 mediate endothelial cytotoxicity. *J. Clin. Invest.*, **96**:2569–2577.

Seifert, P.S. and Hansson, G.K. (1989). Complement receptors and regulatory proteins in human atherosclerotic lesions. *Arteriosclerosis*, **9**:802–811.

Stary, H.C. (1989). Evolution and progression of atherosclerotic lesions in coronary arteries of children and young adults. *Arteriosclerosis*, **9, suppl. I**:19–32.

Steinberg, D. and Witztum, J.L. (1990). Lipoproteins and atherogenesis: current concepts. *J. Am. Med. Assoc.*, **264**:3047–3052.

Stemme, S., Holm, J. and Hansson, G.K. (1992). T lymphocytes in human atherosclerotic plaques are memory cells expressing CD45RO and the integrin VLA-1. *Arterioscler. Thromb.*, **12**:206–211.

Stemme, S., Rymo, L. and Hansson, G.K. (1991). Polyclonal origin of T lymphocytes in human atherosclerotic plaques. *Lab. Invest.*, **65**:654–660.

van der Wal, A.C. (1989). Atherosclerotic lesions in human. In situ immunophenotypic analysis suggesting an immune mediated response. *Lab. Invest.*, **61**:166–170.

van Eden, W., Thole, J.E., van der Zee, R., Noordzij, A., van Embden, J.D.A., Hensen, E.J. and Cohen, I.R. (1988). Cloning of the mycobacterial epitope recognized by T lymphocytes in adjuvant arthritis. *Nature*, **331**:171–173.

Wick, G., Brezinschek, H.P., Hála, K., Dietrich, H., Wolf, H. and Kroemer, G. (1989). The obese strain of chickens: An animal model with spontaneous autoimmune thyroiditis. *Adv. Immunol.*, **47**:433–500.

Wick, G., Huber, L.A., Xu, Q., Jarosch, E., Schönitzer, D. and Jürgens, G. (1991). The decline of the immune response during aging: The role of an altered lipid metabolism. *Ann. NY Acad. Sci.*, **621**:277–290.

Wick, G., Kleindienst, R., Dietrich, H. and Xu, Q. (1992). Is atherosclerosis an autoimmune disease? *Trends Food Sci. Technol.*, **3**:114–119.

Wick, G., Schett, G., Amberger, A., Kleindienst, R. and Xu, Q. (1995). Atherosclerosis-an immunologically mediated disease. *Immunol. Today*, **16**:27–33.

Xu, Q., Oberhuber, G., Gruschwitz, M. and Wick, G. (1990). Immunology of atherosclerosis: cellular composition and major histocompatibility complex class II antigen expression in aortic intima, fatty streaks, and atherosclerotic plaques in young and aged human specimens. *Clin. Immunol. Immunopathol.*, **56**:344–359.

Xu, Q., Dietrich, H., Steiner, H.J., Gown, A.M., Mikuz, G., Kaufmann, S.H.E. and Wick, G. (1992). Induction of arteriosclerosis in normocholesterolemic rabbits by immunization with heat shock protein 65. *Arterioscler Thromb.*, **12**:789–799.

Xu, Q., Willeit, J., Marosi, M., Kleindienst, R., Oberhollenzer, F., Kiechl, S., Stulnig, T., Luef, G. and Wick, G. (1993a). Association of serum antibodies to heat-shock protein 65 with carotid atherosclerosis. *Lancet*, **341**:255–259.

Xu, Q., Kleindienst, R., Waitz, W., Dietrich, H. and Wick, G. (1993b). Increased expression of heat shock protein 65 coincides with a population of infiltrating T lymphocytes in atherosclerotic lesions of rabbits specifically responding to heat shock protein 65. *J. Clin. Invest*, **91**:2693–2702.

Xu, Q., Luef, G., Weimann, S., Gupta, R.S., Wolf, H. and Wick, G. (1993c). Staining of endothelial cells and macrophages in atherosclerotic lesions with human heat-shock protein-reactive antisera. *Arterioscler Thromb.*, **13**:1763–1769.

Xu, Q., Schett, G., Seitz, C.S., Hu, Y., Gupta, R.S. and Wick, G. (1994). Surface staining and cytotoxic activity of heat-shock protein 60 antibody in stressed aortic endothelial cells. *Circ. Res.*, **75**:1078–1085.

INDEX

T - #0269 - 101024 - C0 - 254/178/11 [13] - CB - 9783718658916 - Gloss Lamination